# RISK

## MANAGEMENT

### and the EMERGENCY

### DEPARTMENT

## EXECUTIVE LEADERSHIP

## for PROTECTING PATIENTS

## and HOSPITALS

# RISK

# MANAGEMENT

## and the EMERGENCY

# DEPARTMENT

## EXECUTIVE LEADERSHIP

## for PROTECTING PATIENTS

## and HOSPITALS

Shari Welch

Kevin Klauer

Sarah Freymann Fontenot

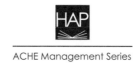

ACHE Management Series

15   14   13   12   11                          5   4   3   2   1

**Library of Congress Cataloging-in-Publication Data**

Welch, Shari J.
  Risk management and the emergency department : executive leadership for protecting patients and hospitals / Shari J. Welch, Sarah Fontenot, and Kevin Klauer.
       p. ; cm.
  Includes bibliographical references.
  ISBN 978-1-56793-417-5 (alk. paper)
  1. Hospitals--Emergency services--Risk management. 2. Hospitals--Emergency services--Administration. I. Fontenot, Sarah. II. Klauer, Kevin. III. Title.
  [DNLM: 1. Risk Management. 2. Emergency Service, Hospital--legislation & jurisprudence. 3. Emergency Service, Hospital--organization & administration. WX 157.1]
  RA975.5.E5W44 2011
  362.11068--dc23
                          2011013846

The paper used in this publication meets the minimum requirements of American National Standard for Information Sciences—Permanence of Paper for Printed Library Materials, ANSI Z39.48-1984. ∞ ™

Acquisitions editor: Janet Davis; Project manager: Amy Carlton; Typesetting: Virginia Byrne; Cover illustration: Scott Miller; Exhibits: Putman Productions.

Health Administration Press
A division of the Foundation of the American
   College of Healthcare Executives
One North Franklin Street, Suite 1700
Chicago, IL 60606–3529
(312) 424–2800

# Contents

## Part I: The Fundamentals of Risk Management in the Emergency Department

## Part II: Healthcare Law and High-Risk Administrative Issues

## Part III: Risk Management Strategies for High-Risk Clinical Entities

## Part IV: Survival Strategies

# Foreword

The emergency department (ED) is the front door to the hospital. More than that, it is the front door to a healthcare delivery system. Every 2 ½ years the equivalent of the entire US population will go through the doors of EDs. Two-thirds of patients occupying inpatient beds at any given moment passed through the ED (McCaig and Nawar 2006). Despite the new and exciting schemes being tested to reform our health system, the need for unscheduled healthcare goes unabated. Emergency medicine will always occupy that important interface between the outpatient and the inpatient universes. Yet the ED continues to be the site of unsatisfactory, inefficient, and unsafe healthcare encounters. According to The Joint Commission (2002), the emergency department is the most common healthcare setting for sentinel events because of waits and delays. Shortages of primary care physicians, lack of health insurance, and an aging population have aligned to create the perfect storm, and that crisis of care will be played out in the ED.

Why is healthcare delivery in the ED so fraught with unsatisfactory and even dangerous events? Shari Welch, Kevin Klauer, and Sarah Freymann Fontenot have set out to dissect the ED, its operations, and its culture to better understand how and why it is so problematic. This book is founded on a new premise: Executive leadership can help clinicians in the trenches do better. Though the clinicians know best how to treat their patients, they often lack the additional training in leadership, implementation, and change management issues needed to improve the ED. The authors believe that executive leadership can embrace, support, and promote these strategies for managing risk in the ED.

Part I highlights the ED's unique operational environment to better understand how it may contribute to medication errors, adverse events, and injuries. The authors have set out to help healthcare executives better understand the environment of the ED. They make the case that the ED is a unique microcosm of healthcare, unlike any other setting. They show how variation in every capacity sets up the ED and its practitioners and patients for bad outcomes. The authors take a 30,000-foot view of teamwork, standardization, and the "just culture" to suggest strategies that improve healthcare delivery in the ED.

Parts II and III look at medicolegal organizational risks and clinical malpractice risks, respectively. Written by physicians and an attorney, these chapters articulate problem areas for easy understanding. Founded on the premise that executive leadership can affect clinical outcomes by helping the clinicians to "get it right," each chapter suggests specific facility and organizational changes to achieve that. Each chapter includes a case study, a defined role for executive leadership, and specific strategies for the healthcare executive. Part IV focuses on the unfortunate circumstance of a legal action against the physician, hospital, or organization and suggests executive responses to such an incident.

This book is no less than a road map for the way top-performing healthcare organizations can establish quality and safety programs for the ED and manage risk through executive leadership. It is a must read for today's healthcare executive with any responsibility for the care delivered in the ED.

Kenneth R. White, PhD, RN, FACHE
Professor, Department of Health Administration
Virginia Commonwealth University
Richmond, Virginia

# Preface

Being a patient can be dangerous, particularly in the emergency department (ED). In 2011 it is still more likely that the bag you checked at the airport will reach your destination than it is that you will have a hospital stay without an adverse event (Nance 2008). In fact it is more dangerous to check into the hospital than to go mountain climbing or bungee jumping (Welch and Jensen 2007). According to The Joint Commission (2008), one-half of sentinel events due to waits and delays in healthcare occur in the ED. According to the National Patient Safety Foundation, one in six Americans has had a personal experience with a medical error (Louis Harris and Associates 1997).

Besides these risks to the patients, the healthcare organization itself is at risk for medicolegal events and malpractice cases. The typical healthcare executive has come to dread phone calls from the ED informing him of an event or a "situation."

The major premise of this book was born in a taxi on the way to the Atlanta airport in 2009. Two of us, Shari Welch (the doctor) and Sarah Fontenot (the lawyer) began exchanging ideas at warp speed. We were both involved with educating physicians about ways to manage risk in the ED. We were intensely focused on quality, safety, and efficiency in the ED. We wondered out loud, "Are we talking to the right people?"

A new and revolutionary concept was born: Executive leadership can play a fundamental role in reducing risk in the ED for patients, providers, and the organization at large. Conservative and slow to adopt standardization, healthcare organizations have been ineffective at embracing strategies to decrease medical error and misdiagnosis. Heretofore this work has been left to the clinicians, who have been woefully ill-equipped to implement strategies that create a safe and fool-proof environment. Clinicians, even medical leadership, are often untrained in change management, so even if they know what needs to be implemented at the front lines to prevent bad outcomes, they have been unable to get there.

We then joined forces with Kevin Klauer, a physician and legal expert who teaches hundreds of physicians each year how to reduce their malpractice risk. We outlined a book that would help the healthcare executive understand how the ED is a unique healthcare setting with factors that create a "laboratory for error." The book would walk through emergency medicine, its operations and processes, its culture and problem clinical scenarios, with a focus on how executive leadership could help the frontline workers to reduce risk.

The result of a shared vision, born in a taxi and growing like the new friendships that paralleled it, this book is a labor of passion and commitment. Making healthcare in the ED safer and more efficient is the mission that gets us up in the morning. Our hope is that this book helps the executives reading it to do that as well.

—Shari J. Welch

# Acknowledgments

We would like to thank Janet Davis and the Health Administration Press team for taking a chance on this book and its rather unconventional premise. We would like to thank Ed Avis for his wise editorial comments and suggestions. But most of all we would like to thank Amy Carlton, whose attention to detail and creative intelligence added to the quality of the manuscript and whose fierce commitment brought the final manuscript home.

# Part I

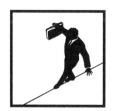

# THE FUNDAMENTALS OF RISK MANAGEMENT IN THE EMERGENCY DEPARTMENT

Nationwide 66 percent of all inpatients passed through the emergency department first (Owens and Elixhauser 2006). In 2008 there were 134 million ED visits, and despite plans for healthcare reform, there does not seem to be a decreased need for unscheduled healthcare on the horizon.

Yet the ED is the place for unsatisfactory patient experiences; there are waits, delays, and inefficiencies. The ED is also inherently unsafe. The Joint Commission (2002) has proclaimed the emergency department as the place in healthcare with the most sentinel events caused by waits and delays. Research has shown that medication errors in the ED are common (Hays 2007). Finally, the emergency department is also one of the healthcare settings with the greatest likelihood of violence.

Part I of this book is a deep dive on the emergency department and all of the elements that contribute to waits, delays, errors, and adverse events. These chapters will help you understand the problems faced daily in the ED and arm you with tools that will be part of the solutions. This 360-degree view will enable you to better understand how the ED micro-cosm differs from other settings and to recognize the constraints to that delivery. From human cognition and human factors engineering to mistake proofing and teamwork, there are real-world cases to illustrate the concepts presented in each chapter and strategies for healthcare leaders to address the myriad problems inherent in ED healthcare.

This section of the book provides a road map for developing both a robust quality improvement program and a comprehensive risk management program for your ED. We make the case that the two disciplines are part of a continuum of safety and should be integrated with data sharing, aligned annual goals, cooperative projects, and a unified report for the board.

Two relatively new concepts in healthcare management are included in Part I: apologies and the role of the board in risk management strategies. All of the topics covered are applied specifically to the ED. Part I is an effort to fully inform healthcare leadership about the problems and the solutions from 30,000 feet up.

# CHAPTER 1

# The Nature of Emergency Medicine

## In This Chapter

- The ED Laboratory
- The Patient
- The Illness
- The Unique Clinical Work
- Sense Making Versus Diagnosing
- The ED Environment
- The Role of Executive Leadership
- Case Study
- Strategies for Healthcare Executives

## THE ED LABORATORY

The emergency department (ED) is a unique clinical environment affected by a number of elements that make the safe and efficient delivery of healthcare seem an impossible proposition. It has been called a "laboratory for error," where time-pressured work is performed in an atmosphere of uncertainty. Devising strategies to improve safety and minimize risk in the emergency department requires a thorough understanding of its unique features and elements:

$$\frac{\text{Time-pressured work} + \text{Environment of uncertainty}}{\text{Laboratory for error}}$$

## THE PATIENT

The patient seen in the ED has characteristics not usually found in patients in other settings. The patient arrives for unscheduled healthcare, and there is little or no information about him. The patient is under stress, is often in pain, and may have conditions that alter his mental status. Language barriers are common in the ED. Many ED patients lack identification, and some are intoxicated and uncooperative. Additionally, patients with mental health problems are a growing burden to the ED. In many communities this accounts for up to 6 percent of all ED volume, which is comparable to the frequency of chest pain presentations (Welch 2006). Mental health patients are among the most difficult patients to manage. But all ED patients share one thing in common: They need urgent if not emergent care. This immediate need requires that all these obstacles be overcome. The challenges of the ED and the constant pressure to deal with them mean the ED is loaded with risk and the possibility of errors.

### The Patient

*Givens*

- Appears randomly, not on a schedule
- Is stressed and in pain
- Requires urgent or emergent care

*Possibilities*

- Is inebriated, intoxicated, or uncooperative
- Carries no identification
- Does not speak English
- Has mental health issues
- Brings along minimal health information

## THE ILLNESS

The patient presenting for emergent or urgent care may have any number of illnesses or injuries. The presentations of these maladies may be atypical and unpredictable, but they generally require some rapid diagnostic and therapeutic intervention. Many critical illnesses can present innocently (e.g., serious infectious diseases that appear minor at first), and minor illnesses can mimic serious illnesses (e.g., acid reflux appearing as an acute myocardial infarction). Serious illnesses and the treatments they require are inherently risky.

## THE UNIQUE CLINICAL WORK

Unlike other clinical specialties, the practice of emergency medicine involves unbounded clinical entities, and there are no limits on the number of patients who can present for care at a given time. The multitasking and interruptions are unique to this setting, and several studies have shown that the intensity of the clinical work is greater in the ED than in other medical office or clinic environments. As Exhibit 1.1 shows, the ED physician has more than three times the number of interruptions in an hour. She also has seven "breaks in task" an hour. The ED doc is almost always caring for three or more patients at once while the office physician spends roughly one minute per hour tending to three patients at once.

There is no context for either the provider or the patient in an ED encounter. Two strangers attempt to find explanations for the patient's subjective complaints in an information vacuum. There is little opportunity to establish a significant relationship in a three-hour ED encounter. These factors make it easy for expectations to be unmet and for patients to be upset and hold the ED accountable for perceived lapses in care. Finally, providers must toggle between the "horizontal patient," who may have serious illnesses that need minute-to-minute management, and the so-called "vertical patient" with high service quality expectations. Compare this to any other specialty: The office physician manages all vertical patients and the hospital-based physician, especially the ICU intensivist, manages all horizontal patients. This variation in the ED is unique and is quite different from other clinical settings.

**Exhibit 1.1: Comparison of Interruptions by Practice Location**

| Interruptions and Multitasking | Office Physician | Emergency Physician |
|---|---|---|
| Interruptions per hour | 9.7 | 23.9 |
| Caring for 3 or more patients | < 0.9 minutes per hour | 37.9 minutes |

SOURCE: Data from Chisholm (2001).

## SENSE MAKING VERSUS DIAGNOSING

Physicians are trained in medical school and residency at *diagnosing,* but the skill that may be even more critical to the practice of emergency medicine is *sense making.* At its most basic, sense making means "how people make sense of events," but it is more complicated than that. Sense making theory looks at how individuals or groups notice and interpret what is happening around them and how they translate this into action. Sense making means asking these two questions: (1) What is going on here? and (2) What do I do next? A key element in sense making is the practice of stopping and incorporating new information again and again to make sense of a situation.

While diagnosing involves choosing among diagnostic possibilities, sense making involves deciding which information even gets considered. In the emergency department, where patients present out of any context and symptoms may evolve over time, the physician must constantly be engaged in sense making and his care plan must be an iterative process. Effective sense making requires that the team engaged in the care of the patient constantly share their assessments and revise their approaches. Communication must be effective and frequent among team members. The physician must articulate his expectations for test results and the patient's responses to treatment. If those expectations are not met, the team—led by the physician—should consider that the earlier sense making was incorrect.

## THE ED ENVIRONMENT

The factors coming to bear on the ED and medicine at large appear to be building into a perfect storm.

---

### The Perfect Storm

The following elements contribute to the perfect storm looming over the ED:

- The changing demographic: EDs are seeing older, sicker, more medically complex patients.
- The fluctuating nursing shortage is threatening staffing levels.
- Many EDs are staffed with younger, less experienced workers who do not stay in one job for long.

---

- A physician shortage, particularly in primary care, is growing; this may cause patients to wait longer to seek care, resulting in sicker people in the ED.
- The on-call crisis affects nearly every medical subspecialty now, which has led to an inability to get timely consultations for patients in the ED.
- There is growing pressure to keep patients out of the hospital.
- More diagnostics can be done in the ED, creating longer ED stays.

Exhibit 1.2 shows a graph from Peter Sprivulis at the Institute for Healthcare Improvement showing the complexity of acute healthcare needs in patients as they age. As the baby boomers become senior citizens—the number of citizens over age 65 will double by 2030 (He et al. 2005)—their healthcare needs will increase: Emergency department personnel will do more to them, for them, and with them.

Though much has been made of the nursing shortage, the physician shortage that is just beginning also will have a significant impact on EDs in the United States. Since the 1980s, when the Association of American Medical Colleges predicted an oversupply of physicians, medical school graduation rates have been flat (Alberti 2011). The curves representing supply and demand suggest a crisis that will know no boundaries: The shortage will cross political and geographic borders and medical specialty boundaries. A 2010 article in the *Journal of the American Medical Association* noted that physicians had decreased their hours worked by 7.2 percent,

**Exhibit 1.2: Complexity of Healthcare Needs in Patients as They Age**

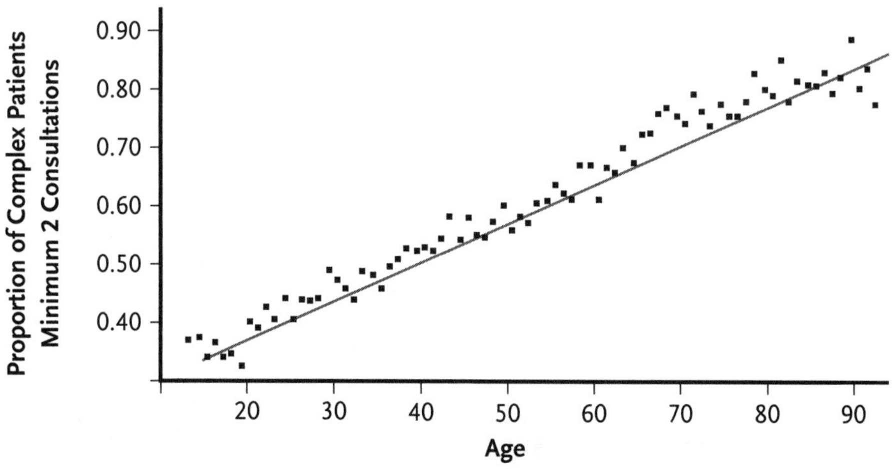

SOURCE: Sprivulis (2004). Used with permission.

**Exhibit 1.3: Healthcare Encounters per Year by Age**

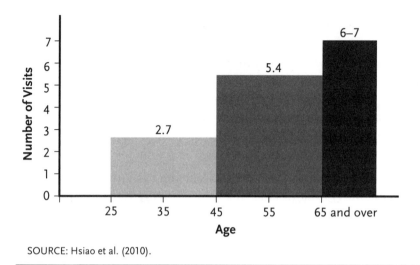

SOURCE: Hsiao et al. (2010).

and the biggest decreases were among the younger physicians (Staiger, Auerbach, and Buerhaus 2010). At the same time the number of physicians retiring is higher than was anticipated. Further, the younger physicians do not want to work the hours that physicians of previous generations worked. This younger workforce has more female physicians, who tend to work fewer hours while balancing medicine and motherhood, and is smaller relative to the patient population.

These trends will compound the already existing shortage of trained emergency physicians. This shortage is particularly acute in rural areas. The shortages across other specialties will exacerbate the on-call crisis and add to the already stressful work environment of the specialty.

The shortage of primary care physicians, the characteristics of younger physicians and their work habits, and the aging demographic requiring more healthcare services will make it even more difficult to obtain routine primary care. Difficulties in seeking primary and preventive care will mean that patients will present to the ED later in the course of their diseases and outcomes will suffer accordingly. Some have predicted that a three- to four-month wait to see a primary care physician is not that far off, considering all of these factors (Ruiz 2008).

Finally, technology has allowed for more diagnostic testing in the ED, and this takes time. The Emergency Department Benchmarking Alliance (EDBA), a non-profit organization with almost 500 ED members, noted in its 2006 survey that the number of CT scans and MRI scans performed in the ED increased 400 percent between 2000 and 2006. Utilization of imaging, and complex diagnostic testing such as cardiac stress testing, continues to rise. This increased diagnostic testing also means the physicians and nurses working in the ED and in other parts of the hospital are in danger of information overload. One study revealed that 61 percent of inpatients and 75 percent of ED patients were discharged without receiving test results (Henson 2011).

## THE ROLE OF EXECUTIVE LEADERSHIP

The role of executive leadership in managing the risk in the ED has not been widely and fully articulated in most healthcare organizations. Yet the effective strategies for managing risk in the ED can't be successfully implemented without this leadership. Many physician and nurse leaders do not have the training or the tools to adequately address these issues. This book explores ways executives can design systems that minimize risk at the front lines. Imagine your organization establishing systems that make it impossible for the front lines to do the wrong thing. Though executives are not healthcare providers, they can influence behavior along many fronts in ways that will lead to a safer, more reliable healthcare environment. With an eye always on systems and processes, not people, and with the will to address these difficult issues articulated from the top of the organization down, gains can and will be made.

In addition to making specific changes at the front lines, the executive leadership should seize the opportunity to influence culture, which not only results in measurable improvements but sets the stage for ongoing improvements in quality, safety, and risk management.

### Case Study

In the 2009 EDBA Benchmarking Survey, hospitals were grouped by volume and studied along operating characteristics such as admission rate, transfer rate, and acuity. It was clear that the census could be stratified into quintiles: volume bands of fewer than 20,000 visits; 20,000–40,000; 40,000–60,000; 60,000–80,000; more than 80,000 visits. Performance on operating characteristics such as length of stay, door-to-physician time, and left-without-being-seen varied among the volume bands. In 2008 the alliance consisted of 172 hospitals. In 2009 Hospital Corporation of America (HCA) joined the alliance, adding more than 150 hospitals to the database. Suddenly the variation in performance at the volume band level dropped. HCA hospitals were performing better than other hospitals within each volume band. How did they do it?

(continued)

An interview with Suzanne Stone-Griffith, vice president of quality at HCA, told the story. "We measure and monitor everything to do with ED performance. We have articulated that we expect EDs to perform well and to constantly be improving. We look for best practices and try to share them among the organization. We have complete alignment from the executives to the frontline workers, and the culture supports the work!"

SOURCE: Stone-Griffith (2011).

**Strategies for Healthcare Executives**

- Understand and recognize the unique factors inherent in the ED that lead to risk.
- By understanding these factors, systems approaches can be adapted to reduce the risk.
- The specifics of new strategies will come from the clinicians and the front lines, but the will must come from the executive suite.
- A cultural change must occur to launch this work successfully.

## Recommended Readings

Botwinick, L., M. Bisognano, and C. Haraden. 2006. "Leadership Guide to Patient Safety." IHI Innovation Series white paper. Cambridge, MA: Institute for Healthcare Improvement.

Croskerry, P. 2009. *Patient Safety in Emergency Medicine*, Chapter 1. Philadephia, PA: Wolters Kluwer/Lippincott Williams & Wilkins.

Pronovost, P. J. 2004. "Senior Executive Adopt-a-Work Unit: A Model for Safety Improvement." *Joint Commission Journal on Quality and Patient Safety* 30 (2): 59–68.

Welch, S. J. 2008. *Critical Decisions in Emergency Medicine: Medical Error and Patient Safety in the Emergency Department.* Dallas, TX: American College of Emergency Physicians.

# CHAPTER 2

# The Emergency Physician's True Liability Risk

## In This Chapter

- Malpractice Risk Versus Other Insurance Risk
- Error and Liability
- Why Patients Sue Physicians
- An Ineffective System
- Impact on Physician Practices
- The Role of Executive Leadership
- Case Study
- Strategies for Healthcare Executives

## MALPRACTICE RISK VERSUS OTHER INSURANCE RISK

According to the Physician Insurers Association of America (PIAA), whose members insure 60 percent of all physicians in private practice in the United States, there is minimal competition in the medical malpractice insurance business (GAO 2003). Insuring physicians against malpractice is not a profitable business, and the number of insurers has steadily declined in the past three decades. Most malpractice companies are owned and operated by physicians not as a money-making endeavor but as a necessity to allow physicians to practice medicine. Medical malpractice insurance is unique in the insurance industry in a number of ways.

### Unique Elements of Malpractice Risk

- Malpractice claims may be delayed.
- Rates are difficult to set.
- Standard of care and causation are ill-defined.
- Pain and suffering are difficult to measure.
- Settlements can vary widely.

Unlike the speedy resolution to the fender bender you have in the parking lot today, there may be a three-year lapse from event to claim in malpractice, and even longer in the case of perinatal or infant care. This arrangement is different from traditional insurance models. The time involved in settling a suit adds to the uncertainty of data for setting rates for particular claims. Will the patient be on disability? Is he a breadwinner? What about pain and suffering?

Unlike other insurance models malpractice is also unpredictable in terms of standards of care and causation. There are few industry standards to quote. Qualified experts can be found to espouse any point of view. Though causation purportedly must be proved in a successful malpractice suit, this is poorly fleshed out in terms of evidence-based medicine. Sometimes the natural course of a disease leads to a bad outcome, but malpractice damages are awarded. Some instances of bad medicine do not lead to litigation. In many ways the system appears ruled by serendipity rather than science.

And the cost of doing this business is high. Remember, whether won or lost, every case costs money to defend. According to PIAA (2006), in 2005 the average cost of defending a case when the defendant prevailed was $110,346.


## ERROR AND LIABILITY

Studies (e.g., Studdert et al. 2006) have shown that doctors have a more than 1-in-100 chance of being tagged with a lawsuit after a patient has an adverse event, even when the doctor was uninvolved (e.g., her name was inadvertently attached to a file even though she didn't see the patient) or did nothing wrong. Although this may seem a low number, when you consider the number of patients who suffer an adverse event in healthcare (4 to 20 percent, depending on how it is defined) this adds up to a lot of cases (Baker et al. 2004). Every physician can expect to be sued at least once in a career, and in some specialties the rate is higher (Zane 2009). Emergency physicians are a high-liability group and face a legal action for every

20,000 to 30,000 ED patients seen (Henry and Bukata 2011). For a full-time physician this means, on average, every five years. There are a number of features of emergency care that predispose it to litigation.

**Factors Contributing to Litigation in Emergency Medicine**

- Doctor and patient are strangers.
- Patients are in pain.
- Patients and their family members are under stress.
- Mistakes are made in the ED.
- The ED environment can affect communication.

## WHY PATIENTS SUE PHYSICIANS

Medicine has made great strides in curing and curbing disease, but that success means patients' expectations are high and their tolerance for adverse events is low. Open heart surgery and organ transplantation have become so common that even the suggestion of an unfavorable outcome is synonymous in the patient's mind with physician failure. In the emergency department patients may have an expectation for a good outcome when one is not possible (e.g., wounds that scar or fractures that heal with decreased mobility).

Informed consent can add a suggestion of liability to the ED encounter. Often patients have time-sensitive injuries or conditions, which means it may not be feasible to present and consider multiple treatment options, get second opinions, or allow for family discussions to take place. Even when time is spent doing bedside teaching and discussion physicians often fail to document the discussions about treatment options that they have had or fail to express on the chart why such discussions did not occur. This is an area in which emergency physicians are particularly vulnerable. Making every effort to inform patients about possible bad outcomes and documenting such discussions can mitigate against this risk. For example, if the patient is informed, "The risk of a wound infection is at minimum 5 percent, and with your diabetes, it is even higher. I want to check you every day to make sure you are not developing an infection," the patient begins to understand early on that there is a possibility of an infection, and should one occur he won't be shocked or surprised. Notifying patients and families of the possibility of complications, worsening conditions, or known adverse outcomes should be considered crucial conversations between an emergency physician and the patient.

Communication is difficult in the noise and chaos of the emergency department. It is hard to create an encounter for the patient that feels safe, caring, and competent. In a healthcare encounter that is between total strangers, this communication element may be even more critical. When physicians improve their communication skills and interpersonal style, they see improvements in patient satisfaction and a decrease in risk management issues and malpractice cases (Press 2005).

When patients decide to sue it is typically a combination of disappointment in the clinical outcome and patient dissatisfaction with the physician, the facility, and/or the encounter. There is a strong correlation between claims and poor communication and rapport with families (Vincent, Young, and Phillips 1994).

## AN INEFFECTIVE SYSTEM

The real risk of malpractice is far less than physicians believe. Despite runaway malpractice insurance premiums, generous settlements, big awards by generous juries, and an epidemic of "defensive medicine," less than 3 percent of patients who experience injuries associated with negligent care actually file claims. Still, the risk is far greater than in comparable first-world nations (Anderson et al. 2005); American physicians are five times more likely to be sued than Canadian physicians, and the cost of malpractice in the United States is 400 percent higher than the cost in Canada.

## IMPACT ON PHYSICIAN PRACTICES

Many physicians today would not encourage their children to go into medicine. According to a 2006 Survey by the American College of Physician Executives 60 percent of physicians have considered leaving medicine because they are concerned about the status of US healthcare in general and the malpractice crisis in particular (Steiger 2006). Ninety-nine percent of American Medical Association (AMA) members surveyed say they are concerned with the medical liability environment (AMA 2008). One third of AMA members reported referring out more complex cases in the past year due to worries over medical liability issues. And 27 percent have stopped doing certain procedures because of medical malpractice pressures. This is bad for healthcare overall, especially in light of the physician shortage.

# THE ROLE OF EXECUTIVE LEADERSHIP

Understanding the link between patient satisfaction, complaints, and litigation is important. Having training mechanisms in place that demonstrate how providers can manage patient problems could mean big payoffs in the future in terms of declining risk. Training in patient satisfaction strategies and techniques, risk management strategies and techniques, and communication skills should be standard. Physicians who consistently garner patient complaints need training in communication skills. All of these activities should have clear support from the executive level, and expectations for all staff should be clearly articulated from the top down.

## Case Study

Baptist Health Care of Pensacola, Florida, was struggling with a malpractice crisis. By the end of 1995 it had faced 60 malpractice claims and paid out more than $200,000 in settlements. At the time its patient satisfaction scores were at the 10th percentile relative to its peers.

Baptist implemented a vigorous, organization-wide effort to improve its patient satisfaction. By the end of 1997 Baptist ranked in the 98th percentile nationally, and in 1998 only 20 claims were made, resulting in a total payout of only $23,000. *Modern Healthcare* awarded Baptist the 1999 Excellence in Healthcare Award.

|  | Number of Claims | Total Dollars Paid Out |
|---|---|---|
| Before 1995 | 60 | >$200,000 |
| After 1998 | 20 | $23,000 |

SOURCE: Press (2005).

## Strategies for Healthcare Executives

- Education of staff and physicians about risk should be an organizational imperative.
- Close monitoring of complaints and establishing a complaint management system are critical.
- Monitoring physician performance on patient satisfaction and coaching outliers can be an effective strategy.
- Empower staff to communicate freely with physicians when they suspect that service recovery may be needed.

(continued)

- Scripting for complaints should be mandated by the leadership of each department.
- Scripting for adverse events should be mandated by the leadership of each department.

## Recommended Readings

Cole, S. A. 1997. "Reducing Malpractice Risk Through More Effective Communication," *American Journal of Managed Care* 3 (4): 649–56.

Mattu, A. 2009. *Emergency Medicine Clinics of North America: Risk Management.* Volume 27 (4) Philadelphia, PA: W. B. Saunders Co.

Press, I. 2005. *Patient Satisfaction: Understanding and Managing the Experience of Care,* Second Edition. Chicago: Health Administration Press.

Thomas, M. O. 2009. *Practicing Medicine in Difficult Times: Protecting Physicians from Malpractice Litigation.* Mississauga, Ontario: Jones and Bartlett Publishers LLC.

# CHAPTER 3

# Setting Up a Comprehensive Quality Improvement Program for Your ED

**In This Chapter**

- Integrating Quality Improvement and Risk Management Efforts
- Volume-Band Behavior and Cohorts
- How to Implement a Simple QI Project
- The Role of Executive Leadership
- Case Study
- Strategies for Healthcare Executives
- Appendix 1

## INTEGRATING QUALITY IMPROVEMENT AND RISK MANAGEMENT

The interconnectedness among quality improvement (QI), patient safety, risk management, and medical malpractice is becoming increasingly clear. By fully integrating these disciplines and infrastructure, organizations can avoid redundancy and each silo can freely share its information and strategies. The Los Angeles County Department of Public Health, the largest county-run health system in the United States, is fully integrated. The central offices share space and personnel. The employees carry a heavy case load effectively and have launched a number of wide-reaching patient safety initiatives. The quality initiatives and their associated data alert leaders to risk management problems and medical malpractice issues before they become manifest via **sentinel events**. This work can be seen as a continuum with quality improvement work at one end and medical malpractice cases at the other (Exhibit 3.1).

---

**The Elements of a Robust QI Program**

- Census data
- Performance metrics
- Operational data
- Provider performance
- Improvement projects

---

**Sentinel event:** Any unanticipated event in a healthcare setting not related to the natural course of the patient's illness resulting in death or serious physical or psychological injury to a patient or patients.

Quality improvement work requires two important elements: data and methodology. QI cannot be done effectively without data, and all QI initiatives should be data driven. The important data elements, as well as low-tech and high-tech mechanisms for obtaining the data, will be presented in this chapter. A methodology should be adopted for improvement projects. There are many methodologies out there, from Juran to Six Sigma, from plan-do-study-act (PDSA) to Lean thinking. Among QI workers, there are devotees of every sort. Each methodology offers a discipline for performing QI work, and each is data driven. The science behind improvement work is often misunderstood by those involved in traditional medical research, but it has been shown to be effective in industry for more than 50 years.

**Exhibit 3.1: Continuum of Patient Safety**

| Quality improvement | Patient safety | Risk management | Medical malpractice |

Opportunity for improvements within each discipline

SOURCE: Welch (2010b).

Back to a discussion of data—there are two ways to get at quality performance. You can count absolute events and report them as a proportion, such as left without being seen (LWBS) percentages, or you can measure time and report an indicator, such as median length of stay (LOS). All improvement work should use a measurement to gauge the success of the change.

There are data that define a department and data that measure its performance. *Census data* describe what is going on in the department. Examples of census data include census by day, month, and year; percentage of admissions; percentage of ICU admissions; percentage of transfers; percentage of pediatric patients; and number of trauma patients. Census data can help a department manage demand capacity and place the department within the right cohort group. Departments with robust QI programs usually have fewer walkaways and often see unexpected growth in census, but most census data do not reflect performance. Instead the data provide a contextual understanding of the operations for a given department. Census data define the ED and what kind of care will be rendered there.

Besides census as a characteristic that defines an ED (reported as patients per day and as annual census), there are operating characteristics such as pediatric volume, admission rate, transfer rate, and current procedural terminology (CPT) coding data, to name a few. Together census data and operating characteristics create a profile of an ED suggesting the acuity of care provided and the services expected by the community. These data help describe a department and help place it in the right comparison group for benchmarking. They are the "genetic makeup" of a department, analogous to height and eye color. By gathering and understanding these data, ED and hospital leaders can seek to characterize each department for appropriate comparative analysis with similar departments. Leaders can also track these characteristics over time to better understand the services being provided to the community and plan for those needed in the future.

### Examples of Census Data

- Census (annual ED volume)
- Acuity by emergency severity index
- Acuity by evaluation and management codes
- Acuity by admission rate
- Census by patient age (pediatric volumes)
- Payer mix

In addition, there are data that measure ED performance. These metrics include *time measures* such as LOS and **door-to-balloon time**, which are typically reported as medians. They also include *proportion measures* such as the "walkaway" categories: LWBS, against medical advice (AMA), and left before treatment complete (LBTC), which are typically reported as percentages. These are the most widely used metrics found in the emergency medicine literature. These metrics have become de facto measures of quality and have been employed in ED benchmarking. Time intervals in the emergency department are currently undergoing feasibility studies by the Centers for Medicare & Medicaid Services (CMS) and are likely to be regarded as quality measures in the proposed value-based purchase model to be employed in the near future.

> **Door-to-balloon time:** The time from arrival at the emergency department to angioplasty in the cardiac catheterization lab for patients with an acute ST elevation myocardial infarction.

### Examples of Performance Measures

- Length of stay (LOS)
- Door-to-balloon time and other core measures
- Walkaways (LWBS, AMA, LBTC)
- Complaint ratios
- Throughput for processes
- Time to pain treatment
- Door-to-physician time

Time measures are becoming increasingly the focus of CMS, payers, and the public. Emergency departments that want to get upstream of the performance measurements that will be used in CMS's value-based purchase scheme (pay for performance) should begin to track time stamps and time intervals of ED visits. In 2010 the Second Performance Measures and Benchmarking Summit defined and clarified the metrics that are in use for emergency medicine (Welch et al. 2010). Exhibit 3.2 shows the increasing granularity of the data that EDs will eventually be reporting via these time stamps and intervals. The appendix to this chapter provides the definitions for these metrics.

The robust QI program should also include operational data. As ED leaders begin to characterize through data the operations and processes that are part of an ED visit, they can improve patient flow through the ED and through the system. As a program develops, the data captures become increasingly granular.

**Exhibit 3.2: ED Timestamps and Intervals**

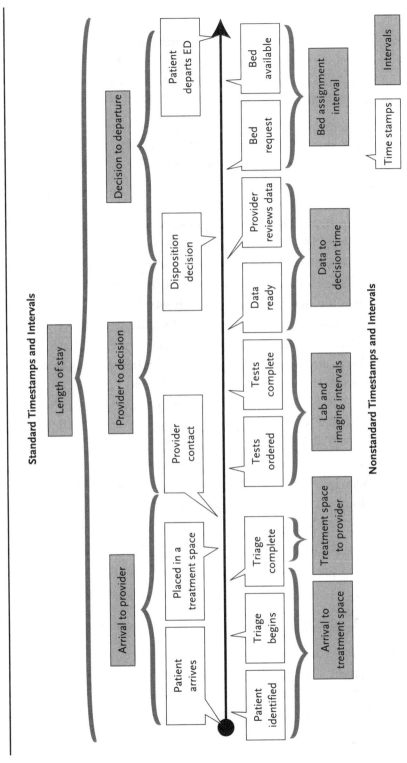

SOURCE: Reprinted from Welch et al. (2010).

As the program evolves, these data get more detailed to help the frontline workers understand and identify the causes of operational delays. For instance, it is not enough to know the interval time from when an x-ray is ordered until the results are available to the provider. More useful would be an examination of the subcycles of radiology operations, which would enable a department to better understand its bottlenecks. For instance, if radiology service is found to be the source of delays in a department and turnaround times for the x-ray or CT subcycles are too long, the next question should be where exactly in the process is the delay occurring? The subcycle time intervals (see Radiology Operational Subcycle Time Intervals box) would help the department to identify whether the delay would be remedied with a transport tech, another radiology tech, another radiologist, or a new IT system.

Two other elements will enhance the QI program: provider performance and QI projects. Provider performance will be discussed at length in Chapter 7 when we focus on the Joint Commission Ongoing Practice Performance Evaluation. Before launching into a basic method for performing QI projects, let's put all of these data elements into perspective in a discussion of something new: volume-band behaviors.

# Exhibit 3.3: Characteristics of ED Census Categories

| | Under 20k (n = 64) | 20k to 40k (n = 146) | 40k to 60k (n = 92) | 60k to 80k (n = 35) | Over 80k EDs (n = 22) | p-value |
|---|---|---|---|---|---|---|
| *Operating Characteristics* | | | | | | |
| Patients per day (n) | | | 131.88 | 188.20 | 273.62 | <0.0001* |
| | | | 54.90 | 55.59 | 54.97 | 0.2017** |
| | | | 20.35 | 21.70 | 23.11 | 0.5980** |
| | | | 19.30 | 20.14 | 20.82 | <0.0001** |
| | | | 1.48 | 0.97 | 1.20 | 0.0151** |
| | | | 17.97 | 18.41 | 21.49 | <0.0001** |
| | | | 44.67 | 46.71 | 44.83 | 0.0025** |
| | | | 65.06 | 62.70 | 60.48 | 0.1322** |
| | | | 712.3 | 1633.6 | 1416.3 | <0.0001* |
| | | | 2.82 | 3.34 | 3.59 | <0.0001** |
| | | | 30.5 | 36.5 | 36.5 | 0.0012* |
| | | | )6.5 | 312.0 | 347.5 | <0.0001* |
| | | | 4.0 | 183.0 | 203.0 | <0.0001* |

*W

**

SO

**DATE DUE**

V(                                              HORTS

Ne                        ___ ___ in a survey by the Emergency Department Benchmarking Alliance (EDBA) suggest a comparison scheme that makes sense based on patterns identified and correlated with census and acuity (Welch et al. 2010). When EDs are grouped into quintiles (volume bands) of 20,000-visit increments based on the number of annual ED visits, several performance patterns emerge. Operating characteristics also differ among EDs based on the volume band occupied. The operating characteristics help to describe and define the work being carried out in the ED. Exhibit 3.3 shows the differences in operating characteristics and performance as a function of ED volume.

Statistically significant trends can be seen in the data. As annual census and daily arrivals increase, the percentage of high-acuity patients rises, the admission rate rises, and the transfer rate falls. In addition, as census increases, the percentage of patients arriving by EMS and the rate of admission of these patients go up, while the percentage of admissions originating in the ED decreases. In general terms: Size matters, and performance capability on metrics is dependent upon the ED annual volume. This will be important when CMS begins rolling out its pay-for-performance program. Like departments should be compared to like departments.

## HOW TO IMPLEMENT A SIMPLE QI PROJECT

Each focused audit/QI project involves the following five steps in sequence:

1. Development of an aim statement (including stretch goals)
2. Identification of data measures with baseline data and method of measurement
3. Development of a change package, usually through teamwork
4. Planning and execution of a pilot study
5. Full implementation or rollout

The *aim statement* lays out the goal of the focused audit or project. It is specific in terms of what is to be measured (How will we know that a change is an improvement?) and the time frame in which the project will take place. *Data measures* are data points that can be used to monitor and evaluate the quality of the processes that affect patient care. These are the metrics to be measured and tracked to demonstrate whether an implemented change is truly an improvement. Well-implemented QI projects do not run on intuition. The data tell the team whether or not the change has been an improvement. Where there is no IT support for data collection, an ED can get rudimentary data from the ED patient log and spot audits. If needed, charts may be audited each month for these census data and metrics. Sometimes smaller EDs with little or no IT support are the most creative in terms of their quest for data. For example, a smaller ED working as part of the IHI Innovation Community in 2006 set up a simple mechanism to find how many bags of IV fluid were being used by day and by shift. As a nurse or tech pulled the rubber plug off the IV bag and pierced the bag with the tubing, the plug went into a tin can next to the cupboard housing the bags. At the end of the day, the plugs were counted to determine how many bags were used (Welch 2009b). Still, it is noteworthy that the complexity of patient care being delivered and the amount of data being generated in the ED are no longer manageable without IT support.

The *change package* is typically crafted by a team, such as a task force of stakeholders interested in successful change around a process or project. Unlike the traditional medical research model in which variables are controlled and one intervention is made, often many small changes will occur simultaneously in the department as part of the change package. The *pilot study* is critical to managing change during an improvement project. Rather than rolling out change widely before identifying problems with the new process, a smaller-scale trial is done to identify glitches before the process is introduced to the department at large. One important strategy recognized by experts in change management is to pilot the innovation with "A-Team" members, people who want the pilot to succeed. You can demonstrate success with data and present the pilot results to the rest of the department to generate enthusiasm for the change.

Following the pilot (or two) and other preparations, the change is rolled out. Educating staff through e-mails, posters, and even slogans and T-shirts can help launch a successful improvement project.

## THE ROLE OF EXECUTIVE LEADERSHIP

The Institute for Healthcare Improvement has long recognized the notion that sponsorship from the executive level is critical to the success of improvement work. This calls for clear and unqualified sponsorship of each project from the C-suite. The CEO should come to the clinical unit to support the changes early in the piloting. She should be concerned with the success and let the rank and file see her concern. Clever leaders find small ways to reward the change agents in the project and the staff workers who will be making sacrifices as the project unfolds. Change is rarely easy, and this type of executive-level sponsorship can keep morale up and momentum going during difficult change projects.

### Case Study

Patients who are ill with septic shock do best when they are taken as quickly as possible to the ICU and a number of simultaneous interventions now called "the septic shock bundle" are begun. These interventions are difficult to fully execute in a busy emergency department. The necessary one-on-one physician and nurse care and other resources are easier to provide in the ICU than in the ED. After spending more than four hours in his emergency department caring for a critically ill patient with septic shock, Dr. Steve Souter, a 20-year veteran emergency room physician, decided to tackle the delays in admission to the ICU for critically ill patients head on.

He met with the intensivists, nurses, managers, and administrators at Intermountain Medical Center and headed up a process change that enables the ED physician to expedite the admission process of critical care patients. Following the rapid response team model used so successfully elsewhere, the team developed this simple process: When a patient meets critical care criteria, an "ED-ICU Priority 1" is called. A conference call using a special call-in system is arranged, and the physician gives a report to the ICU team including respiratory therapy, the intensivist, the charge nurse, and the nursing supervisor. Immediately following the call the critical care service sends down a team to accept the hand-off in person and transports the patient to the ICU. The whole admission process is expedited for the good of the patient and the emergency department.

This process model succeeded and is an example of how process improvement does not occur by committee but rather by innovation at the front lines. It also shows how one committed individual, organizing a team or task force of stakeholders, can move an institution!

*Results:*

LOS admitted patients     300 minutes
LOS "Priority 1" patients    <1 hour

When patients are admitted using the old admission process, the LOS is 300 minutes, which is just too long for an unstable ICU patient. After implementation of the Priority 1 process, patients are admitted to the ICU in well under an hour.

SOURCE: Welch (2009b).

---

### Strategies for Healthcare Executives

- Understand the elements of a robust QI program and how it provides the platform for risk management work.
- Commit the technology and personnel resources necessary for such a program.
- Lend sponsorship and support for each innovation in the ED so there is never any question of your commitment to the quality and safety culture.
- Encourage the integration of the QI department and the risk management department to increase cost effectiveness and allow risk to be identified before a sentinel event.

## Recommended Readings

Jensen, K. 2007. "The Science of Flow." In *Leadership for Smooth Patient Flow.* Chicago: Health Administration Press.

Spath, P. L. 2000. "Measuring Performance of High Risk Processes." *Error Reduction in Health Care.* San Francisco: Jossey-Bass.

Welch, S. J. 2009. "Launching a Quality Improvement Program for the Emergency Department" and "Quality Improvement Methodologies." In *Quality Matters: Solutions for a Safe and Efficient Emergency Department.* Chicago: Joint Commission Resources Publishing.

## APPENDIX 1

### Timestamps

- **Arrival time:** The date and time that the patient first arrives at the institution for the purpose of requesting emergency care should be recorded as the arrival time. This is the first contact, not necessarily the registration time or the triage time.
- **EMS offload time:** The date and time that the patient is transferred from the EMS stretcher, placed in a treatment space, and care is assumed by the ED staff. This is typically recorded in the EMS run report.
- **Treatment space time:** The date and time of placement in a treatment space. "Treatment space" refers to any space the hospital or facility designates as a space to render emergency care.
- **Provider contact time:** The date and time of first contact between the patient and the physician or the provider (defined as an institutionally credentialed provider but specifically not the triage nurse) to initiate the medical screening exam.
- **Data-ready time:** The date and time when all relevant data—test results, image interpretations, and treatment responses—are available to the provider for decision making regarding patient disposition. (Most EDs do not have IT to enable the capture of these data yet, but we anticipate it will eventually be available routinely in future IT systems.)
- **Disposition decision time:** The date and time that the order regarding the disposition of the patient (transfer, observe, discharge) is documented.
- **Admit decision time:** The disposition decision time applied to admitted patients. The date and time that the admit order is documented by the provider.
- **Departure time:** The date and time of physical departure of a patient from the ED treatment space for all categories of patients, including admitted, discharged, observed, and behavioral health patients.

## Time Intervals

- **Arrival-to-provider time** (a.k.a. "door to doc")
- **ED length of stay**: Arrival time to departure time. This is tracked for the following subsets of patients:
  - Admitted patients
  - Discharged patients
  - Observation patients
  - Behavioral health patients
- **Arrival-to–treatment space time**
  - Treatment space to provider time
  - Provider to data-ready time
  - Data ready to decision time
- **Decision-to-departure time**: Disposition decision time to the actual departure time of the patient.
- **Admit decision-to-departure time**: The decision-to-departure time applied to admitted patients. This metric is undergoing testing as a trial for CMS Hospital Inpatient Quality Measures.

## Subcycle Intervals

For clarity and consistency the term "turnaround time" has been replaced with "interval" in the subcycles definitions. Turnaround time was used inconsistently in the literature and in practice and so was abandoned.

- **EMS offload interval**: Arrival time to EMS offload time.
- **Triage interval**: The time from the initiation to the completion of rapid or comprehensive triage or intake by an institutionally credentialed provider.
- **Laboratory interval**: The time from the order for laboratory testing until the time the results are available.
- **ED consultation interval**: The time from the order for an ED consult until the time the patient is evaluated by the consulting service and the final recommendation is communicated to the ED provider.
- **Imaging interval**: The time from the order for an imaging test until the time that the results are available. Institutions are recommended to track for each modality:
  - Plain radiography
  - CT scans

- Ultrasound
- MRI
- **Bed assignment interval**: The time from the order or request for an inpatient bed to the time a bed is assigned (empty, clean, and staffed) and the ED receives notification.

## Proportion Metrics

A number of measures reported as percentages or rates can capture elements of performance in the ED. The proportion metrics are well established in the literature and in hospital operations. Patient complaints and walkaways correlate with timeliness in the ED (Welch et al. 2006). Think of them as indirect markers for timeliness and efficiency.

- **LWBS**: All patients who leave the ED before being seen by a provider.
- **LBTC**: All patients who leave the ED after being seen by a provider but before formal disposition is made.
- **AMA**: All patients who leave the ED against the advice of the provider and after the risks and benefits of further care have been explained and documented. AMA patients are a subset of LBTC patients.
- **Complaint ratio**: All spontaneous written, phoned, or spoken expressions of concern brought to the attention of the ED management or hospital staff. There must be a mechanism for recording these expressions, and the mechanism will be institution-specific. Complaint ratios are tracked by convention as complaints per 1,000 ED visits.

SOURCE: Welch et al. (2011).

# CHAPTER 4

# Reliability in Emergency Medicine

**In This Chapter**

- The Concept of Reliability
- How Reliable Is Healthcare?
- Reason's Swiss Cheese Model
- Strategies to Improve Reliability
- The Three Tiers of Reliability
- Information Technology: The String Around Your Finger
- The Role of Executive Leadership
- Case Study
- Strategies for Healthcare Executives

## THE CONCEPT OF RELIABILITY

According to Thomas Nolan, one of the leading authorities in healthcare performance improvement and a senior fellow at the Institute for Healthcare Improvement, *reliability* is defined as "failure-free operations over time" from the point of view of the patient (Nolan et al. 2004). In other words, it is the capability of a process, procedure, or health service to perform its intended function in the required time under existing conditions. Reliability is measured in the following manner:

$$\text{Reliability} = \frac{\text{Number of actions that achieve the intended result}}{\text{Total number of actions taken}}$$

As we'll discuss later in this chapter, the use of standardized procedures greatly improves reliability in healthcare. Many standardized procedures evolve from the application of clinical evidence. Thus, how often clinical evidence is applied is an important measure of reliability. Almost all studies that investigate the reliability of the application of clinical evidence conclude that the reliability level is only at 1 or 2 defects for every 10 attempts; 80 to 90 percent reliable, in the jargon of reli-

> **$10^{-1}$:** A reliability level of 80 to 90 percent; referred to as "ten to the minus one."

ability speak, or "ten to the minus one" (Baker et al. 2004). For example, if 90 percent of surgery patients receive antibiotics within an hour of surgical incision (which is shown by clinical evidence to be a good way to reduce infection), the reliability of that process is **$10^{-1}$**. When we talk about a process having a reliability of $10^{-2}$, we mean fewer than 5 defects per 100 attempts (this is not mathematically accurate, but the Institute for Healthcare Improvement has taken liberties with the math to establish these standards). To take a process to a higher level of reliability (for example, fewer than 5 failures out of 1,000 opportunities, or $10^{-3}$), a vigorously applied methodology can and must be implemented. If a process fails more than 20 percent of the time, it is considered a "chaotic process." Exhibit 4.1 includes examples of varying reliability in medicine and the associated terminology.

## HOW RELIABLE IS HEALTHCARE?

Although emergency physicians in the United States take comfort in the knowledge that they practice in one of the most advanced healthcare systems in the world, this system is highly unreliable and fraught with error. In his landmark article "Error

---

**Exhibit 4.1: Examples of Varying Reliability in Medicine**

| Chaotic Process | > 20 percent failure | Outpatient urine culture follow-up |
| --- | --- | --- |
| | | Breast cancer screening |
| $10^{-1}$ | 80 to 90 percent success | Hospital-acquired infection |
| | (one or two failures in 10 tries) | Adverse drug events |
| $10^{-2}$ | < 5 failures per 100 | ED wound infections |
| $10^{-3}$ | < 5 failures per 1,000 | Missed intubations hospitalized |
| | | Patients injured through negligence |
| $10^{-4}$ | < 5 failures per 10,000 | Anesthetic-related fatalities |

SOURCE: Welch and Jensen (2007).

---

in Medicine," Lucian Leape (1994) recounted a number of disturbing statistics, demonstrating how flawed the healthcare we deliver can be. Autopsy studies have shown that 35 to 40 percent of deaths are caused by missed diagnoses. Leape quotes one study showing the average intensive care unit had 1.7 errors in treatment per patient, per day.

When looking at operational errors, the data are worse. Positive urine cultures were either untreated or not followed up on 52 percent of the time. More sobering, according to The Joint Commission (2002), more than half of sentinel events involving death or permanent injury over a seven-year period occurred in the emergency department.

Roger Resar (2006), a physician from the Mayo Clinic actively involved in research applying reliability tools to healthcare, has suggested that any process with a reliability of $10^{-1}$ (80 to 90 percent efficacy rate) has no common process articulated, meaning no standardization in care. This includes many procedures and processes in medicine, from **DVT** prophylaxis of inpatients to follow up of outpatient urine cultures. A randomly chosen healthcare worker is unlikely to be capable of articulating this process. A process or procedure with $10^{-2}$ reliability has medium to high variation. Ten to the minus three reliability indicates a well-designed system with low variation and cooperative relationships. For comparison, aviation passenger safety is measured at $10^{-6}$. Nuclear power plants must demonstrate a design capable of operating at $10^{-6}$ before they can be built.

> **Deep venous thrombosis (DVT):** Blood clots, typically in the legs, sometimes developed by postoperative patients. By applying compression stockings and getting patients moving early in the post-op period, this risk is reduced.

Reliability is a cousin to patient safety, a discipline well developed in the industrialized world. Reliability has a methodology and a set of definitions, tools, and concepts that can be applied to healthcare settings, particularly emergency medicine.

## REASON'S SWISS CHEESE MODEL

Dr. James Reason (2000) first proposed the "Swiss cheese model" of organizational errors (Exhibit 4.2), describing how a series of breached defenses and small mistakes that pass undetected could lead to catastrophic outcomes. An easy way to think of these accidents is to look at airline crashes. Typically, a crash does not occur because of a single event. Rather, a series of factors (usually undetected) combine to breach the system's defenses, which results in an accident. Reliability science and strategies are a way to prevent such breaches.

**Exhibit 4.2: Swiss Cheese Model of Organizational Errors**

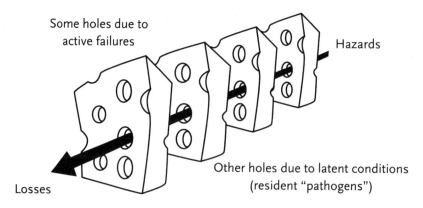

*Successive Layers of Defenses, Barriers, and Safeguards*

SOURCE: Adapted from Reason (2000).

Here is a good example from the world of emergency medicine. Mr. Smith is an elderly man brought to the ED with confusion. His family is with him but leaves temporarily. His nurse leaves the department to get lunch, and there is a hand-off to a nurse who is less familiar with the patient. Though the patient is confused and undergoing testing, he is stable and is moved to a different room when a patient in respiratory distress arrives. The CT technician is looking for the patient who needs a CT pulmonary angiogram (a high-radiation test) looking for blood clots in the lung. She asks Mr. Smith, "Are you Mr. Johnson?" and in his confusion he answers yes. The patient inadvertently gets the high-radiation test that was not intended for him.

There was not one cause of this adverse event. All of the following contributed to the mistake: a confused patient, an absent family member, his regular nurse out of the department, a room change, and a CT tech who did not check the patient's arm band. This series of breaches in the normal safety mechanisms led to the "organizational accident."

## STRATEGIES TO IMPROVE RELIABILITY

What should be our goal in emergency medicine, indeed, in healthcare? Would it be a worthy goal to have our patients receive the appropriate care in a timely fashion 99.9 percent of the time? Would that be good enough? To put this reliability into perspective, let's take a look at other service industries. If other industries had a reliability of 99.9 percent (and very little in medicine reaches that level), then we

---

**Exhibit 4.3: Three-Tier Approach to Increasing Reliability**

- $10^{-1}$: Prevent initial failure
- $10^{-2}$: Identify failure and mitigate
- $10^{-3}$: Redesign processes

SOURCE: Resar (2006).

---

would be looking at 84 unsafe plane landings a day, a plane crash every third day, 16,000 pieces of lost mail per hour, and 37,000 ATM errors per hour (Welch and Jensen 2007).

Reliability principles are used successfully in other industries (such as aviation and nuclear power) to improve the overall performance of complex systems and to compensate for the limits of human ability. Reliability principles can improve safety and the rate at which a system consistently produces desired outcomes.

## THE THREE TIERS OF RELIABILITY

Even with the eventual standardization of most medical processes in emergency medicine, the specialty will not get the reliability of those processes to better than 95 percent without further effort. Resar (2006) and his team propose a three-tiered strategy for moving from $10^{-1}$ to $10^{-3}$ reliability (Exhibit 4.3). They observed that increasing reliability does not occur by accident. It takes a clearly articulated vision, a strategy, and a methodology to implement the necessary change.

Resar's first step involves preventing the initial failure, which can be done by articulating the intended behaviors and using standardization. Make the standardization process work for the majority of patients by instituting training, using common equipment and procedures, and providing regular feedback on compliance to staff. This should bring the process to 80 to 90 percent efficacy.

**Strategies for $10^{-1}$ Reliability: Basic Failure Prevention**

- Common equipment
- Standard orders
- Personal checklists
- Feedback on compliance
- Awareness and training

The second step involves identifying the common failures that might occur and mitigating them through error proofing. Design procedures to include redundancies and other safeguards to make failures visible so they can be intercepted. These actions should bring reliability close to $10^{-2}$.

---

**Strategies for $10^{-2}$ Reliability: Identifying and Mitigating the Failures**

- Building decision aids and reminders into the system
- Making the desired action the default
- Instituting redundancy (double checks)
- Making interventions happen by default and automatically
- Taking advantage of existing habits and patterns
- Standardizing processes

---

The final step in the three-tiered approach involves identifying critical failures inherent in the process and trying to remedy those by process redesign. This step will anticipate the outliers—the cases that physicians might point to as exceptions to a protocol—and then design fail-safe measures around them.

---

**Strategies for $10^{-3}$ Reliability: Critical Failure Mode Function and Redesign**

- Identify the failure modes of the standardized process
- Focus on structure: transitions of care, information transfer
- Failure mode and events analysis (FMEA)

---

A good analogy from the banking industry involves research around errors in the use of ATMs. A common error in early ATM operations involved the customer leaving without his card. ATMs were redesigned to anticipate the error by returning the customer's debit card before dispensing cash, or having the card never leave his hand by using a swipe process. Other industries quickly caught on. For example, is there a gas station now that keeps a credit card while gas is pumped? Could we identify common errors in the ED and design processes aimed at failure prevention?

Efforts at improving a clinical pathway or process should start with small pilot studies and a carefully selected target sample. This methodology is vastly different from the medical research model. Instead of random sampling with large populations of patients, choose a subset of patients that is easy to target for success. At this stage the process is not designed for the outliers, or as Resar (2006) calls them, "onesies and twosies" (referring to the 1 to 2 percent of a population that will fail in a process). Rather, the design is for the overall population. Then refine the process by making small changes, measuring the results, and conducting small repetitive audits to monitor the responses to the changes. Over time, the reliability of the process will increase, and it is all done at the local level.

Resar urges that strategies and tools need not be confined to one tier at a time. Processes can be improved by using tools from all tiers at once and several changes can be implemented at once for maximum impact.

## INFORMATION TECHNOLOGY: THE STRING AROUND YOUR FINGER

Imagine an emergency physician is evaluating a young female patient with abdominal pain. The computer recognizes this pattern and combination of clinical data: A female patient of childbearing age, plus abdominal pain, plus a positive pregnancy test. The physician's communication device goes off and asks him, "Doctor, do you want an Rh factor sent? Would you also like an ultrasound?" Another critically ill patient might distract him, or he might be eating a ham sandwich, but *the system* makes the care he renders more reliable. (Note: In evaluating female patients with abdominal pain, ectopic pregnancy is one of the high-risk diagnoses that needs to be ruled out. An Rh factor is frequently forgotten in cases like this and is a diagnostic imperative.)

Imagine a system that alerts the physician when her patient has pneumonia and the time window for antibiotics is about to close, or a patient shows appendicitis on the CT scan and needs immediate attention. The system could improve compliance with the latest evidence-based medicine by prompting the physician regarding critical actions. The technological equivalent of a string tied around your finger, a comprehensive reliability program with information technology at its heart is our future. Ultimately, we can expect that reliability in emergency medicine will be increased with the help of information technology and clinical decision support. Providers will be able to achieve 95 percent reliability with standardized

> **Core measures:** A set of quality indicators defined by The Joint Commission. There are 33 core measures in 4 categories (acute myocardial infarction, community-acquired pneumonia, congestive heart failure, and surgical care improvement project). Under each category, key actions are listed that represent the most widely accepted, research-based care processes for appropriate care in that category.

order sets prompted through technology. Leadership should encourage providers to embrace this vision of the future of emergency medicine.

## THE ROLE OF EXECUTIVE LEADERSHIP

High-reliability organizations do not get that way by accident or by intuition. Executives need to show their understanding about reliability principles and strategies and how they may be applied throughout the organization. Executives should familiarize themselves with the language and the strategies of reliability and encourage the front lines to identify organizational reliability gaps and craft system fixes for them.

### Case Study

Northeastern Vermont Regional Hospital in St. Johnsbury boasts 100 percent compliance with **core measures** for community-acquired pneumonia. How did the organization get there?

First, the hospital provided education, training, and feedback to all physicians and staff about pneumonia care. Second, it standardized the process so that the ED would be responsible for all first doses of antibiotics and the other core measures. Prior to the project it was never clear whether the hospitalists or the ED was accountable for these things. By articulating the who, what, where, and how, the hospital was able to improve compliance. The hospital achieved that kind of reliability by being certain that everyone performed his task in a timely fashion every time.

|  | Before | After |
|---|---|---|
| Documentation of $O_2$ saturation | 87% | 100% |
| Blood cultures before antibiotics | 75% | 100% |
| Antibiotics within four hours | 68% | 100% |

SOURCE: Welch (2008a).

## Recommended Readings

Baker, G. R., P. G. Norton, V. Flintoft, R. Blais, A. Brown, J. Cox, E. Etchells, W. A. Ghali, P. Hébert, S. R. Majumdar, M. O'Beirne, L. Palacios-Derflingher, R. J. Reid, S. Sheps, and R. Tamblyn. 2004. "The Canadian Adverse Events Study: The Incidence of Adverse Events Among Hospitalized Patients in Canada." *Canadian Medical Association Journal* 170: 1678–86.

Botwinick, L., M. Bisognano, and C. Haraden. 2006. "Leadership Guide to Patient Safety." Cambridge, MA: Institute for Healthcare Improvement. www.ihi.org/IHI/Topics/LeadingSystemImprovement/Leadership/Literature/LeadershipGuidetoPatientSafety.htm

Davis, P., R. Lay-Yee, R. Briant, W. Ali, A. Scott, and S. Schugs. 2002. "Adverse Events in New Zealand Public Hospitals I: Occurrence and Impact. *New Zealand Medical Journal* 115: U271.

Leape, L. L. 1994. "Error in Medicine." *Journal of the American Medical Association* 272: 1851–57.

Nolan, T., R. Resar, C. Haraden, and F. Griffin. 2004. "Improving the Reliability of Healthcare." Cambridge, MA: Institute for Healthcare Improvement. www.ihi.org/IHI/Results/WhitePapers/ImprovingtheReliabilityofHealthCare.htm.

Welch, S., and K. Jensen. 2007. "The Concept of Reliability in Emergency Medicine." *American Journal of Medical Quality* 22 (1): 50–58.

# CHAPTER 5

# Human Cognition and Human Factors Engineering

**In This Chapter**

- Slips, Mistakes, and Errors in Medicine
- Human Factors Engineering
- Designing Effective Systems
- The Night Warriors
- The Role of Executive Leadership
- Case Study
- Strategies for Healthcare Executives

## SLIPS, MISTAKES, AND ERRORS IN MEDICINE

The human mind is prone to slips and mistakes. To understand and anticipate these failures is to begin down the road to solving the problem of medical errors. Here's what we know about human cognition—thought occurs at three different levels: schemata, rule-based thought, and knowledge-based thought.

---

**Three Tiers of Thought**

1. Schemata
2. Rule-based thought
3. Knowledge-based thought

---

We spend most of our time functioning at the first two levels. With *schemata*, we use preprogrammed responses that require little higher-order functioning. Driving to the office and filling out forms by rote are examples of schemata at work. With *rule-based thought*—thinking at the next level—the brain makes analogous comparisons: if X then Y. If a patient has a cough and a fever, we order a chest x-ray. Lastly, there is *knowledge-based analytical functioning*. We use this highest level of thought with difficult diagnostic cases to organize data into different patterns, which helps us to solve problems. Superimpose upon this the fact humans make slips and mistakes predictably. In fact, slips and mistakes are a normal part of cognitive functioning.

Errors we make while functioning at the schemata level are called "slips" and fall into four general categories.

**Slips: Unintended Acts**

- Capture
- Description error
- Associative activation
- Loss of activation

**Done nomogram**: A chart used to predict serious aspirin overdose using blood levels of aspirin and the time from ingestion.

Let's look at some examples and think about how these might come into play in the emergency department. With *capture*, frequent schemata take over. For example, you get into the car and drive to work when you intended to go to the dentist's office. In the ED this might mean ordering a chest x-ray when you intended to order a CT pulmonary angiogram instead. With *description error* the right action is attempted with the wrong object, like trying to eat soup with a fork. In the ED examples of description error might include looking up the **Done nomogram** for a Tylenol overdose or using absorbable suture when you meant to use ethilon (non-absorbable nylon). With *associative activation* incorrect mental associations occur—for instance, answering the phone when the doorbell rings. In the stress of the ED many auditory and visual cues might be wrongly associated. A commonly occurring slip is to grab the Vocera transmitter when a cell phone rings. Finally, *loss of activation* involves simple memory lapses, such as walking into a room and forgetting why you came or, in the fast paced ED, logging onto a database and forgetting what you came to retrieve.

Slips are more likely to occur in certain environments. Fatigue, activity, heat, noise, and visual stimuli all lead to slips. Research reveals that the ED is typically challenged by all of these factors (Croskerry and Sinclair 2001). In particular, the noise level creates distractions and interruptions, which all but guarantee slips.

In contrast to slips, mistakes involve more complicated cognitive functions and are more difficult to understand. There are rule-based mistakes, which involve misapplied expertise and misinterpreted situations. There are also knowledge-based mistakes, which involve the wrong pattern matching or the influence of bias.

Two major mechanisms that lead to mistakes have been recognized as frequent sources of medical error in the emergency department (Croskerry 2003): availability heuristic and confirmation bias.

In *availability heuristic* the physician or staff are biased, either because of other patients they are seeing or because some information about the patient results in bias (Davis and Jacques 2008). For example, you assume that a patient with **rales** and **dyspnea** has pneumonia because you have diagnosed two other cases today, but you don't consider congestive heart failure. In another example a confused homeless man (known to be an alcoholic by the staff) whose diagnostic workup consists only of alcohol level is allowed to sleep in the department, but eight hours later he is found to have a subdural hematoma.

The second mechanism, *confirmation bias,* is common in the emergency department (Pines 2006). ED physicians are good at "blink" responses and judgments about patients. In fact numerous articles have found that experienced ED physicians are 85 to 95 percent accurate at predicting the outcomes of patients, which is high reliability in medicine (Sinuff et al. 2006; Rocker et al. 2004; Dent et al. 2007). Unfortunately this capability can pervert the diagnostic process. In the ideal diagnostic process model, the physician listens to the patient's complaints and performs a physical exam. Then she works out a differential diagnosis and uses labs and imaging studies to make the final diagnosis. In contrast, the ED physician is prone to jumping to the diagnosis in that brief initial assessment and then ordering tests to confirm that early hunch. She forgets to consider the full differential. This leads to diagnostic errors.

> **Rales:** A recognizable sound on pulmonary exam indicating fluid in the lungs.

> **Dyspnea:** Difficulty breathing, shortness of breath.

Experts are just beginning to recognize how human error translates into medical errors.

Certain environmental factors increase the likelihood of mistakes:

---

**Factors Increasing the Risk of Mistakes**

- Distractions
- Time pressures
- Multiple caregivers
- Lack of callbacks and repeat-backs (The most reliable verbal orders are volleyed back and forth for confirmation.)
- Lack of clear standardization
- Sound-alike drug names (e.g., mag sulfate and morphine sulfate)
- Documentation delays

---

## HUMAN FACTORS ENGINEERING

Human factors engineering (HFE) is a technical discipline that is concerned with understanding the capabilities and limitations of people, equipment, and environments. Human factors engineers are concerned with six factors:

---

**Human Factors Engineering**

- Things are built to serve humans and should be designed with the user in mind.
- Differences in individuals (variation) must be appreciated and factored into design.
- The design of things influences human behavior.
- The scientific method can be used to generate data about human behavior.
- Data are used to evaluate design.
- A systems orientation is sentinel to this work.

SOURCE: Fairbanks and Gellatly (2009).

---

Human errors are predictable, and certain types of errors occur at predictable rates. Performing simple arithmetic will result in a 3 percent error rate. Ten percent of the time the inspector will not be able to find the error. Errors of commission (such as misreading a label) occur at a rate of about 0.3 percent. Errors of omission (forgetting a step without reminders) occur about 1 percent of the time. A number of reports suggest that medication errors occur in the ED at a rate of 1 to 3 percent (Weant 2010). If you look at error rates in high-stress situations with dangerous activities occurring rapidly, that number soars to 25 percent.

## DESIGNING EFFECTIVE SYSTEMS

A basic premise of HFE is that systems can be designed to overcome the limits of human performance. Here are ten tips on how to design effective ED systems, adapted from the book *Achieving Safe and Reliable Health Care* (Leonard et al. 2004).

1. Have simple rules: Complex environments are best handled by simple rules. The rules in the ED for all processes and operations should be easy to articulate, understand, and follow.
2. Be consistent and predictable: Systems should provide staff with a common foundation as they approach work.
3. Include redundancy: Build multiple layers of defense against errors into work flow.
4. Force functions: Institute mechanisms that make it easy to do the right thing and impossible to do the wrong thing (e.g., oxygen tubing that cannot be hooked into an IV port).
5. Prohibit work-arounds: Investigate why staff are engaged in workarounds, particularly if they are unsafe, and design better systems.
6. Minimize reliance on memory: A great example in the ED is IT support that gives and calculates the dose of medications at order entry.
7. Allow expertise: Good systems allow clinicians to use their best judgments; departing from protocols should be an option.
8. Maximize technology support: Ensure it is fast, easy, and reliable at the user interface.
9. Centralize workflow: The system should be easier and more effective than what came before, and the advantages should be apparent to the frontline workers.
10. Be prepared for failure: Occasionally at implementation a system fails. Be prepared to acknowledge this and either revise or withdraw the system.

## THE NIGHT WARRIORS

Healthcare, in particular emergency healthcare, is a 24/7 proposition, which creates a propensity for error. Further, the well-being of persons working night hours under sleep deprivation is just now being studied. Recent research performed at the State University of New York in Albany (Vinogradova et al. 2009) demonstrated that rats deprived of sleep at night (analogous to night-shift workers) aged more quickly, had a shorter lifespan, and demonstrated more tumorigenesis than rats that were not sleep deprived. Other studies suggest that working the night shift may increase the risk of developing breast cancer and other cancers, though other research is contradictory and inconclusive. On the other hand, we know that the night shift does take a toll on its workers. A recent study published in *Chronobiology International* showed that night-shift workers had an increased odds ratio of obesity, central obesity (suggesting endocrine dysfunction), and hypertension (Odle-Dusseau, Bradley, and Pilcher 2010). Investigators also have found an increased risk for cardiovascular disease in night-shift workers (Thomas and Power 2010). Other studies have shown a shortened life expectancy, an increased risk of diabetes, anxiety and depression, eating disorders, and sleep disturbances (Scheer and Bass 2009). Night-shift workers eat fewer calories but more fat and sugar, often resorting to fast food, caffeinated drinks, and energy drinks (Strangely 2009); the long-term consequences of this are only beginning to be studied. Suffice it to say that night-shift work is hazardous to your health.

Experts also now recognize that the sleep deprivation inherent in night-shift work has effects on human performance. In a recent edition of the journal *Sleep*, investigators at the Henry Ford Hospital reported on the effects of sleep deprivation on attention and memory (Gumenyuk et al. 2010). The researchers found the limits of human performance are tested when subjects are forced to challenge their natural circadian rhythms. Sleep restriction experiments also have shown that the ability to multitask and to perform psychomotor tests falters when subjects are sleep deprived. Another study done at Stanford University noted that night-shift workers get less sleep overall, are prone to sleep attacks (suddenly falling asleep, often at work), and are at increased risk for motor vehicle collisions (Ohayon, Smolensky, and Roth 2010). Should night-shift workers be chauffeured to work?

Are there recommended strategies to make night shifts more healthful? One of the largest studies of shift work and scheduling strategies was reported in *Ergonomics* (Klein Hesselink, de Leede, and Goudswaard 2010). The study involved more than 4,600 steel workers, and a number of scheduling models were tested. The model found to be associated with the least illness and absenteeism was one in which shifts were rotated forward (day to evening to night), with extra time off allotted after the night shift. The extra time off allowed the night workers to catch up on sleep, rather than forcing them to do so in an irregular pattern. Of particular note, the older workers demonstrated the most benefit from that model, a finding that has implications for our aging workforce.

Other strategies to help workers manage the difficulties of the night shift include trying to get more "prime sleep." Studies have shown that the most restful sleep is stage 4 REM sleep, which is most prevalent between 9 p.m. and 3 a.m. (Brandt 2003). This prime sleep is the hardest to come by when challenging normal circadian rhythms. These findings have led to experimentation with schedules that involve shorter shifts staggered around the prime sleep hours.

Most experts agree that night-shift workers should be encouraged to get normal durations of sleep when off shift. Avoiding caffeine and using room-darkening shades and earplugs to limit sensory interruptions can help facilitate sleep (Trimble 1998). If the worker will be switching back to a normal circadian sleep pattern, he should be encouraged to rise from sleep by noon the next day to "reset" his clock. Making exercise central to the night-shift lifestyle will have positive effects on weight management, mood disorders, and high blood pressure. As noted earlier, night workers have a tendency to eat fast food and sugars. However, a low-carbohydrate diet may provide higher energy levels and less post-meal drowsiness.

---

**Successful Strategies for Night-Shift Work**

- Prime sleep
- Forward-rotating schedules
- Extra recovery time after night shifts
- Monitoring for well-being
- Exercise
- Low-carbohydrate, high-protein diet
- Monitoring for diabetes, hypertension, and obesity

---

## THE ROLE OF EXECUTIVE LEADERSHIP

Night-shift work is part of many healthcare careers, especially emergency medicine. Recent research in this field should command our full attention for reasons of performance, safety, and general health. Emerging evidence supports that the night warriors in emergency medicine deserve a model of health-based work scheduling and "combat pay." This model should be structured to optimize performance and health, with more time off to minimize sleep deprivation. Night-shift personnel should be paid in a way that acknowledges the hardships implicit in night-shift work. We in healthcare, including executives, physician leaders, human resources personnel, risk managers, and patient safety officers, are responsible for the proper education and treatment of night workers. This responsibility is not being met in most organizations. By attending to the needs and realities of night-shift workers, we can help ensure their longevity in the workforce.

## Case Study

A large hospital system saw three episodes in which newborn infants inadvertently received tube feedings through an IV system. Each sentinel event occurred at a different location. After careful root cause analysis was performed, the following factors were identified as contributing to the errors:

1. All errors occurred on the night shift and after the nurseries began a trial of dimming lights to create circadian rhythms in the nursery.
2. All errors were with experienced career nurses, not inexperienced or float nurses.
3. All errors occurred after an equipment change. Prior to the equipment change the equipment was incompatible; the tube feedings could not be hooked up to the IV hubs.
4. After the organization switched the equipment back there were no further events.

SOURCE: Welch, unpublished risk management case review

## Strategies for Healthcare Executives

- Educate staff about the limits of human performance.
- Build a rigorous system for capturing errors and near misses.
- Build out mechanisms—including alerts, cues, and redundancy—for preventing or mitigating against errors.
- Recognize the problems inherent in work that causes sleep deprivation, and craft policies, including scheduling strategies, to minimize them.
- Provide resources, education, and training for night-shift workers, and value their contributions.

## Recommended Readings

Croskerry, P. 2009. "Human Factors Engineering and Safe Systems." In *Patient Safety in Emergency Medicine,* edited by P. Croskerry, K. S. Cosby, S. M. Schenkel, and R. L. Wears. Philadephia, PA: Wolters Kluwer/Lippincott Williams & Wilkins.

Kohn L. T., J. M. Corrigan, and M. S. Donaldson, editors. 2000. *To Err Is Human: Building a Safer Health System.* Washington DC: National Academies Press.

Leonard, M., A. Frankel, T. Simmonds, with K. Vega. 2004. *Achieving Safe and Reliable Healthcare.* Chicago: Health Administration Press.

# CHAPTER 6

# Error Proofing and Mistake Proofing the ED

**In This Chapter**

- How Safe Is Healthcare?
- Human Cognition and Human Error
- Mistake Proofing by Design
- The Role of Executive Leadership
- Case Study
- Strategies for Healthcare Executives

## HOW SAFE IS HEALTHCARE?

More people die each year from medical error than from breast cancer, motor vehicle accidents, or AIDS. In fact, according to the Harvard Medical Practices study, which estimates medical injuries in hospitals, mortality from **iatrogenic** causes likely approaches 100,000 deaths a year in the United States (Leape et al. 1991). (Such projections were the basis for the 100,000 Lives Campaign organized by the Institute for Healthcare Improvement in 2004.) In addition, the National Patient Safety Foundation revealed in a study (Louis Harris and Associates 1997) that roughly one in six Americans had a personal experience with a medical error.

> **Iatrogenic:** An illness or symptoms induced in a patient as the result of a physician's words or actions (e.g., as a consequence of taking a prescribed drug).

As you can see in Exhibit 6.1, the chances of an adverse event even in routine healthcare encounters make it as dangerous as mountain climbing or bungee jumping. The chance of a fatality

**Exhibit 6.1: How Hazardous Is Healthcare?**

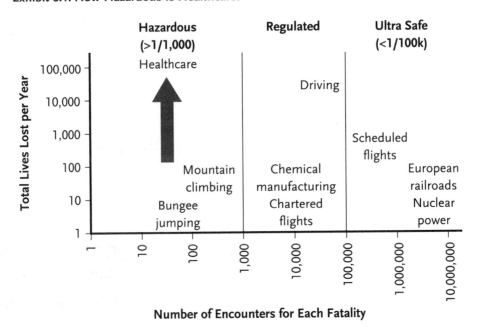

**Number of Encounters for Each Fatality**

SOURCE: Welch and Jensen (2007).

makes healthcare much more risky than driving a car. In the preceding chapter we discussed how unreliable our healthcare system is, but now we see it may actually be quite dangerous.

The culture and craft of medicine, which emphasize the skill and character of the physician as the main weapons against medical error, contribute to the problem. The suggestion is that if the physician has integrity, cares about his patient, and works and studies hard, quality and safety will be achieved. Meanwhile a growing body of research has shown that the vast majority of medical errors (more than 80 percent) are system-derived (Leonard et al. 2004; National Quality Forum 2003, 2009), meaning system flaws set good people up to fail. In fact, most experts suggest that only 5 percent of medical errors are due to incompetent or poorly rendered care.

## HUMAN COGNITION AND HUMAN ERROR

Cognitive psychologists have shown that humans err regularly and predictably (see Chapter 5). One scheme for understanding how we turn thought into action (and therefore where we make mistakes) notes that a task inherently involves two steps (Grout 2007):

1.  Determining the intent of the action
2.  Executing the action based on that intent

Slips and mistakes can occur at either step. Mistakes occur when the wrong intent is formulated. Slips can also occur when the intent is correct but the action does not occur as intended. So we can think of mistakes as *errors of intent* versus *errors in execution.* To mistake proof your ED, you need to know whether an error is one of intent or one of execution to design around it. A great example of mistake proofing in the ED is the end tidal $CO_2$ device or monitor. In this task the correct intent is to put a tube into the trachea, but the execution can fail in many ways. Some end tidal $CO_2$ devices use colorimetric information to cue the user that the ET tube is in the esophagus, while others use digital readouts. These devices detect the error in execution before damages ensue. This safeguard does not address errors of intent, such as a clinician not recognizing a patient's pending respiratory failure.

D. A. Norman's (1989) book *The Design of Everyday Things* divides knowledge into two categories:

1.  *Knowledge in the head* is information contained in the human memory. Historically efforts at mistake proofing in healthcare have involved putting more knowledge in the head.
2.  *Knowledge in the world* is information provided by the environment in which a task is performed.

Too often in the ED we try to remedy errors with retraining: putting more information in the user's head when knowledge in the world is more effective. A good example involves look-alike medications. For instance, eye preparations that contain pupillary dilating drugs are dangerous in some settings and inappropriate in others. After a nurse inadvertently puts a dilating medication in the eyes of a patient with acute angle closure glaucoma—which makes acute angle closure glaucoma worse and can be particularly painful for the patient—the traditional paradigm would involve retraining. Making the labels on these preparations visibly red—putting knowledge in the world—has been shown to prevent this error.

Another example involves instruction manuals of any sort in a work environment. Often the tasks being performed have many steps that are not familiar to the user. One sensible piece of advice is to use single-sided copying. This way the user can't inadvertently go to the wrong page when a manual is open to two pages and get the steps out of sequence. Another simple change is to do away with manuals altogether and have real-time cues in place. When computer technology is employed, pop-up screens provide the user with immediate feedback that an action has been performed incorrectly.

Increasingly in healthcare we realize, as manufacturing and service industries have realized before us, that knowledge in the head and safety measures that depend on people are far less effective than using knowledge in the world and safety that depends on systems or design.

## MISTAKE PROOFING BY DESIGN

Mistake proofing is the use of process or design features to prevent errors or prevent the negative impact of those errors. One of the oldest examples is the Otis elevator brake, introduced in the 1850s, which stopped the elevator between floors when a cable broke. Another example is the everyday filing cabinet. The early cabinets would tip over if more than one drawer was open. The mistake-proof design prevents tipping by only allowing one drawer to open at a time. Human creativity and ingenuity have been used in the environment to prevent or mitigate mistakes that humans make.

One common problem in EDs is that as patients lift themselves up from a wheelchair, with or without assistance, the wheelchair begins to roll and the patient falls. The wheelchair has a brake, but human error means the brake won't be set consistently. Newer chairs have been designed to engage the brakes when the patient pushes down on the armrests, creating a secure chair to balance against.

The problem of mislabeled lab specimens plagues emergency departments every day. One root cause is that specimens are often obtained before the patient has been fully registered. These specimens often go unlabeled or incorrectly labeled. Further, asking staff to label a rainbow collection of blood tubes by hand is time consuming and difficult to enforce. One solution, the Bloodloc system, uses a wristband with preprinted labels and a unique ID number. As the blood is drawn the labels are peeled from the patient's wristband and applied to the tubes. These tubes may be sent to the lab as is for stat results or held until full registration allows the patient's permanent ID number to be assigned. Reconciliation of the data can occur at any time.

In general, mistake proofing is inexpensive, and reduced errors save EDs money and time. Emergency department workers have a long history of improvisation and "jury rigging" the world to help their patients, such as using a foley catheter balloon as a posterior nasal packing, using bed sheets as levers to relocate a shoulder, or using lidocaine to get a cockroach out of a patient's ear. It is now time to unleash that ingenuity to make our work foolproof and make our departments safer for our patients.

# THE ROLE OF EXECUTIVE LEADERSHIP

Just as anesthesiologists were able to virtually eradicate mistakes and errors in their specialty, so can your organization strive for safety and reliability. It means putting systems in place to capture the sentinel events and the near misses. It will involve a profound and sweeping cultural change and the creation of a "just culture" discussed in Chapter 9. It will not happen without the highest levels of the organization being visibly on board.

---

### Case Study

In 1848 an 18-year-old girl visited her physician to have a problem toenail removed. Hannah Greer received an anesthetic of chloroform to sedate her for this procedure. She was overdosed and sustained cardiac arrest. Efforts at resuscitation (consisting of pouring brandy and water down the unconscious girl's throat) were unsuccessful. This was the first recorded death due to complications of anesthesia. The Hannah Greer case has been debated and discussed for 150 years.

In 1954 Henry Beecher, an anesthesiologist at Massachusetts General Hospital, began to examine the safety of anesthesia. In his study he concluded that anesthesia was "twice as deadly as polio."

In 1984 J. B. Cooper looked at the management of errors and equipment failures in the OR. He noted that 70 percent of the errors were due to humans. Anesthesiologists began an open dialogue about how to prevent harm and standardize care, using technology to prevent accidents.

Some of the innovations that have been instrumental in improving the reliability and safety of anesthesia are:

- Pulse oximetry
- End tidal $CO_2$ monitoring
- Ultrasound for line placement
- Continuous ECG monitoring
- Frequent BP monitoring
- Intraoperative documentation standards

Anesthesia has become safer as a result of these innovations and standardizations and, in fact, is the most reliable subspecialty in medicine. In 1954 one out of 1,500 patients died of anesthetic complications. In 2001 that number had fallen to one in 250,000 patients.

SOURCE: Cooper, Newbower, and Kitz (1984).

**Strategies for Healthcare Executives**

- Design systems that make the wrong thing the impossible thing to do.
- Design systems that capture mistakes, errors, and near misses in a nonpunitive way.
- When errors are recognized, look for system causes and solutions.
- Articulate a strong patient safety mission.

## Recommended Readings

Cooper, J. B., R. S. Newbower, and R. J. Kitz. 1984. "An Analysis of Major Errors and Equipment Failures in Anesthesia Management Considerations for Prevention and Detection." *Anesthesiology* 60 (1): 34–42.

Grout, J. 2007. "Mistake Proofing the Design of Health Care Processes." AHRQ Publication No. 07–0020. Rockville, MD: Agency for Healthcare Research and Quality.

Kohn, L. T., J. M. Corrigan, and M. S. Donaldson, editors. 2000. *To Err is Human: Building a Safer Health System.* Washington DC: National Academies Press

Leonard, M., A. Frankel, T. Simmonds, with K. Vega. 2004. *Achieving Safe and Reliable Healthcare.* Chicago: Health Administration Press.

Spath, P. 2000. *Error Reduction in Healthcare: A Systems Approach to Improving Patient Safety.* Chicago: Health Forum Inc.

# Standardization in the Emergency Department

**In This Chapter**

- Standardization in Aviation
- The Case for Standardization in Emergency Medicine
- The Pushback Against Standardization
- The Conservative Medical Culture
- Designing for Process Failures
- The Role of Executive Leadership
- Case Study
- Strategies for Healthcare Executives

In Chapter 6, we outlined the opportunities for information technology and design to improve reliability in healthcare. The two other keys to improving reliability, safety, and quality are standardization and teamwork. We'll address standardization here and teamwork in Chapter 8.

## STANDARDIZATION IN AVIATION

While standardization in emergency medicine has a long way to go, the commercial aviation world has embraced standardization and systems to offset human error. Mistakes are expected, the limits of human performance are recognized, and the system includes processes and mechanisms to compensate for error. It all starts with standardization. Commercial aviation now has less than one fatality per million take-offs. In fact there have been fewer commercial airline deaths over the past 60 years than there are motor vehicle deaths in the United States every three months (Borowsky and Gaynor 2002). A traveler could fly once a day for 11,000 years without an accident!

Processes in aviation are clearly articulated with checklists, redundancies, checks and double checks, and call-backs and repeat-backs. Communication is airtight, common processes are performed by protocol, and all activities are standardized. Aviation has made standardization a fundamental element of operations and the cornerstone of the aviation industry's culture.

For healthcare as a whole to become safer and more reliable, it must work to duplicate this same culture of safety. It will need to build systems that compensate for human error with safeguards and redundancies to improve human performance. It will also need to take gags off of frontline workers and encourage a climate of open disclosure about near misses and an anticipation of these errors.

## THE CASE FOR STANDARDIZATION IN EMERGENCY MEDICINE

The majority of common ED operations are chaotic (meaning there are defects more than 20 percent of the time) with no standardized process. For example, abdominal pain is one of the most common chief complaints presenting to the ED, and urine analysis is considered a critical part of the workup for abdominal pain. Urine samples are also required for toxicology screens, pregnancy tests, and the evaluation of flank pain. Despite the sheer magnitude of the number of urine samples collected every day across the country, the typical ED has no clearly articulated process for collecting the specimens, no timeline, and no definition of process failure. Without a definition for process failure or a way to measure failure, how can a solution for the problem be found? This failure frequently causes delays in the diagnosis of abdominal pain, and yet no one has tackled the issue with a standardized order set and process that could be universally adopted.

### Benefits of Standardization

1. Decreases medical error
2. Improves reliability
3. Improves staff training

(continued)

4. Improves defect detection
5. Encourages frontline staff ownership
6. Cuts costs

First and most compelling, standardization helps reduce error. Outpatient anticoagulation therapy is wholly lacking in standardization and is one of the most common areas of outpatient serious adverse medication events. This makes it nearly impossible to train healthcare workers and to track defects in the process. Standardization would reduce errors and make it easier to recognize them when they occur.

Second, standardization improves the reliability of processes and operations, as demonstrated in nuclear power, on flight decks, in cockpits, and closer to home, in anesthesia. Standardized order sets and standardized processes are two important tools in the reliability toolbox. Since the 1980s the specialty of anesthesia has moved toward universal standards of care and has become one of the most reliable specialties in medicine. The Anesthesia Patient Safety Foundation has tracked and disseminated data on safe anesthesia administration for more than 20 years, which has led to standards of care for the specialty.

Third, staff training is easier when a single treatment approach is adopted. Increasingly we are appreciating that a team approach to medical care is safest and also efficient. Note that in the most critical medical situations (cardiac arrest, trauma resuscitation) protocol utilization and a med teams approach were long ago accepted. Most Level I trauma centers run a trauma code like a military operation with assigned positions and responsibilities. Training personnel using these standardizations is easier than if each resuscitation were run in a random fashion.

Fourth, an important step on the pathway to increased reliability, safety, and efficiency is the recognition of defects in a process. By recognizing where mistakes might occur, systems can be adapted to compensate for them. When there is no standard process as a baseline, the recognition of these defects is slower and uses more resources. Many processes in the emergency department have no clearly articulated procedures. Vomiting is a common chief complaint in the emergency department. If it is in conjunction with abdominal pain, most patients will receive an IV and a medication to stop the vomiting. Yet few emergency departments have standardized this process and adopted order sets that allow a vomiting patient to receive an IV and anti-emetic medications by default. Instead patients suffer delays before relief is given while nurses interrupt doctors seeing other patients, asking "Can I start an IV in room 3 and give some Zofran (an anti-emetic)?" These interruptions can in turn lead to medical errors, and the lack of standardization results in unnecessary delays in care. To the patient vomiting in the ED, a wait of 30 minutes or more would be viewed as a process failure or defect. When processes become standardized it is easier to recognize and remedy the defects.

Fifth, the front lines can take ownership of the standardization process. Because there is not enough evidence-based knowledge about ED operations, most standardization will need to be locally developed. This is a good thing. Standardization developed by frontline workers who best know the processes and constraints of the institution (as opposed to being imported by an outside regulatory body) is more likely to be successful and encourage staff ownership of the process. In the 2006 Institute for Healthcare Improvement's (IHI) Emergency Department Innovation Community (the ED Collaborative) a dozen EDs participated in the Protocols and Process Improvement Workgroup. These teams began testing protocols for various ED processes, such as urine collection and CAP (community-acquired pneumonia) treatment. They were encouraged to take a protocol "off the shelf" from the IHI website and to customize it locally for their department and institution. Though their work went largely unpublished, these teams showed improved performance with the implementation of standardization, and success began building upon success (Welch 2009b). The Collaborative ended in 2008, but the participants continue their work in this area, pushing the limits of performance in the ED through standardization.

And finally, the financial case for standardization is easy to make. Standardized processes save money for a variety of reasons. First, standardization reduces defects. Second, increasing efficiency increases the number of bed turns, which increases revenue. While fixed costs remain the same, more patients processed through the system means higher profit margins. In addition, and as many ED managers can attest, when a physician group commits to a single treatment plan, supplies and medications can be ordered in bulk. Lastly, when waits and delays occur due to operational inefficiency, what is the cost of such delays? What is the cost of a complaint?

## THE PUSHBACK AGAINST STANDARDIZATION

Frequently, physicians and staff object to standardization in a process because they have a mind-set of designing for perfection (with 100 percent of patients being successfully treated). This is the approach physicians take with their patients—one at a time—in the delivery of care. When asked to devise a standardized process, physicians can always think of outliers and exceptions to a protocol and use them as an objection to standardization. Although the 100 percent goal is admirable for clinical outcomes, it becomes a stumbling block in reliability and patient safety efforts. The goal is to make the process foolproof for the majority of patients, then refine it for higher levels of reliability. Providers can then study failures to learn how to make the process more reliable. This concept is important for healthcare workers to accept. Letting go of the perfection goal is a necessary first step on the road to reliability.

## The Concepts Behind Standardization

- Let go of the perfection goal.
- Design for the majority.
- Recognize its effect on other high-reliability organizations.
- Decrease variation.

Some of the pushback regarding standardization may have to do with earlier approaches to the process. Experts devised a protocol with little staff input, customization was infrequent, there was no plan to ensure compliance, and there was little leadership to draw from. The newer approach to standardization begins with good evidence-based medicine or system-based knowledge and encourages customization. Changes are monitored, and as the flaws in a protocol are recognized (unwanted, undesired, unexpected, or unplanned outcomes), the team sets out to improve on the protocol by learning from the defects. Leadership drives the expectation of compliance. Instead of hoping that physicians will opt into the standardization, the new model requires an explanation for why the physician opted out.

Once again, it may be worth comparing medicine to the aviation model. The aviation industry assumes that errors and failures are inevitable, and it designs systems to "absorb" them, building in multiple buffers, automation, and redundancy. A glance in a cockpit sheds light on the extensive feedback given to the pilot in duplicate and triplicate. In addition, procedures are standardized to the maximum extent possible. Specific protocols must be followed for trip planning, operations, and maintenance. Pilots also go through checklists as well as regular proficiency examinations.

Physicians, who have been trained and rewarded through physician culture to be autonomous, often balk at a model where every action is prescribed and monitored. Physicians are taught to disdain protocols as "cookbook" medicine and likely have never been exposed to the positive contributions made by protocols and standardization.

## THE CONSERVATIVE MEDICAL CULTURE

It has been suggested that medicine lags behind other industries that are safety-critical (Von Thaden et al. 2006). Medicine needs to shift from a culture of blame in the face of adverse events to a culture of learning. Replacing the traditional incident report model of tracking sentinel events for a new model with emphasis on system fixes and near-miss identification would be a good first step. Research points to cultural differences between other high-reliability operations and medicine (Sexton, Thomas, and Helmreich 2000). Healthcare workers are more likely to deny the effects of stress and fatigue, find it more difficult to discuss errors, and have a harder time accepting personal susceptibility to error when compared with cockpit crews.

Ironically, it has been noted that physician pilots, who have no trouble accepting standardization and protocols in the cockpit, rail against them in the hospital, clinic, or emergency department (Welch 2007). Why is that?

Part of it is cultural. The mental model physicians have operated under is this: If the physician cares, studies, and tries hard, quality healthcare will be the result. As healthcare becomes increasingly complex and data driven, the old model of care does not deliver. In fact, the more we learn about human cognition, the limits of human performance, and the functioning of complex systems, the more we appreciate how error-prone the old paradigm really is.

## DESIGNING FOR PROCESS FAILURES

As care for individual patients becomes more complex, ED visits will involve longer stays with more diagnostic and therapeutic interventions, more information to be managed, and more opportunities for individual errors to accrue. *Errors of commission* (doing something incorrectly, such as misreading a label) occur three times out of 1,000. *Errors of omission* (not doing something, such as failing to follow up on abnormal lab tests) occur one time in 100 (Nolan 2000).

Now consider the compounding effects of these human errors in healthcare processes that involve multiple steps. For example, fulfilling a physician's medication order for a patient has been estimated to have between 40 and 60 steps. If each step in a 50-step process has a 1 in 100 chance of error, the chance that the process will be completed successfully and error free for all 50 steps is .61, or only 61 percent of the time (Botwinick, Bisognano, and Haraden 2006)!

System changes can increase the likelihood of success for each step and for the overall process. Examples of system changes include medication repeat-backs by nurse and physician, built-in alarms using information technology to indicate allergies and incompatibilities, marking high-risk medications with red or making their administration systems incompatible with routine administration systems, standardized doses, or premade IV solutions. The idea is to change the system by changing steps in the process or the environment in which we carry out the process. We use these types of strategies instead of relying on humans to carry out such tasks flawlessly every time, which we know can't happen!

Standardization helps protect against these kinds of operational and process failures. Some of the most innovative, progressive, and operationally efficient EDs have standardized order sets, sometimes called **advanced triage protocols**, for the top five to ten chief complaints. Some innovative departments are also standardizing the processes for urine collection and radiology operations, common sources of bottlenecking and delays in the ED.

Another example is to set triggers on the electronic tracking system to cue the following:

> **Advanced triage protocols:** Chief complaint-based, nurse-driven order sets that allow the nurse to begin diagnostic and therapeutic interventions from triage, before the physician sees the patient.

- More than 30 minutes for a nurse to clear a medication order, in particular orders for pain medication
- More than 30 minutes for the lab to receive specimens, in particular urinalysis
- More than one hour for x-ray results

These are random time frames, though loosely anchored in benchmarking data collected by VHA and best practices suggested by the Abaris Group (McGrayne 2005).

By setting a definition of a process failure with a time frame, and using standardization and cueing for the staff, you can improve routine ED processes. The system can be changed to make the work occur with fewer delays and errors. By the way, low-tech departments without sophisticated IT support can do many of these things using markers and a whiteboard. The staff use the whiteboard to note the time the urine is ordered, and the charge nurse polices this whiteboard for delays and defects.

---

**A Few Tips on the Successful Design and Implementation of Standardized Order Sets in General**

1. Individual protocols should be developed locally or modified from other organizations and approved by the physician group.
2. Early input from other stakeholders can eliminate problems later.

(continued)

3. The medical executive committee should make the protocols the standard of care for the organization.
4. All protocols may be preempted at the individual physician level.
5. Deviation from standardized protocols must be justified.
6. An individual's signature on a medical record authorizes the protocol use.
7. Protocols should be periodically reviewed and adjusted based on changes in the medical literature or the needs of the individual department.

# THE ROLE OF EXECUTIVE LEADERSHIP

The most progressive healthcare organizations with the strongest mandates for patient safety make standardization an organizational imperative. Standardization requires a top-down articulation from the highest levels of leadership, programs for incentivizing physician and staff behavior to follow protocols and standardization, and wholesale cultural change.

## Case Study

The University of Utah in Salt Lake City has a history of research focusing on pain management in the ED. Dr. David Fosnocht has studied pain management and patient preferences for pain control (oral over parenteral). His team recently conducted a study in which nurses were empowered by protocol to medicate patients orally when they had a high index of suspicion for extremity fractures. When triage protocols allowing nurses to administer pain medication were implemented, performance on time-to-pain-management improved:

|  | Before | After |
|---|---|---|
| Time to analgesic | 76 Minutes | 40 Minutes |
| Rate of administration | 45% | 70% |

SOURCE: Fosnocht and Swanson (2007).

## Strategies for Healthcare Executives

- Understand and support the development of protocols in the ED.
- Let standardization be developed by the clinicians but articulated and implemented with executive leadership and support.
- Encourage and support nurses' participation in protocols.
- Allow practitioners to "opt out" of protocols, but they must be prepared to explain why.
- Make standardization a part of the organizational culture.
- Encourage the approval of protocols through the medical executive committee so that they become the institutional gold standard of care.
- Build standardization into everyday workflow.
- Standardize between units as much as possible.


## Recommended Readings

Botwinick, L., M. Bisognano, and C. Haraden. 2006. *Leadership Guide to Patient Safety.* Cambridge, MA: Institute for Healthcare Improvement.

Nolan, T., R. Resar, and C. Haraden. 2004. *Improving the Reliability of Healthcare.* Cambridge, MA: Institute for Healthcare Improvement

Pronovost, P. J., C. G. Holzmueller, E. Martinez, C. L. Cafeo, D. Hunt, C. Dickson, M. Awad, M. A. Makary. 2006. "A Practical Tool to Learn From Defects in Patient Care." *Joint Commission Journal on Quality and Patient Safety* 32 (2): 102–8.

Resar, R. 2005. "Why We Need to Learn Standardization." *Australian Family Physician* 34 (½): 1–2.

Welch, S. J. 2009. "Intake." *Quality Matters: Solutions for a Safe and Efficient Emergency Department.* Oakbrook Terrace, IL: Joint Commission Resources Publishing.

# CHAPTER 8

# Teamwork in the ED

**In This Chapter**

- Crew Resource Management
- Communication Errors
- Teamwork Training Applied
- Group Work Versus Teamwork
- Improving Communication
- Advantage of Teamwork and Med Teams
- The Role of Executive Leadership
- Case Study
- Strategies for Healthcare Executives

## CREW RESOURCE MANAGEMENT

In the late 1970s a series of commercial airline mishaps led to several exhaustive studies looking for the root causes of these errors. One of the sentinel events involved a United Airlines plane heading into Portland, Oregon, after a shock absorber broke and the landing gear descended prematurely. Though the crew had contingency plans for landing safely, the pilot was preoccupied with the malfunction; while waiting for instructions from the ground, the plane ran out of fuel. The pilot failed to verbalize his problems, and the crew did not voice their concerns about fuel. Because of this lack of communication and teamwork, the plane crashed in a wooded area six miles from the runway and seven people died. A sequence of similar mishaps and an investigative study by Helmreich (1997) led to the conclusion that 70 percent of commercial airline accidents were the result of communication errors.

In 1978 a report by the military inspector general identified poor teamwork as a factor in many aircraft accidents. In 1979 a NASA workshop looking at the problem coined the term "crew resource management." In 1980 United Airlines became the first airline to develop crew resource management (CRM) training for its flight crews (Cooper, White, and Lauber 1980). By 1989 all three branches of the US military had developed crew resource management training. Finally, in 1997 the Federal Aviation Administration required all airline carriers to provide this training to all flight crews (Helmreich, Merritt, and Wilhelm 1999).

Research suggests that CRM training has led to heightened safety-awareness attitudes; improved communication, coordination, and decision-making behaviors; and enhanced error-management skills (Helmreich and Foushee 1993; Oser et al. 2001; Smith-Jentsch et al. 2001). CRM training also has demonstrated consistently positive results across a wide range of team structures, including flight crews, maintenance teams, dispatchers, and air traffic control teams. It was applied to healthcare settings in the late 1990s and is now seeing a resurgence in interest, particularly in hospital-based healthcare delivery units like the OR, labor and delivery, the ED, and the ICU (Brooks-Buza, Fernandez, and Stenger 2001).

---

**Crew Resource Management Principles**

- Teamwork behaviors are teachable.
- Team behaviors do not replace clinical skills.
- Superb individuals may not perform well in teams.
- ED staff may not be skilled in team behaviors.

---

## COMMUNICATION ERRORS

Interestingly, The Joint Commission (2011) has concluded that, as in aviation, about 70 percent of adverse events in healthcare are due to communication failures (Exhibit 8.1). Communication in healthcare, in particular in settings such as the ED, is casual, imprecise and undisciplined, and on the fly. Unlike other high-risk settings, there are few standards for the transmittal of critical information from one team member to another. Much information is expected to be transferred "by intuition." One strategy to effectively improve communications involves training in teamwork.

**Exhibit 8.1: Root Causes of Sentinel Events**

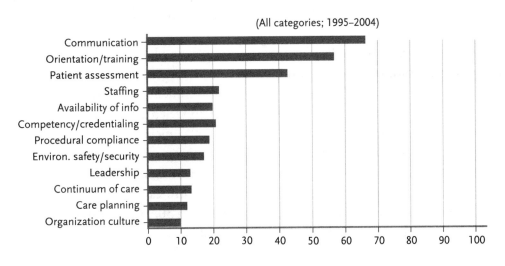

(All categories; 1995–2004)

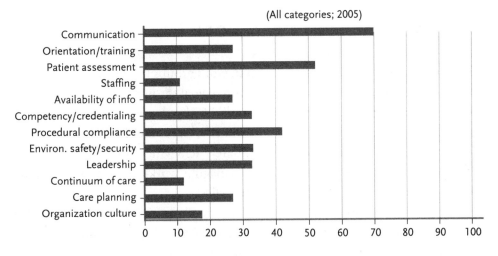

(All categories; 2005)

SOURCE: The Joint Commission (2011).

## TEAMWORK TRAINING APPLIED

Other industries, such as aviation and nuclear power, and high-risk settings, such as aircraft carriers and military medical units, have embraced this ideology. In the late 1990s CRM, also called "med teams training," was making its way into hospital healthcare units such as the ED, labor and delivery, and operating suites, but for reasons that are unclear it never became mainstream. The early data suggested promise for these principles in healthcare settings. It is no surprise that clinicians interested in improving healthcare delivery, quality, and safety have turned again to the subject and that there has been an increase in reported research using med teams approaches.

With its needs for quick decision making using incomplete data, and its demand for effective coordination of groups of caregivers, emergency medicine has much in common with aviation. Armed with a large government grant, Morey and colleagues in 2002 embarked on an ambitious study modeled after aviation research. The yearlong multicenter study included almost 700 clinicians (physicians, nurses, and technicians) who received formal CRM training (the Emergency Teams Training Course) and were assigned to work teams in nine community hospital EDs. The study tracked clinical errors and observed statistically significant improvement in team behaviors. The clinical error rate fell from 30.9 percent to 4.5 percent over eight months, though the workload remained the same.

## GROUP WORK VERSUS TEAMWORK

Healthcare workers typically function well in work groups but less well as teams. A team is two or more people who achieve a mutual goal through interdependent and adaptive actions. A group is two or more individuals who achieve a goal through individual independent contributions. In the ED, personnel function reasonably well as a group with independent tasks ultimately achieving a goal. The adaptation and flexibility of teamwork lends itself to managing workload, planning, solving problems, and developing improvement strategies.

The medical teams approach teaches team members a high level of **situation awareness** (Artman 2000). Situation awareness (SA) is the perception of environmental elements with respect to time and/or space, the comprehension of their meaning, and the projection of their status after some variable has changed, such as time. Lacking SA or having inadequate SA has been identified as one of the primary factors in accidents attributed to human error.

> **Situation awareness (SA):** Being aware of what is happening around you and understanding what the information means to you now and in the future.

Being in tune with the idiosyncrasies and aberrations in healthcare and being aware of the status and work of other team members are critical features of situation awareness. Cooperation is essential. Team members are taught to balance immediate tasks with situation awareness and to monitor the work and progress of others to ensure smooth healthcare delivery. The teamwork system is designed to improve workflow and reduce clinical errors. It encourages team members to coordinate and support each other in clinical tasks. A basic advantage of this model over work groups is the ability to manage workloads more effectively.

**Essential Elements of a Team**

- A common purpose
- Shared goals
- Interdependent actions
- Centralized communication
- Accountability
- Situation awareness
- Flexibility and dynamism

## IMPROVING COMMUNICATION

Another important feature of the medical team approach involves communication. Medical teams are taught to communicate using rigorous communication tools such as SBAR (situation, background, assessment recommendation). Exhibit 8.2 shows an example of such a communication tool.

Other important elements in communication associated with medical teams training include call-backs and repeat-backs. In this form of disciplined communication the caregivers articulate back and forth with one another to be certain that no misunderstanding has occurred, in particular with medication administration. Here is an example of a repeat-back exchange:

Doctor: "I would like 75 mgs. of Lidocaine administered IV push on Mr. Wilson in Bed 2."

Nurse: "Doctor, that is 75 mgs. of Lidocaine IV push on Mr. Wilson in Bed 2."

Doctor: "That is correct."

One communication technique promoted enthusiastically by the Institute for Healthcare Improvement has been dubbed "The Two Challenge Rule." This technique encourages and empowers the nurse to question an order that he has concerns about. The second challenge is a nod to the fact that in the multitasking,

**Exhibit 8.2: SBAR Communication Tool**

## S SITUATION

❑ I am calling about ____<patient name and location>____ .

❑ The patient's code status is ____<code status>____ .

❑ The problem I am calling about is _____ .

❑ I am afraid the patient is going to arrest.

❑ I have just assessed the patient personally:

  ❑ Vital signs are:

    ❑ Blood pressure ____/____ ❑ Pulse ____ ❑ Respiration ____ ❑ Temperature ____

❑ I am concerned about the:

  ❑ Blood pressure because it is over 200 or less than 100 or 30 mmHg below usual.

  ❑ Pulse because it is over 140 or less than 50.

  ❑ Respiration because it is less than 5 or over 40.

  ❑ Temperature because it is less than 96 or over 104.

## B BACKGROUND

❑ The patient's mental status is:

  ❑ Alert and oriented to person, place, and time

  ❑ Confused and ❑ cooperative ❑ noncooperative

  ❑ Agitated or combative

  ❑ Lethargic but conversant and able to swallow

  ❑ Stuporous and not talking clearly and possibly not able to swallow

  ❑ Comatose. Eyes closed. Not responding to stimulation.

❑ The skin is:

  ❑ Warm and dry

  ❑ Pale

  ❑ Mottled

  ❑ Diaphoretic

  ❑ Extremities are cold

  ❑ Extremities are warm

❑ The patient is not or is on oxygen.

  ❑ The patient has been on _____ (l/min) or (%) oxygen for _____ minutes (hours)

  ❑ The oximeter is reading _____%

  ❑ The oximeter does not detect a good pulse and is giving erratic readings.

**Exhibit 8.2: SBAR Communication Tool (continued)**

## A ASSESSMENT

❏ **This is what I think the problem is:** ____<u><say what you think is the problem></u>____ .

❏ **The problem seems to be** ❏ **cardiac** ❏ **infection** ❏ **neurologic** ❏ **respiratory**
   ❏ _____

❏ **I am not sure what the problem is but the patient is deteriorating.**

❏ **The patient seems to be unstable and may get worse; we need to do something.**

## R RECOMMENDATION

❏ **I suggest or request that you** ____<u><say what you would like to see done></u>____

   ❏ Transfer the patient to critical care.

   ❏ Come to see the patient at this time.

   ❏ Talk to the patient or family about code status.

   ❏ Ask the on-call family practice resident to see the patient now.

   ❏ Ask for a consultant to see the patient now.

❏ **Are any tests needed?**

   ❏ Do you need any tests like ❏ CXR ❏ ABG ❏ ECG ❏ CBC or ❏ BMP?

   ❏ Others?

❏ **If a change in treatment is ordered then ask:**

   ❏ How often do you want vital signs?

   ❏ How long do you expect this problem will last?

   ❏ If the patient does not get better, when would you want us to call again?

SOURCE: Bonacum and Leonard (2004).

---

interruption-filled environment of the ED, a physician may not recognize her own error on the first pass. Here is an example:

Doctor: "I want 50 mgs. of morphine IV push given to Mr. Wilson in Bed 2."

Nurse: "Doctor, you want 50 mgs. of morphine IV push given to Mr. Wilson in Bed 2?"

Doctor: "That is what I ordered."

Nurse: "Doctor, you really want 50 mgs. of morphine IV push? I don't think his blood pressure or respirations would like it!"

## ADVANTAGES OF TEAMWORK AND MED TEAMS

Dynamics Research Corporation and investigators from Brown University and Madigan Army Medical Center looked at team behavior in different litigation cases (Risser et al. 1999). Most cases involved a chain of errors involving poor organizational structure, poor task prioritization, poor communication, and a lack of cross- monitoring of other caregivers' work. They identified an average 8.8 team errors (mostly in communication) per case. They concluded that 50 percent of the harm done could have been averted with med teams training and implementation. In studies on caregivers who had received med teams training, they observed an 80 percent decrease in observed errors and fewer cases referred to risk management. Staff satisfaction by survey improved, suggesting that the work environment was not only safer but better for the frontline workers.

## THE ROLE OF EXECUTIVE LEADERSHIP

There are great opportunities for leaders to champion teamwork training. Bringing in formal med teams training for the acute care units such as the OR, the ER, and labor and delivery and disseminating this new knowledge throughout the organization has been shown to be effective in a number of studies. In some models a core of trained individuals teaches others in the organization. Executive leaders may champion team drills on these acute care units, which often identify flaws in existing procedures and policies.

### Case Study

A 32-year-old Hispanic male who speaks little English presents to the emergency department complaining of right-sided flank pain. He has had some nausea, and though he has not taken his temperature, he has felt chills and sweating. He is also having difficulty passing his urine. He has no personal or family history of kidney stones.

On physical exam he is an ill-appearing man. Vital signs: Pulse 118 BP 105/80 Resp 22 unlabored Pulse Oximetry 98%. He is lying quite still on his stretcher and periodically grimaces in pain. His abdominal exam is inconsistent, and it is unclear whether there is reproducible abdominal or flank tenderness. A bedside UA reveals a trace of blood. He receives IV hydration, antiemetic, and ketorolac

(continued)

for pain. A CBC and chemistry panel are sent, and a spiral CT without contrast is performed. The nurse later informs the physician that a small kidney stone is noted on the scan.

Over the next few hours the patient seems minimally improved. His CBC shows a WBC of 14k with a left shift. His urinalysis shows 3 WBCs, 10 RBCs, and no bacteria or casts. The physician plans to send him out with a diagnosis of renal colic, with symptomatic care and a urine strainer. As he is dictating the chart and preparing the discharge paperwork he takes note of the full CT reading by the radiologist. Although a small kidney stone was indeed noted, the radiologist also remarked on inflammatory changes in the vicinity of the appendix and recommended that a full-contrast abdominal CT be performed to ascertain whether or not appendicitis was present. The patient begins the long process of ingesting contrast for an abdominal CT, and three hours later the diagnosis of appendicitis is confirmed. The patient makes it to the operating room almost nine hours after arrival and at laparoscopy, a perforated appendix is found.

A breakdown of the case suggests that lack of teamwork contributed to delays and a near-miss diagnosis:

1. The nurse and physician are not communicating well or often regarding the patient's status.
2. There is no redundancy (double checks) via the various team members. A true med teams approach would have all team members (physician, nurses, and techs, even unit clerks) monitoring for test results and pushing the information to the provider.

There is a communication breakdown between ED providers and radiology. Because a diagnosis of appendicitis should be considered a critical alert, radiology could provide a double check by alerting the ED of a possible appendicitis case.

With situation awareness (each team member aware of the others' workload and progress) there could be more cooperation, which would expedite care. For example, if the nurse recognizes the physician is busy, she could watch for test results and push them to him.

SOURCE: Welch (2008c).

### Strategies for Healthcare Executives

- Map out a plan to bring formal teamwork training to high-risk clinical units.
- Encourage and mentor physician leaders in teamwork.
- Publish and promote successes of teamwork initiatives.

## Recommended Readings

Adams, J. G., and J. S. Bohan. 2000. "System Contributions to Error." *Academy of Emergency Medicine* 7 (11): 1189–93.

Croskerry, P. 2009. "It's About the Team, It's About Communication." In *Patient Safety in Emergency Medicine*. Philadelphia, PA: Lippincott Williams & Wilkins.

Helmreich, R. L. 1997. "Managing Human Error in Aviation." *Scientific American* (May) 62–67.

Morey, J. C., R. Simon, G. D. Jay, et al. 2002. "Error Reduction and Performance Improvement in the Emergency Department Through Formal Teamwork Training: Evaluation Results of the MedTeams Project." *Health Services Research Journal* 37 (6): 1553–81.

Risser, D. T., M. M. Rice, M. L. Salisbury, et al. 1999. "The Potential for Improved Teamwork to Reduce Medical Errors in the Emergency Department." *Annals of Emergency Medicine* 34 (3): 373–83.

Wears, R., and L. Leape. 1999. "Human Error in Emergency Medicine." *Annals of Emergency Medicine* 34 (3): 370–72

Shapiro, M., J. Morey, S. Small, et al. 2001. "Simulation-based Teamwork Training for Emergency Department Staff: Does It Improve Clinical Team Performance When Added to an Existing Didactic Teamwork Curriculum?" *Quality and Safety in Health Care* 13 (6): 417–21.

# CHAPTER 9

# The Just Culture

**In This Chapter**

- The Bad Apple
- The Patient Safety Culture
- No Blame Versus Accountability
- Attitudes Toward Safety
- Safety Attitudes Questionnaire
- The Role of Executive Leadership
- Case Study
- Strategies for Healthcare Executives

## THE BAD APPLE

A widely used model for managing errors in healthcare involves "finding the bad apple." This system functions by identifying individuals as the cause of bad outcomes and becomes active only after a mistake or sentinel event has been made. Instead of anticipating and expecting human errors and designing a system to prevent them, this "blame and shame" model has been used with little success for several decades. The incident reports, retrospective investigations conducted in whispers, and individual punishments are known to be flawed and ineffective strategies for creating a safety culture. Yet these methods are still commonly used at hospitals for dealing with adverse events. Even if weeding out healthcare's bad apples this way were successful, medical errors would only decrease by 5 percent, given that 95 percent of errors are due to system flaws and failures (Leonard et al.

2004). Good people trying hard to work in a bad system results in medical errors and adverse events. So how do we build a safety culture?

## THE PATIENT SAFETY CULTURE

Most current models for managing error in healthcare have no system for tracking near misses, and at most institutions the incident report model itself has become a deterrent to reporting. For example, on a busy night shift the ED staff recognize that the wrong patient was about to be transported to radiology for a CT scan. Diligence and situation awareness on the part of the team prevented this from occurring. But the staff members are fatigued, and reporting such an event would require extra paperwork, keeping them there after the shift should end. In addition, they know from experience a report will likely mean interviews with patient safety personnel and perhaps even the department manager. Sometimes such interviews are done on the worker's own time without compensation. Implicit in the encounter will likely be the suggestion that somehow the worker or the department was at fault.

Could you imagine an entirely different scenario? Could a worker be rewarded for identifying a near miss? Could he quickly and with little trouble put the wheels in motion to investigate the episode? Could the act of coming forward be rewarded and the time spent on investigation be compensated to encourage reporting? Could the worker be treated as a hero instead of a culprit?

---

### Elements of the Safety Culture

- Uses a nonpunitive approach to error
- Rewards people for identifying latent error
- Fosters a preoccupation with error
- Fosters a preoccupation with near misses
- Looks for system fixes
- Institutionalizes standardization

---

## NO BLAME VERSUS ACCOUNTABILITY

In 2001 attorney David Marx first wrote about the "just culture." He had spent his career focusing on the interface among systems engineering, human factors, and the law. Marx describes a precarious balance between creating an environment that encourages workers to come forward with medical errors and having zero tolerance for "reckless behavior." He describes three categories of fallibility:

1. Inadvertent error (The physician on the night shift is tired and accidentally orders a CT pulmonary angiogram when he intended to order a chest x-ray.)
2. At-risk behavior (Because the patient asked the nurse to turn out the lights, the nurse violates protocol and carries the blood specimens to the nurses' station to label them, where an error occurs.)
3. Reckless behavior (The physician orders a high-radiation test on a female patient without a pregnancy test.)

Reckless behavior in healthcare is extremely rare, but when it occurs should it be punished? Marx says yes. Marx (2001) notes that in the old model healthcare turned a blind eye to reckless behavior. At the system level we waited for harm to come to a patient and then, depending on how much damage occurred, someone might be blamed and punished. In the just culture everyone is accountable for certain behaviors, whether there is harm done or not. For instance, hand washing and surgical time-outs are considered imperatives, and to refuse to do either is considered reckless. This is a much more tenable model for patient safety: Judge people on the quality of their choices.

## ATTITUDES TOWARD SAFETY

Interest in developing a culture based on safety has increased in recent years, particularly in safety-critical industries such as nuclear power, space, aviation, and medicine. Within this context, attitudes such as morale and job satisfaction have been correlated with performance (Weakliem and Frenkel 2006). Meta-analyses have demonstrated a consistent correlation between happy and satisfied workers and better performance.

### Attitudinal Surveys

- Diagnose organizational strengths and weaknesses.
- Evaluate the effect of organizational change.
- Improve communication with employees.
- Provide context for other variables (absenteeism and turnover).
- Develop targeted interventions.

Workers in a culture of teamwork and collaboration whose contribution is valued tend to be more productive. How safety factors into this equation is only newly being investigated. Many organizations are attempting to get a handle on this by using structured interviews, focus groups, and attitudinal surveys. By surveying frontline workers, an organization can become familiar with their opinions and impressions and in turn get a snapshot of the organization's climate.

Research done in the aviation industry suggests that the safety climate is quantifiable to the extent that individuals can perceive a genuine and proactive commitment to safety by their organization (Sexton et al. 2001). Attitudes about the safety climate reflect the organizational importance of safety and can influence how aviation crew members practice safety. When the safety climate is poor, threat and error management in flight can suffer. The research project, dubbed LOSA (line operations safety audit), showed that crews with positive perceptions of the safety climate trapped more errors, managed threats better, made fewer violations, and committed errors that were less consequential than crews with negative perceptions of the safety climate. In other words, crews' attitudes toward safety had a direct impact on their performance and thus the safety of the environment.

High-reliability organizations see management's role as creating and maintaining optimal work conditions, removing obstacles to safe and efficient workflow, and fostering an environment in which safety is valued and safe practices are widely endorsed and followed. If workers perceive management to be accomplishing these goals, they can be motivated to conform to the norm of being safe. If workers perceive management to be placing obstacles in their paths, they can be demotivated and may undermine the culture of safety. All of these observations and corollaries are applicable to the emergency department and its workers.

## SAFETY ATTITUDES QUESTIONNAIRE

Bryan Sexton and colleagues (2006) developed the SAQ (safety attitudes questionnaire) to assess the attitudes of frontline healthcare workers about their work environment. The survey used aviation's approach but generated and tested new items after talking to focus groups, reviewing the literature, and conducting round-table discussions with experts. The questionnaire features 60 survey items in six scales using a five-point Likert scale (disagree strongly, disagree slightly, neutral, agree slightly, agree strongly).

The Institute for Healthcare Improvement administered the questionnaire to more than 300 hospitals across 200 different clinical areas, and the work environments varied by more than tenfold. The surveys often identify issues and areas for improvement, and researchers have observed an astonishing pattern. Improvement in the safety climate has been associated with improvements in medication error rates, lengths of stay, nursing turnover rates, and the fiscal bottom line. This shows a clear return on investment in patient safety.

In addition, the safety climate is not a fixed construct. It can be altered and improved with commitment and targeted interventions.

## THE ROLE OF EXECUTIVE LEADERSHIP

One of the most difficult challenges in improving patient safety is changing an organization's culture to one that is blameless but holds practitioners accountable for rare instances of at-risk or reckless behavior. This change has to come from the executives, not the clinicians. The executive leadership needs to incorporate patient safety in the mission, vision, and values of the organization and include it in strategic planning. This means articulating at every level of the organization the importance of this work and the culture that supports it. Leaders must also carry out specific initiatives and a master work plan for safety with one-, two-, five-, and ten-year goals.

On a busy ED shift two female pediatric patients register at the same time. Their last names are similar but not identical. They are placed in adjacent rooms. One is a three-month-old brought by her parents with a chief complaint of "fussiness." The other is a three-year-old being evaluated for "coughing that makes her vomit." The same physician is evaluating both pediatric patients. After several hours of evaluation the toddler is found to have bronchitis but continues to have episodes of coughing and vomiting. To facilitate a few hours of sleep for the toddler and parents the physician orders a weight-appropriate dose of phenergan with codeine elixir.

The nurse caring for the toddler prepares the dose of phenergan with codeine. As the nurse leaves at the end of her shift she asks the nurse taking over her patients, "Could you give this phenergan with codeine to my baby girl?" She mentions the room number and the name of the physician. The new nurse verifies on the tracking system and finds a female patient with the same treating physician, and she administers the medication. Some time later the parents of the infant appear panicky and ask the physician to check their baby again.

On physical exam the infant is lethargic with poor color and is difficult to arouse. The physician immediately recognizes deterioration and calls a pediatric code in the ED. The infant is being bagged when the new nurse asks, "Doctor, could this be a medication reaction?" The physician remarks, "I haven't ordered any meds for this baby." They realize that the medication error has occurred.

*Case Analysis*
Several factors contributed to the error in this case. They are identified in the following list along with steps taken to remedy the problems. Most important, there was no blaming, shaming, or retraining.

1. The tracking board: Patient names had been removed from the tracking system the month before. It is believed that this contributed to a number of near misses regarding patients' identities. Since HIPAA clearly states that patient safety trumps privacy, the names were again placed on the tracking board to provide more identifiers.
2. Pediatric medication procedure: Medication errors are 20 times as common in pediatric patients as in adults, in part due to extreme variations in dosing. The hospital developed a new "two nurse check" standard in which every pediatric medication dose is double-checked by another RN.
3. Two patient identifiers: This was the standard procedure for the organization, but staff were often using only one identifier. An improvement initiative was designed to ramp up compliance that included observation for this at-risk behavior. In addition the name tags were made more legible, with name and age in large readable print.

(continued)

4. Repeat-backs: The department pediatric medication policy now includes a requirement for repeat-backs of medications to the provider before administration. The staff are considering making it a practice for all patients receiving medications.
5. An ED pharmacist: The organization is considering a trial placing a pharmacist in the ED.

SOURCE: Welch and Fontenot (2011).

### Strategies for Healthcare Executives

- Implement a nonjudgmental reporting system.
- Reward the identification of near miss events.
- Simplify and streamline the reporting process.
- Administer SAQ at regular intervals on each clinical unit.

## Recommended Readings

Institute of Medicine. 2001. *Crossing the Quality Chasm: A New Health System for the 21st Century.* Washington, DC: National Academies Press. (The second IOM report dealing with how to build a safe and reliable healthcare system.)

Leonard, M, A. Frankel, T. Simmonds, with K. Vega. 2004. *Achieving Safe and Reliable Healthcare: Strategies and Solutions.* Chicago: Health Administration Press.

Sexton, J. B., and J. R. Klinect. 2001. "The Link Between Patient Safety Attitudes and Observed Performance in Flight Operations." Proceedings of the Eleventh International Symposium on Aviation Psychology, 7–13. Columbus, OH: Ohio State University Publishing.

Spath, P. 2000. *Error Reduction in Healthcare: A Systems Approach to Improving Patient Safety.* Chicago: Health Forum Inc.

Wears, R., and L. Leape. 1999. "Human Error in Emergency Medicine." *Annals of Emergency Medicine* 34(3): 370–72 (This is an early article addressing human error in the ED, factors and remedies.)

# CHAPTER 10

# Patient Satisfaction as a Risk Management Strategy

## In This Chapter

- Patient Satisfaction Versus Customer Service
- Why Pursue Patient Satisfaction?
- Demographics and Patient Satisfaction
- The Five Correlates of Satisfaction
- The Role of Executive Leadership
- Case Study
- Strategies for Healthcare Executives

## PATIENT SATISFACTION VERSUS CUSTOMER SERVICE

Although emergency medicine attempts to follow the course of other service industries, its customer service model is unique. First, patients can report great personal satisfaction when poor clinical care was rendered and vice versa. In addition, patients are not necessarily reliable assessors of clinical quality. Another challenge involves the time frame for satisfaction measures. Patients frequently view their healthcare through episodes of a particular illness and not by the services provided. The heart patient will recall the ED, the cardiac catheterization lab, the operating room, and the critical care unit as a continuum of healthcare, without clearly distinguishing the differing elements or venues of care. Finally, measuring patient satisfaction has proved a formidable task. While an eating establishment may count patrons or profits to evaluate customer satisfaction, in healthcare there are no such easy measures.

A working definition of patient satisfaction includes overall satisfaction (usually by survey), likelihood to recommend, and willingness to return. Indeed, these three overall measures as practical indicators of patient satisfaction abound in the literature. Early patient satisfaction surveys were seldom validated instruments. Surveys were mailed to patients after discharge, and response rates were often only 25 percent, subjecting them to selection bias (Sun, Adams, and Burstin 2001). The past 15 years have seen improvements in this area with the development of survey instruments specifically for ED patients.

---

### Customer Service Defined

- Overall satisfaction (by survey)
- Likelihood to recommend
- Willingness to return

---

Other quantifiable measures have been developed to clarify the elusive patient satisfaction picture, including door-to-doctor times, which correlate well with satisfaction, or the ultimate indicator of patient dissatisfaction, leaving without being seen. Researchers are regularly using continuous quality improvement tools to measure the response to particular process improvement changes—all in an effort to improve the patient experience in the ED.

## WHY PURSUE PATIENT SATISFACTION?

From a risk management perspective, patient satisfaction makes sense. Caregivers who participate in a system of good customer satisfaction experience fewer malpractice suits than their counterparts do (Vincent, Young, and Phillips 1994). From a clinical perspective, patient satisfaction also makes sense. Patients who are satisfied with their care are more likely to be compliant with treatment plans and respond better to their treatment. In addition, there is a connection between patient satisfaction and staff satisfaction (Miaoulis, Gutman, and Snow 2009). Results of Press Ganey surveys of patient and staff satisfaction show a clear relationship between the two; at one hospital, while customer satisfaction increased, employee turnover decreased by 57 percent (Press 2002).

Finally, patient satisfaction translates into fiscal improvement. "An ED visit is a significant encounter between the patient and hospital, and one that affects 'repurchase' decisions for future health care," note researchers Mack and File (1995) in an analysis of ED choices among Medicare patients. Ninety-seven percent of patients in this study had a choice of emergency departments, and more than half had been referred by others. Despite the elderly being disproportionate users of healthcare, approximately half of this population have no regular physician and choose the ED for routine primary care. This verbal networking and utilization of services by the elderly have huge implications for patient satisfaction efforts. Geriatric services including home health aides, equipment (walkers and bedside commodes), and consultants, should be available in the ED to improve services rendered to seniors and enhance their experience of care in the ED.

### Reasons for Pursuing Patient Satisfaction

- Compliance
- Malpractice and risk management
- Staff satisfaction and retention
- Fiscal improvement

## DEMOGRAPHICS AND PATIENT SATISFACTION

Research has helped us understand how the characteristics of the person in the bed affect patient satisfaction. Patients who are older were more likely to express satisfaction than those who are younger (Boudreaux et al. 2000). Young patients and minority patients tend to be less satisfied with care, which is consistent with data from outpatient and in-hospital settings (Sun et al. 2000). In one study (Boudreaux and O'Hea 2004), patients who were insured were more likely to recommend the ED to others, while the uninsured/indigent patients were less likely to do so. Another variable that correlates with good patient satisfaction is acuity. The higher-acuity patients are more satisfied, as are patients receiving multiple treatments (Boudreaux et al. 2004). A large review also showed weak correlation with marital status, diagnosis, daily census, and satisfaction with tests, presence of chronic illness, number of previous visits, and type of treatment (Boudreaux and O'Hea 2004). Other non-correlative or weak predictors of patient satisfaction include satisfaction with the registration process, mode of arrival, and admission status (Hall and Press 1996).

Characteristics that did not influence patient satisfaction in the ED setting were gender (although other health surveys had shown men to be harder to please), weekday versus weekend, time of day, and disposition (Hall and Press

1996; Soremekun, Takayesu, and Bohan 2011). In addition, patient volume per se did not affect satisfaction, although typically higher-volume teaching hospitals and trauma centers do not perform well on patient satisfaction surveys. This is perhaps due to longer wait times at these types of facilities.

### Demographic Variables That Correlate with Patient Satisfaction

- Increasing age
- Insurance coverage
- Increasing acuity/more care
- Non-teaching hospital

### Demographic Variables That Correlate with Patient Dissatisfaction

- Younger age
- Uninsured
- Lower acuity
- Minority

## THE FIVE CORRELATES OF SATISFACTION

The growing body of research on patient satisfaction in the ED shows five major correlates of patient satisfaction: empathy/attitude (bedside manner), acceptable wait times (particularly perceived times versus actual wait times), technical issues (both technical skills and available technology), pain management, and information dispensation.

### The Five Correlates of Patient Satisfaction

- Empathy
- Acceptable wait times
- Technical issues
- Pain management
- Information dispensation

## Empathy

The "art of caring" for patients correlates with patient satisfaction. Seven to 13 percent of ED complaints cite a provider's uncaring attitude (Chande, Bhende, and Davis 1991; Schwartz and Overton 1987; Vukimer 2006). Caring physicians and nurses are variables that show up repeatedly in satisfaction data and occasionally override wait times as predictors of patient satisfaction. Simply stated, speed cannot compensate for rudeness, disrespect, or an uncaring attitude.

Healthcare organizations that embark on customer service training programs to improve interactions between the healthcare provider and patient have seen positive results. The most successful and sustained programs involved organizations that are committed to the principles of customer service and satisfaction (Mayer 2004). Other service variables that correlate with patient satisfaction and the perception of care include an organized staff, staff introductions, and satisfactory discharge instructions (Worthington 2004). Overall, when physicians display more concern, give more information, and encourage dialogue with their patients, the result is higher satisfaction.

Call-back systems are also being used as a patient satisfaction intervention (Jones et al. 1997). Patients who have left before completing treatment are called to determine why they left and to check on their clinical course. In addition, patients who may have had a poor ED experience due to delays or unmet expectations can be called back. This system provides a chance to salvage the ED encounter, it is an effective risk management tool, and it moves the patient satisfaction program forward.

## Acceptable Wait Times

Patients presenting to the ED typically do not understand the triage system and interpret patient flow in the department as somehow being unfair (Rehmani and Norain 2007). They overestimate the urgency of their need for healthcare. These perceived factors set up the patient to view their wait time as too long. A team at Kaiser Permanente's Southern California Region (Bursch, Beezy, and Shaw 1993) has shown that perceived wait time, not actual wait time, is the most important variable contributing to patient satisfaction.

Just as customers are pleased when the wait for a table at a restaurant is less than they originally thought, higher patient satisfaction has been shown to correlate with shorter-than-expected ED wait times (Hedges, Trout, and Magnusson 2002). Other studies suggest that focusing on appropriate expectations for wait times should also have a positive effect on patient satisfaction. Some EDs post wait times in the waiting room or on billboards. Other options include signs explaining the triage system and pamphlets explaining the average length of stay for common chief complaints. Informing patients of wait times at the outset and then performing better than the time estimates given can be a great patient satisfier (Soremekun, Takayesu, and Bohan 2011).

## Technical Issues

Clinicians and healthcare providers think little when a patient requires two or three attempts at a blood draw or an IV placement. However, for the patient multiple attempts can be traumatic and color her perceptions of the ED encounter. Perceived technical skills correlate with positive perception of staff and have been found in two studies to be the best predictor of global satisfaction (Mack, File, and Horwitz 1995; Rhee and Bird 1996).

This realization may be troublesome for ED physicians at our nation's teaching hospitals. If technical skills are highly correlated with patient satisfaction and an enhanced patient experience, should we have the less-experienced staff among us learning their technical skills on ED patients? The data on this topic are somewhat mixed. One study found that ED patients would allow medical students to perform simple, noninvasive procedures (IVs, splints, and suturing) (Santen et al. 2005).

**Radiology ultrasonography:** A procedure performed by a technician in the ultrasound department and read by a trained radiologist.

**ED ultrasonography:** Also called "bedside ultrasound," this procedure refers to testing done in the ED with a machine trundled to the bedside.

On the other hand, another study concluded that patients are reluctant to have medical students perform a first procedure on them, and many would not allow medical students to perform some procedures at all (Graber, Pierre, and Charlton 2003). This is actually an international dilemma—one study from Ireland found patients reported feeling pressured to have students involved in their care. However 78 percent reported the experience with students as positive (Kuan and O'Donnell 2007). This presents dilemmas in medical education and informed consent. Scripting could help, as could guidelines for effectively enrolling patients in such learning encounters.

Bedside ultrasound has an impact on patients' perceptions of technical skill in the ED and seems to influence patient satisfaction favorably. In one study, patients received **ED ultrasonography** instead of **radiology ultrasonography**. Those receiving ED ultrasonography viewed the physician as having a more caring attitude, rated the physician as having better skills and abilities, and rated the overall satisfaction with the ED visit higher (Durston, Carl, and Guerra 1999). The scores improved as the physician skills progressed.

---

**Ultrasound in Transition**

ED ultrasound is in transition. Originally ultrasound in the ED was meant for quick diagnosis, seen as a tool much like a stethoscope. Some hospitals, typically at academic centers, have been promoting the use of the more complicated and difficult-to-operate radiology machines, overly detailed examinations and stored images, and exhaustive documentation requirements because they improve the ability to bill for ultrasound procedures. However, this switch makes bedside ultrasound less efficient for the physician in the ED. But one study shows patient satisfaction improves with the introduction of bedside ultrasound into a department (Durston, Carl, and Guerra 1999).

---

## Pain Management

One of the major symptoms that cause patients to seek emergency medical care is pain, and the complexities of pain management in the ED are only beginning to be unraveled. While there is a general correlation between pain relief and satisfaction, cultural factors, the intensity of the original pain experience, and differing pain scales all work to confound an understanding of this area of medical research. A few themes relating to pain management and satisfaction in the ED are emerging and are worth noting.

Patients appear to have preferences and expectations regarding pain management in the ED that can easily be met. In general, patients under 54 years old prefer oral analgesia. Though oral medication is preferred by all age groups, of the patients who prefer IV analgesia, the majority will be senior citizens. The more severe the pain intensity reported, the more likely the patient will prefer parenteral medication. For example, senior citizens with long bone fractures, such as broken hips, will prefer IV pain medication, which has the quickest onset. In several studies, intramuscular analgesia was the least preferred route of administration for analgesia in the ED (Fosnocht, Hollifield, and Swanson 2004; Miner et al. 2008). Pain management in children correlates highly with patient satisfaction and should be the focus for departments seeing high pediatric volumes. Earlier studies suggested differences in management of pain in the ED with undertreatment of ethnic minorities and women as specific patient populations (Todd, Samaroo, and Hoffman 1993; Todd 1996; Tanabe et al. 2007). Timely alleviation of adverse symptoms has also been shown to deter patients from leaving before being seen by a doctor (Arendt et al. 2003).

In short, an ED should have a well-stocked selection of oral analgesics and be liberal with their dispensation. In addition, it should be easy to assess in triage which patients may need parenteral medications and to expedite IV placement.

### Information Dispensation

Studies have shown that information can have a greater effect on patient satisfaction than perceived wait times and that staff overestimate the amount of information they give patients (Allshouse 1993). Unexplained and uncertain waits feel longer and have a negative effect on the patients' perceptions of wait times (Maister 1985). Some EDs have set service goals for staff to give informational updates at specified time intervals to patients and their families.

Other informational dispensation techniques are currently being investigated, including videos, closed circuit television, and pamphlets. However, nothing may be better for patient satisfaction than human interaction and verbally delivered updates. The practice of ED rounding protocols with scheduled information updates from staff to patients and families has been shown in one study to reduce LWBS by 23.4 percent, leaving against medical advice by 22.6 percent, falls by 58.8 percent, and call-light use by 34.7 percent (Meade, Kennedy, and Kaplan 2010).

These findings have given rise to a new position in the ED—the patient advocate. The patient advocate can be a licensed practical nurse, a social worker, or a volunteer. The patient advocate makes frequent contact with the patient and family members, keeping them informed of delays and progress, and may also be trained to assist with noninvasive comfort measures, such as getting blankets, telephones, or ice chips. An additional benefit of having a patient advocate in the department is to free the professional staff for the more pressing technical tasks for which they are trained.

## THE ROLE OF EXECUTIVE LEADERSHIP

A strong culture of customer service necessarily originates with executive leadership. Physicians still push back against the idea of patient satisfaction tracking and measurement. As recently as September 2010 one of the emergency medicine trade papers began a series of columns challenging Press Ganey in particular and patient satisfaction surveys in general on methodological grounds and attempted to lead a backlash against them (Sullivan and DeLucia 2010). Executive leadership can make its expectations clear by requiring levels of performance to be articulated in contracts with emergency physician groups.

LDS Hospital in Salt Lake City, Utah, began a comprehensive quality improvement program with customer service initiatives in 2000. It focused on improving throughput times. Its efforts were rewarded and are demonstrated in the graphic display that follows. As length of stay was reduced the percentage of patients who walked away without being seen and the absolute numbers of complaints also declined. In-house patient satisfaction scores improved concurrently.

**Mean Turnaround Time (minutes) by Quarter: 4-Year Trend**

**Complaints per 1,000 ED Visits per Year**

(continued)

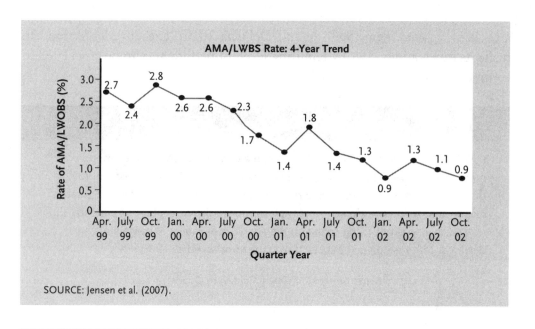

**AMA/LWBS Rate: 4-Year Trend**

SOURCE: Jensen et al. (2007).

---

**Strategies for Healthcare Executives**

• Understand the five correlates of patient satisfaction, and design processes and operations that incorporate that understanding into patient care.
• Articulate an organization-wide commitment to patient satisfaction.
• Set up a system of rewards for staff and departments that perform well on patient satisfaction surveys.
• Incorporate your patient complaint management into patient satisfaction efforts.

---

## Recommended Readings

Cunningham, L. 1991. *The Quality Connection in Health Care: Integrating Patient Satisfaction and Risk Management.* San Francisco: Jossey-Bass.

Press, I. 2002. *Patient Satisfaction: Defining, Measuring and Improving the Experience of Care.* Chicago: Health Administration Press.

Vincent, C., M. Young, and A. Phillips. 1994. "Why People Sue Doctors: A Study of Patients and Relatives Taking Legal Action." *Lancet* 343: 1609–13.

Welch, S. J., and S. Freymann Fontenot. 2010. "Quality Matters: The Painful Truth: Cutting-Edge ED Protocols Blunt Patients' Pain." *Emergency Medicine News* 33 (1): 12–13.

Welch, S. 2010. "Twenty Years of Patient Satisfaction Research Applied to the Emergency Department." *American Journal of Medical Quality* 25 (1): 64–72.

# CHAPTER 11

# The Apology in Emergency Medicine

**In This Chapter**

- The Apology: Healing Words
- Apology and Disclosure
- The Five Rs of Apology
- Apologies and Risk Management
- Scripting for Adverse Events and Medical Error
- The Role of Executive Leadership
- Case Study
- Strategies for Healthcare Executives

## THE APOLOGY: HEALING WORDS

The notion of apology in medicine and the surrounding debate over its place in clinical practice followed on the heels of great revelations: Medicine is practiced and delivered by humans, and humans make mistakes. Therefore there are mistakes in medicine. This new dialogue began with Lucian Leape's (1994) groundbreaking article "Error in Medicine." On its tail came the Institute of Medicine's books and a different kind of vision for healthcare.

In his book *Healing Words: The Power of Apology in Medicine*, Michael Woods (2007) suggests that when something unexpected or untoward occurs in medicine, the act of apology is sentinel for providers, patients, and family. The phrase "I'm sorry" is one of the most commonly used in any language, and people reflexively speak it throughout the day.

The power of an apology is enormous if sincerely done in any context. An apology has the power to heal humiliations, free the mind from deep-seated guilt, remove the desire for vengeance, and ultimately restore broken relationships (Lazare 2004).

Leape (2005) has applied the characterization of the therapeutic power of an apology to medical errors:

- Apology begins to restore the patient's dignity and respect. Injury is humiliating and unfair. An apology can mitigate the humiliation: "You respect me enough to acknowledge my hurt."
- Apology provides an assurance of shared values, reaffirming the patient's and doctor's mutual commitment to the rules of the relationship and re-establishing trust. "I really am the person you thought I was."
- Apology assures patients that they are not at fault—a common and often unappreciated response to mishaps.
- Apology assures patients that they are now safe and that the caregiver recognizes the hurt and is committed to taking every possible measure to prevent further injury.
- Apology shows the patient that the doctor is also suffering. In this sense it levels the playing field, helping to restore the patient's self-respect.
- By making amends, such as providing extra attention or attending to the patient's immediate needs, apology demonstrates that the doctor understands the impact of the patient's suffering and loss of trust.

For reasons that we explore in the next section, practitioners and workers in healthcare have been effectively gagged by the culture of healthcare and kept from speaking these healing words. "I'm sorry" can express respect, regret, compassion, and caring, yet we have disallowed such expressions in healthcare when patients and providers need to exchange them most.

### Constraints to "I'm Sorry"

- Physician culture
- Legal advice
- Risk management
- The culture of the organization

The biggest constraint to apology is cultural and begins with the physician. The "deny and defend" approach to bad outcomes was created by attorneys and the malpractice insurance industry. Lawyers are prone to warning doctors that patients and families may see an apology as an admission of guilt. It becomes hard to show that apology may reduce risk: How do you measure lawsuits that do not occur? Of course an apology in no way guarantees avoidance of a lawsuit (Croskerry et al. 2009). In an effort to defuse potential liability for an apology, 29 states have adopted "apology laws" (Exhibit 11.1). These statutes make an apology or statement of sympathy expressed by a physician in the setting of medical error inadmissible as evidence to prove negligence.

The taboo on apologizing is not driven by data but by fear and anecdote. Though apologizing and admitting mistakes are becoming more culturally accepted, behind

---

**Exhibit 11.1 States with Apology Laws**

1. Arizona: A.R.S. § 12-2605 (2005)
2. California: Evidence Code § 1160 (2000)
3. Colorado: Revised Statute § 13-25-135 (2003)
4. Connecticut: Public Act No. 05-275 Sec. 9 (2005)
5. Delaware: HB 412 (2006)
6. Florida: Stat § 90.4026 (2001)
7. Georgia: Title 24 Code GA Annotated 24-3-37.1 (2005)
8. Hawaii: HRS § Sec. 626-1 (2006)
9. Illinois: Public Act 094-0677 Sec. 8-1901 (2005)
10. Louisiana: R.S. § 3715.5 (2005)
11. Maine: MRSA § 2908 (2005)
12. Maryland: MD Court & Judicial Proceedings Code Ann. § 10-920 (2004)
13. Massachusetts: ALM GL ch.233, § 23D (1986)
14. Missouri: HB 393 (2005)
15. Montana: H.R. 24 59th Leg., (2005)
16. New Hampshire: RSA § 507-E:4 (2005)
17. North Carolina: General Stat. § 8C-1, Rule 413
18. Ohio: ORC Ann § 2317.43 (2004)
19. Oklahoma: 63 OKL. St. § 1-1708.1H (2004)
20. Oregon: Rev. Stat. § 677.082 (2003)
21. South Carolina: Ch.1, Title19 Code of Laws 1976, 19-1-190 (2006)
22. South Dakota: H.R. 1148 8th Leg., (2005)
23. Tennessee: Evid Rule § 409.1 (2003)
24. Texas: Civil Prac and Rem Code § 19.061 (1999)
25. Vermont: S 198 Sec. 1. 12 V.S.A. § 1912 (2006)
26. Virginia: Code of Virginia § 8.01-52.1 (2005)
27. Washington: Rev Code Wash § 5.66.010 (2002)
28. West Virginia: HB 3174 (2005)
29. Wyoming: Wyo. Stat. § 1-1-130

closed doors the old dialogues continue. Insurers tell their physician clients, "Never use the words 'I'm sorry.'"

Risk management has also contributed to the constraints to apology. Most risk managers have subscribed to the notion that it isn't appropriate to apologize unless something bad has happened that could have been prevented and that the organization is responsible for. Risk managers are less supportive of providing a full apology than physicians are willing to offer one (Loren et al. 2010). But, as Woods (2007) points out, we say "I am so sorry" when we learn of a death in the family or other bad news even though we have no connection to it or liability for it. Apology has nothing to do with causation.

Remember, apology is most effective at the front lines and in the clinical trenches. In fact, the likelihood of being sued falls by 50 percent when an apology is offered immediately (Pelt and Faldmo 2008). More than 70 percent of malpractice claims are due to poor patient–provider relationships (Beckman et al. 1994). Providers who have good communication skills and talk to their patients in an authentic way are sued less often (Vincent, Young, and Phillips 1994). Risk has everything to do with the interpersonal relationships between patients and providers and relatively little to do with the quality of the care that was rendered.

## APOLOGY AND DISCLOSURE

Healthcare organizations are increasingly moving toward early disclosure of a medical adverse event or error with full disclosure of the facts. Patients and their families want information, particularly reassurance that they will recover and that efforts are being made to prevent the problem from occurring again. Patients want an apology as part of the disclosure of a harmful medical error (Gallagher and Lucas 2005). Organizations that have processes in place outlining how such episodes should be managed are helping patients and their families cope and helping staff recover as well.

Provider training and leadership in how to apologize and disclose have been successful at both the University of Michigan Health System (Boothman 2006) and the VA Hospital in Lexington, Kentucky (Woods 2007) (see the case study on page 104). Although the organization and insurers can't micromanage the interpersonal relationship between provider and patient, they can get out of the way and provide basic principles and approaches.

# THE FIVE Rs OF APOLOGY

According to Beverly Engel's (2001) book *The Power of Apology*, an authentic apology has three elements: regret, responsibility, and remedy. Woods (2007) feels that in healthcare there are two added critical elements: recognition and remaining engaged. The five Rs are:

1. Regret. An expression of regret tells the patient you recognize her fear, anxiety, and pain. It should go something like this: "I am sorry this happened. It is not what either of us wanted or expected, and I need to tell you how sorry I am."

2. Responsibility. This is the step that your insurer and your organization are most worried about. You need to convey that you are responsible for your patient's care, you will get to the bottom of how this error happened, and you will work to ensure it doesn't happen again. This is surprisingly important to patients and their families. Woods (2007) recommends first-person singular, not plural, for these expressions (see the scripting section on page 102 for more examples).

3. Remedy. This element includes discussing both medical and financial remedies. Risk management should help you assure the patient that if a longer stay or another surgery is required, your organization will provide aid. For example, "Please do not worry about your condition or the expenses associated with whatever care you need. The hospital will take care of you and any consequences of this event." Evidence is mounting that when the patient does not face a financial burden after a medical error, he is less likely to seek compensation in the courts (Woods 2007).

4. Recognition. Caregivers must understand when an apology is needed and not become defensive, withdrawn, or evasive. Providers must learn to recognize early when the patient's or family's expectations have not been met.

5. Remaining engaged. Too often after an adverse event, complication, or medical error the providers want to disengage from the patient and the family. Yet this is the time when the patient needs to feel the physician or provider is there to help her deal with the looming consequences. The patient must not feel abandoned by the provider. This can be particularly difficult for the emergency physician whose scope of care ends at the ED doors. Phone calls to the family or patient to check on progress are important.

# APOLOGIES AND RISK MANAGEMENT

There are now growing examples of the effectiveness of incorporating apology into a risk management strategy, effectively reducing risk and the costs incurred after adverse events (Peto et al. 2009; Cox 2007; Wojcieszak, Banja, and Houk 2006). The University of Michigan Health System crafted a policy in 2001 that incorporated apology into its risk management strategy. The core of this program was to enhance patient safety and provider–patient communication. The policy had three basic tenets:

1. Compensating patients quickly and fairly when unreasonable medical care caused a bad outcome
2. Rigorous defense of the staff and hospital when treatment and management met the standard of care or did not cause an injury
3. A focus on learning from mistakes and the patient experience

In the first year of the program dramatic improvement could be seen. Of the seven cases that went to trial, all but one case was won. The lost case was ultimately settled for a smaller sum than was anticipated. The system saved $2.2 million in the first year.

---

**Communication During the Apology**

- Make full eye contact.
- Place hands relaxed at the sides (do not cross arms across the chest).
- Sit down and consider sitting on the edge of the bed after asking the patient's permission.
- Use open hand gestures.
- Give the patient and family ample time to ask questions.

---

# SCRIPTING FOR ADVERSE EVENTS AND MEDICAL ERROR

Scripting, in which staff are provided with positive dialogue for specific situations in the ED, shows promise in improving the communication and interpersonal interaction of the physician–patient encounter (Handel et al. 2010; Robert Wood Johnson Foundation 2006; Mustard 2003). The following examples are taken directly from Woods (2007) and illustrate the language and dialogue that should take place when adverse events occur. Your organization's risk management department could develop and teach similar scripts. Some providers will also need coaching in the delivery of the script.

---

### Examples of Scripting

- "I'm sorry this has happened to you, and I want to assure you I'll do everything possible to get at how this happened." (Recognition)
- "I'm sorry you are upset—I am upset about this, too. I am doing everything I can to understand how and why this happened." (Recognition)
- "I really regret this happened. I know it is not what either of us wanted or expected, and I want you to know how sorry I am for what you are going through." (Regret)
- "I am responsible for your care, and I will find out what happened and if possible why it happened. I will keep you posted of what I learn and how it can be used to prevent this from happening again. At this point I am not sure if I would have done anything differently, but I intend to explore this thoroughly." (Responsibility)
- "I am responsible for your care and for this regrettable outcome. The drug reaction you experienced has been reported, but it is very uncommon. I'm looking into matters to see if your reaction could have been anticipated. I will keep you posted of what I have learned." (Responsibility)
- "While it is still early to tell, I don't think you will have any long-term health problems, but I will verify this over time. I want you to know the problem occurred because of a communication error, and I am looking into changes that will keep it from happening again." (Remedy)
- "I am responsible for your care and will be completely available to you. Here is my card. Please call me directly if you have any problems." (Remaining engaged)

---

## THE ROLE OF EXECUTIVE LEADERSHIP

Incorporating apology and disclosure into the culture of the organization is the responsibility of executive leadership. Both the risk management department and the legal department will have to align with the goals and culture change expressed by the executive leadership. This will take finesse at best and high-level staff changes at worst if these individuals resist these changes. As long as there is one attorney or one risk management professional promoting fear over apology, the program will not be allowed to grow.

---

### Case Study

The VA Medical Center in Lexington, Kentucky, had one of the worst records for malpractice claims in the system. In 1987, after losing two large lawsuits totaling more than $1.5 million, the risk management committee decided that a new approach was needed. The goal was to change the culture to foster a more empathetic attitude among clinicians, particularly after a patient had been harmed. Rather than respond with a defensive or adversarial approach, the committee wanted caregivers to respond in a caregiving way.

As the new policies and program were implemented the risk management committee mapped out the details of timing and disclosure at the organizational level. They opted for a rapid full disclosure of adverse events and ramped up their patient safety efforts. All employees were now expected to report not only errors but near misses to the hospital risk management committee. The committee acts promptly to determine the root cause, and if a patient is harmed it makes quick recommendations for remedy, including financial compensation. At a face-to-face meeting representatives of the hospital apologize for the event and explain what is being done to correct the system that allowed the error, and the chief of staff answers all questions from the patient and his or her family. The hospital attorney offers a fair settlement.

The VA Medical Center in Lexington found that this approach helped diffuse the anger of the patient and family members and effectively curbed the motivation for litigation. Legal fees decreased. Following implementation of this program the VA Medical Center in Lexington reported 88 malpractice claims in seven years, but the average cost of each claim was one-twentieth of the average cost reported by the National Practitioner Data Bank.

*Results:*
VA Lexington average cost of claim: $15,622
National Practitioner Data Bank average: $270,854

SOURCE: Woods (2007).

**Strategies for Healthcare Executives**

- Support training for staff at all levels that includes apology as part of a response to medical error.
- With the legal and risk management departments, develop and train staff using scripts for major adverse events.
- Integrate this program with a robust patient safety program that seeks to get upstream of latent errors and patient safety issues.
- Demand that your risk management and legal departments have 24/7 on-call capability to quickly address ED adverse events and make rapid offers of compensation when needed.
- Cultivate a culture of apology and disclosure that is timely and patient-centered, and iterate these goals often and at all levels of leadership.

## Recommended Readings

Engel, B. 2001. *The Power of Apology*, New York: John Wiley & Sons.

Lazare A. 2004. *On Apology*. New York: Oxford University Press.

Leape, L. L. 1994. "Error in Medicine." *Journal of the American Medical Association* 272: 1851–57.

Woods, M. 2007. *Healing Words: The Power of Apology in Medicine.* Oakbrook Terrace, IL: Joint Commission Resources.

# The Role of the Board in Risk Management

**In This Chapter**

- Hospital Governance 101
- The Emerging Role of the Board in Quality, Safety, and Risk
- The Patient Safety Committee
- The Data and Examples
- The Role of Executive Leadership
- Case Study
- Strategies for Healthcare Executives

## HOSPITAL GOVERNANCE 101

The governing board of a hospital represents the stakeholders and makes decisions on their behalf (Griffith and White 2006). Being a board member for a healthcare organization is no longer an "in name only" position. Much is required of hospital boards, and the appointment is anything but casual. In today's regulatory environment, boards of not-for-profit organizations are being held accountable for appropriately fulfilling their fiduciary duties. The primary fiduciary duty of oversight requires, among other things, that boards help management set and monitor the organization's strategic direction. Aside from these fiduciary duties, the board is also responsible for oversight in other areas.

**The duty of oversight requires that boards:**

- Select and work with the CEO.
- Establish the mission, vision, and values.
- Approve strategies and an annual budget to implement the mission.
- Maintain the quality of care.
- Monitor results for compliance to goals, laws, and regulations.

Boards succeed at the critical decisions they make because they follow carefully designed processes for educating themselves, managing their agenda, and monitoring and improving their own performance. Most boards measure their own success using a balanced scorecard that includes financial, market performance, operational share, customer satisfaction, and staff satisfaction dimensions.

Although boards can have any number of members, most high-functioning boards have between 10 and 20 members, chosen from the community for both the particular expertise each brings and the constituents each represents. The CEO is typically a member of the board. Most board members serve three to four years, and most healthcare organizations have self-perpetuating boards, with members nominating and vetting their successors. Monetary compensation for not-for-profit board members is rare and declining.

Most well-functioning boards have several standing committees:

**Standing Committees of the Governing Board**

- Executive (officers: chair, vice chair, secretary, treasurer, other standing committee chairs; CEO; CFO; and medical staff representatives)
- Nominations (senior board officers)
- Board performance (often the same as the nominations committee)
- Quality (the newest standing committee for most governing boards and often led by a respected clinician)

Each board and its CEO must determine what level of board participation is sufficient and appropriate; however, with the increasing emphasis on accountability of nonprofit boards expect to see more board engagement in the strategic planning process in the future.

The board's level of engagement should be consistent with its oversight role. Board members should provide input on the critical strategic issues and the proposed strategic direction; they should not attempt to usurp management's implementation role. More specifically, boards should be engaged in conversations about what will be accomplished (the mission, values, vision, and strategic goals), not how to achieve the results (the objectives and tactics).

---

### Strategic Planning Activities

- Assessing the internal and external environments, using qualitative and quantitative analyses
- Drawing conclusions about the implications of the situational assessment for the hospital or health system
- Stating assumptions about the future
- Identifying the critical strategic issues that must be addressed over the longer term
- Articulating or refining the mission
- Agreeing on a set of core values or guidelines for behavior for all internal stakeholders
- Creating a concrete vision of what will be accomplished in the future
- Choosing a limited number of measurable strategic goals or areas of priority and focus
- Developing objectives or shorter-term, organization-wide initiatives that describe how to accomplish the mission, vision, and goals
- Developing plans for communicating, monitoring, and updating the strategic plan

---

## THE EMERGING ROLE OF THE BOARD IN QUALITY, SAFETY, AND RISK

Until recently discussions about quality, safety, and risk involved the focus and commitment of the CEO and physician leaders. But the role of the board can be decisive in agenda setting and resource allocation. Traditionally boards have surrendered these domains to the hospital medical staff and have focused on their fiduciary responsibilities. Most board members are lay people and often did not feel qualified to understand the clinical elements of quality and safety. In addition, there were few useful measures to help boards understand the safety of their institutions.

The safety movement has catapulted boards into action. Emerging evidence (laid out in the next section) indicates that an engaged board can help promote safety, especially when it devotes a quarter of its time to quality and safety issues. IHI suggests the following strategies for involving the board in quality and safety efforts:

**Six Things All Boards Should Do to Improve Quality and Reduce Harm**

1. Set aims. Set a specific aim to reduce harm this year; make an explicit, public commitment to measurable quality improvement.
2. Get data and hear stories. Select and review progress toward safer care as the first agenda item at every board meeting, grounded in transparency—and putting a "human face" on harm data. For example, track the rate of medication errors and near misses in the ED. Present the data at each board meeting along with a story about a real patient who experienced a medication error.
3. Establish and monitor system-level measures. Identify a small group of organization-wide patient safety measures that are continually updated and are made transparent to the entire organization and its customers.
4. Change the environment, policies, and culture. Commit to establishing and maintaining an environment that is respectful, fair, and just for all who experience pain and loss because of avoidable harm and adverse outcomes: the patients, their families, and the staff at the sharp end of error.
5. Learn, starting with the board. Develop the board's capability and learn about how the best boards work with executive and medical staff leaders to reduce harm.
6. Establish executive accountability. Oversee the effective execution of a plan to achieve aims to reduce harm, including executive team accountability for clear quality improvement targets.

SOURCE: Institute for Healthcare Improvement (2003).

## THE PATIENT SAFETY COMMITTEE

Whether or not there is a patient safety officer, most institutions have a patient safety committee, which is often a medical staff committee. This committee reviews adverse events and incident reports, helps enforce safety-related policies, develops safety initiatives, and disseminates information about patient safety to providers. The committee generally includes a diverse group of clinicians (physicians, nurses, pharmacists), hospital administrators, and in some cases lay people.

Patient safety committees face two particular challenges. The first is how to integrate their work and domain into the work of the quality committee and risk management. We have observed that most organizations operate in an ad hoc fashion relative to the overlapping functions of each discipline and domain, making each operation less effective than it could be. The best models provide clearly identified areas of exclusivity as well as areas of overlap and cooperation.

The second challenge for the patient safety committee is to find time and energy to focus on patient safety projects. Often the committee becomes encumbered by endless compliance mandates and reacting to sentinel events. The truly effective patient safety committee gives its members the time and resources to get upstream of patient safety problems and craft proactive solutions.

If the board has a quality committee, the patient safety committee (along with the medical staff quality committee and risk management) should report to it. If there is no quality committee the patient safety committee should send regular reports to the chair of the governing board and the CEO, who together set the agenda for the board.

## THE DATA AND EXAMPLES

Hospital governing boards assume an important role in improving delivery of quality care. Having more knowledge about the prevalence and impact of particular board activities can help them perform this role more effectively. A 2008 study reported in the *Journal of Healthcare Management* drew from a survey of hospital and system leaders (presidents and CEOs) on various aspects of board engagement in quality. More than 80 percent of the responding CEOs indicated that their governing boards were working to establish strategic goals for quality improvement, use quality dashboards to track performance, and follow up on corrective actions related to adverse events. Only 61 percent of the respondents indicated that their governing boards had a quality committee (Jiang et al. 2008).

The existence of a board quality committee was associated with higher likelihood of adopting various oversight practices and lower mortality rates for six common medical conditions measured by the Agency for Healthcare Research and Quality's inpatient quality indicators and the state inpatient databases (Joshi and Hines 2006). Hospital governing boards that appear to be actively engaged in quality oversight do so particularly through the use of internal data and national benchmarks. Having a board quality committee can significantly enhance the board's oversight function. Other potentially useful activities—such as board involvement in setting the agenda for the discussion on quality, inclusion of the quality measures

**Exhibit 12.1: Perceived Effectiveness of Board Oversight Function for Quality**

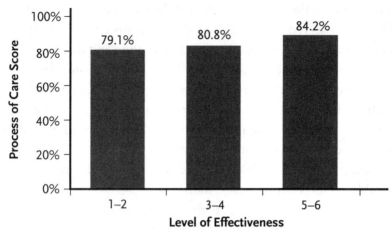

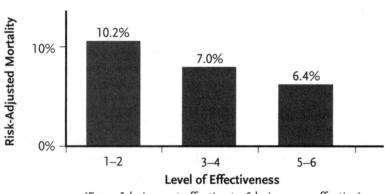

SOURCE: Data from Jiang et al. (2009).

in the CEO's performance evaluation, and improvement of quality literacy of board members—are performed infrequently.

In 2009 another compelling study related the existence of particular board practices with outcome measures such as mortality (Exhibit 12.1). Based on the previous survey of hospital presidents and CEOs, this study examined differences in hospital quality performance associated with the adoption of particular practices in board oversight of quality (Jiang et al. 2009). Quality was measured by performance in process of care and risk-adjusted mortality, using the Hospital Compare data from the Centers for Medicare & Medicaid Services and the Healthcare Cost and Utilization Project inpatient databases of the Agency for Healthcare Research and Quality. When hospital boards were engaged in establishing strategic goals for quality improvement and setting the quality agenda for the organization, these hospitals showed higher scores in process of care and lower risk-adjusted mortality rates.

---

**Board Practices Found to Be Associated with Better Performance in Process of Care and Mortality**

1. Having a board quality committee
2. Establishing strategic goals for quality improvement
3. Being involved in setting the quality agenda for the hospital
4. Making quality improvement an agenda item in board meetings
5. Using a dashboard with national benchmarks that includes indicators for clinical quality, patient safety, and patient satisfaction
6. Linking senior executives' performance evaluation to quality and patient safety indicators

---

Involvement of physician leadership in the board quality committee further enhanced the hospital's quality performance. Taken together, these findings seem to support the notion that activist boards that are engaged in strategic goals for quality and safety will see quantifiable improvement in clinical benchmarks.

## THE ROLE OF EXECUTIVE LEADERSHIP

One of the most important roles for the executive leadership is to support board members who may be skittish about entering the realm of quality and safety. Including board members on patient safety walkarounds, bringing in educators to do tutorials, and making the board feel welcome to contribute in these areas are critical to engage them in this work.

---

### Case Study

In 2008 the CEO of a western Pennsylvania health system was not sleeping at night—and with good reason. The number of risk management cases and sentinel events occurring in his emergency department was soaring. The department had been a top performer by most national benchmarking standards. The busy emergency department, which was seeing more than 50,000 patients a year, was efficient. There was no apparent reason for the sudden surge. The board held the

(continued)

CEO accountable for patient safety in the organization, and he in turn engaged the board to determine a course of action. He brought the data and each case from the emergency department to the board so that it was informed and understood the stories. The board approved the funds to bring in an outside consultant to assess the emergency department and identify causes for some of the safety and quality lapses that had been witnessed.

The consultants noted that the emergency department was staffing mid-level providers in a ratio (to physicians) that was aberrant relative to the rest of the country. The ED physician medical director had been having trouble recruiting physicians. Gradually nurse practitioners had been assuming more and more emergent care, and the physician oversight was now strained. The consultants recommended a change in leadership and a change in the staffing model.

The board approved a plan by the CEO that included financial incentives for recruiting physicians, and both the leadership and staffing model were changed. This is a perfect example of engaging the board in quality and safety efforts while leaving the management details to the CEO.

### Strategies for Healthcare Executives

- Work to educate the board—particularly the board chair—about patient safety and risk management efforts.
- At each meeting, share stories involving patient safety and risk management from within the organization to "put a face" on particular issues.
- Promote patient safety and risk management in the mission, vision, and values statements of the organization.
- Include patient safety and risk management in the strategic planning of the organization.
- Implement a patient safety leadership walkaround program, and include board members on a rotating basis.

## Recommended Readings

Conway, J. 2008. "Getting Boards on Board: Engaging Governing Boards in Quality and Safety." *Joint Commission Journal on Quality and Patient Safety* 34 (4): 214–20.

Jiang, H. J., C. Lockee, K. Bass, and I. Fraser. 2009. "Board Oversight of Quality: Any Differences in Process of Care and Mortality?" *Journal of Healthcare Management* 54 (1): 15–29.

————. 2008. "Board Engagement in Quality: Findings of a Survey of Hospital and System Leaders." *Journal of Healthcare Management* 53 (2): 121–34.

Joshi, M. S., and S. C. Hines. 2006. "Getting the Board on Board: Engaging Hospital Boards in Quality and Patient Safety." *Joint Commission Journal on Quality and Patient Safety* 32 (4): 179–87.

Knecht, P. R. 2007. *Engaging the Board in Strategic Planning: Rationale, Tools and Techniques.* San Diego, CA: The Governance Institute.

# CHAPTER 13

# A Comprehensive Risk Management Program for the ED

**In This Chapter**

- Risk Management Defined
- Eight Components of a Robust Risk Management Program
- Progressive Steps
- Integrating Quality Improvement and Risk Management
- Risk Management Tools and Reporting
- The Role of Executive Leadership
- Case Study
- Strategies for Healthcare Executives

## RISK MANAGEMENT DEFINED

Risk management is an organized effort to identify, assess, and reduce risks to patients, visitors, staff, and organizational assets. The scope of risk management work includes risks related to patient care, medical staff, employees, property, finance, and other areas.

## EIGHT COMPONENTS OF A ROBUST RISK MANAGEMENT PROGRAM

In *Risk Management for Health Care Institutions* (Kaveler and Spiegel 2003), the authors suggest that a comprehensive risk management program includes the following elements:

1. A designated, trained, and experienced risk manager
2. Access to credentialing, management, and medical data
3. A written policy committing resources to risk management
4. A system for identifying, reviewing, and analyzing adverse outcomes
5. Centralized and integrated data collection
6. An annual report to a governing body
7. Educational programs for providers and staff
8. Data on adverse events and medical malpractice passed along to appropriate committees

## PROGRESSIVE STEPS

Kaveler and Spiegel (2003) provide a "progressive steps" framework for risk management in healthcare organizations: risk identification, risk analysis, risk control, and risk financing. All of these can be applied to the ED to help develop a comprehensive program.

### Progressive Steps

- Risk identification
- Risk analysis
- Risk control
- Risk financing

### Risk Identification

Many sources are used to identify risk in a healthcare setting. In the ED, incident reporting, occurrence screening, patient complaints, patient satisfaction surveys, professional liability claims data, workers' compensation data, Joint Commission surveys, consultants' assessments, infection control data, QI data, and staff surveys can be important tools for identifying risk.

For example, if a patient's family member complains that her husband had a kidney stone and did not get anything for pain, this can be a red flag that pain is not being managed well in the ED. Insufficient pain management has recently become an area where patients may seek recourse from the institution. In another example, The Joint Commission monitors the use of restraints in the ED and the adherence to restraint policies. A citation regarding policy adherence could uncover the potential for a patient liability issue involving restraints. Just as the robust QI program should involve ongoing data capture and study, so should a comprehensive risk management program.

### Risk Identification

- Incident reporting
- Occurrence reporting
- Liability claims data
- Patient complaints
- Workers' compensation data
- Joint Commission surveys
- Patient satisfaction surveys
- Staff surveys
- QI data
- Consultants' assessments

Incident reporting systems range from paper reporting to sophisticated point-of-service electronic systems. Occurrence reporting is typically done retrospectively through chart reviews and is part of a performance improvement program. Patient complaints, liability reporting, and satisfaction surveys can all provide insight into the patient experience in the ED. More will be said about reporting later in this chapter.

## Risk Analysis

Once a risk has been identified, risk analysis determines the potential severity of the loss and the probability that such a loss will occur. Typically risk management professionals give priority to the areas of greatest risk of financial loss (such as missed MI cases) instead of minor claims, such as wound infections, which occur in approximately 5 percent of lacerations.

## Risk Control

Risk control involves preventing losses or mitigating the magnitude of the loss. Risk control techniques include the following.

### Exposure Avoidance
An ED can reduce the possibility of a loss to zero. For example, a hospital might decide to no longer be a trauma center to avoid the risk inherent in treating multiple trauma patients.

## Loss Prevention

| Elopement: Unauthorized departure of a patient. |
| :-- |

An ED can decrease the likelihood of an untoward event occurring and reduce the frequency of the loss. For example, after a lawsuit and several incident reports surrounding the **elopement** of a psychiatric patient, a hospital introduced a program whereby patient safety attendants observed all dangerous psychiatric patients and prevented elopements.

## Loss Reduction

An ED develops strategies to minimize the consequences of a given risk. For instance, if a patient falls or has some other adverse event in the ED, having risk management immediately involved and developing a rapport with the injured patient and family may limit the severity of a loss that has already occurred (Witman, Park, and Hardin 1996). A robust risk management program can limit the losses once a sentinel event has occurred, but targeted interventions can also prevent the event—and the lawsuit.

---

**Risk Control Techniques for the ED**

- Exposure avoidance
- Loss prevention
- Loss reduction

---

## Risk Financing

Risk financing generates funds to pay for losses that risk control strategies do not eliminate. These techniques can involve risk retention (assuming losses and setting aside funds to cover them) and risk transfer (shifting the financial obligation for a loss—by buying insurance—but not the legal responsibilities).

# INTEGRATING QUALITY IMPROVEMENT AND RISK MANAGEMENT

James Orlikoff first suggested the interrelationship between risk management and quality improvement in an article for the American Hospital Association, but little

**Exhibit 13.1: A Comparison of Risk Management and Quality Improvement Functions**

| Risk Management | Quality Improvement |
|---|---|
| Protects the institution's assets | Reflects the institution's caring philosophy |
| Protects human and intangible resources | Improves the performance of all professionals and protects patients |
| Prevents injury to patients, visitors, staff, and property | Focuses on the quality of care delivered by the organization |
| Reduces loss by focusing on individual loss or on single accidents | Sets the quality of care rendered according to standards and measurable criteria |
| Prevents incidents by improving the quality of care through ongoing monitoring activities | Prevents future losses or patient injuries by continuous monitoring of problem resolution areas |
| Reviews each incident and the pattern of incidents through application of risk management processes: risk identification, risk analysis, risk control, and risk financing | Searches for patterns of failure using QI processes: problem identification, problem assessment, corrective action, follow-up, and report |
| Concerned with acceptable levels of care from a legal standpoint | Concerned with optimal level of care |
| Directed toward all persons, events, and environs in the healthcare setting | Directed toward patient care |
| Focused on legal, insurance, and risk financing activities | Focused on improving care |

SOURCE: Adapted from Orlikoff and Landau (1981).

progress toward that goal has been made (Orlikoff and Landau 1981). Exhibit 13.1 compares the functions of risk management and quality improvement.

# RISK MANAGEMENT TOOLS AND REPORTING

Prompt identification of injuries, accidents, and adverse outcomes to staff, patients, and visitors has been a primary concern of risk management programs since hospitals began using them. Institutions address potential problems and correct their causes before they can occur again, but risk management processes are only as good as their reporting capability. In addition administrators can take immediate action to avoid or lessen the impact of a lawsuit. Three reporting systems are typically used.

**Risk Management Reporting Systems**

- Incident reporting
- Occurrence reporting
- Occurrence screening

Incident Reporting

In use since the 1940s, incident reporting identifies events that were not consistent with routine operation of the hospital or care of patients or visitors. Equipment malfunction, falls, and medication errors are common incident reports. Analysis of adverse events increases awareness and improves clinical practice. Incident reports should only be filed by the person witnessing or discovering the adverse event. The report should be filed with risk management, not in the patient's chart. Staff should be instructed in the proper documentation of such events to minimize risk.

What is included in an incident report?

- The name of the person(s) affected and the names of any witnesses to an incident
- Where and when the incident occurred
- The events surrounding the incident
- Whether an injury occurred as a direct result of the incident
- The response and corrective measures that were taken

The incident report should be signed and dated prior to handing it in to the appropriate person, such as a supervisor.

What situations should be reported? Examples include:

- Injuries both physical (falls, needle sticks) and emotional (verbal abuse)
- Errors in patient care and medication
- Patient complaints, including any episodes of aggression
- Faulty equipment or product failure (such as running out of oxygen)
- Any incident in which patient or staff safety is compromised

## Dos and Don'ts of Filing an Incident Report

- Do record the details in objective terms—describe exactly what was seen and heard and nothing else.
- Do describe what actions were taken at the scene.
- Do document the time of the incident, the name of the doctor, and the time the doctor was notified.
- Don't include names and addresses of witnesses in the report (it is easier for attorneys to sue the institution).
- Don't enter the incident into the patient's chart; send the report to the person designated by the institution, such as the director of risk management.
- Don't blame anyone, and don't admit liability.

SOURCE: Hazen and Cookson (1990).

## Occurrence Reporting

Some insurers require that institutions develop a list of adverse patient occurrences for reporting, such as infant death or allergic reaction to medication. The best of these reporting systems grant immunity to the person reporting them and cultivate a "just culture," mentioned in Chapter 9. Most states have occurrence reporting policies, procedures, and forms. The Joint Commission also has a list of adverse events that it considers reportable. There is considerable overlap with what should be reported as an incident and what should be reported as an occurrence or APO (adverse patient occurrence). Although lists vary at the discretion of the organization, the insurers, or the state, simply specifying the reportable events increases their identification by 40 to 60 percent (Kaveler and Spiegel 2003).

## Examples of Sentinel Events That Are Voluntarily Reportable Under The Joint Commission's Sentinel Event Policy

- Any patient death, paralysis, coma, or other major permanent loss of function associated with a medication error
- Any suicide of a patient in a setting where the patient is housed around the clock, including suicides following elopement from such a setting

(continued)

- Any elopement of a patient from an around-the-clock care setting resulting in a temporally related death (suicide or homicide) or major permanent loss of function
- Any procedure on the wrong patient, wrong side of the body, or wrong organ
- Any **intrapartum** (related to the birth process) maternal death
- Any perinatal death unrelated to a congenital condition in an infant having a birth weight greater than 2,500 grams
- Assault, homicide, or other crime resulting in patient death or major permanent loss of function
- A patient fall that results in death or major permanent loss of function as a direct result of the injuries sustained in the fall
- Hemolytic transfusion reaction involving major blood group incompatibilities

SOURCE: The Joint Commission (1998).

Occurrence Screening

This system identifies variations in normal operating procedures even if no adverse event has occurred. This ongoing surveillance is typically done with retrospective reviews. More progressive and mature programs make occurrence screening easy and reward staff for reporting these situations, which allows EDs to get upstream of incidents before they occur. An occurrence screening system uses criteria to identify APOs but does not require reporting to capture these events. Types of APOs that can be identified this way include:

> **Intrapartum:** Related to the birth process.

> **Nosocomial infections:** Hospital-acquired infections.

- Transfers to higher levels of care
- **Nosocomial** infections
- Emergency return to the operating room

Peer review determines whether a deviation from standards has occurred or whether the occurrence might be naturally associated with the disease or illness. This methodology can identify an estimated 80 to 85 percent of APOs and, when combined with other methodologies, an organization can identify 90 to 95 percent of APOs (Kaveler and Spiegel 2003).

Once an adverse event or incident has occurred you will need to analyze why and how it occurred. This should be done without looking for individuals to punish—the "name, blame, shame, and train" approach, which has been shown to be a notoriously ineffective way to address incidents and encourage reporting (Cohen 2007).

The two most common analytical methodologies are root cause analysis (RCA) and failure mode and effect analysis (FMEA).

### Root Cause Analysis

RCA is a systematic approach to identifying the underlying causes of an adverse occurrence so that effective steps can be taken to modify processes to prevent future occurrences.

### Failure Mode and Effect Analysis

FMEA is a method of analyzing processes associated with high-risk procedures to identify weaknesses before a problem occurs. The Joint Commission now requires that healthcare organizations select one high-risk process a year and subject it to an FMEA using flow charts and RCA strategies to change and improve processes.

## THE ROLE OF EXECUTIVE LEADERSHIP

The Institute for Healthcare Improvement has long recognized that sponsorship from the executive level is critical to the success of quality improvement and risk management (Botwinick, Bisognano, and Haraden 2006). The CEO should come to the clinical unit to support the changes early in the piloting of each patient safety and risk management project. The executive leadership can and should set the expectation that the QI, patient safety, and risk management workers perform in an integrated and cooperative manner and demonstrate clear results from their work. Each year goals should be articulated for this unified group and each subgroup should share its work with the others in regular meetings. Many risk management projects are triggered from QI work. Occurrences and incidents can provide the foundation for process improvement.

A seven-year-old boy with severe asthma was brought in with a critically low oxygen level. He had been placed on a respirator many times before. The physician, nurses, and respiratory therapist tried inhaled medications to improve his breathing, but there was no improvement. The physician decided to intubate the child and place him on a ventilator.

The patient was given medication to paralyze him, and the physician performed an endotracheal intubation. The respiratory therapist attempted to push oxygen into the child's lungs, but for reasons that were unclear, there was no oxygen getting to the child. The physician performed the intubation again, but again there was no oxygen inflating the lungs. In the room other physicians, critical care nurses, and respiratory therapists were stumped and could not figure where the problem was occurring. The child's oxygen kept dropping, and soon his heart rate was only 30. He was headed for a cardiac arrest.

Serendipitously a young resident from the University Hospital walked by and told the providers in the room, "It is a new type of ambu bag with a pop-off valve. You have to disable the pop-off valve to ventilate the child." He showed the professionals in the room how it worked. The child was ventilated and recovered uneventfully.

FMEA revealed the incident was due to equipment failure. These new devices had been introduced without proper staff training. The practitioners discovered that even in a quiet room without clinical pressure and the instructions in front of them, the equipment's pop-off valve was difficult to disable. Further analysis and investigation concluded that this equipment was not appropriate for the ED.

SOURCE: Unpublished report. Intermountain Medical Center, Salt Lake City (2008). Used with permission.

### Strategies for Healthcare Executives

- Encourage the integration of the QI departments and the risk management departments, because this will be cost effective and allow risk to be identified before a sentinel event.
- Locate the QI staff, the patient safety officer, and the risk management department in contiguous offices; hold regular joint meetings; and encourage collaborative projects to bring about this integration.

(continued)

- Commit the necessary technological and personnel resources for such a program.
- Openly promote the just culture in your organization.
- Set expectations for annual reports with clear evidence of success through initiatives and projects with tangible results that can be shared throughout the organization.

## Recommended Readings

Carroll, R. 2009. *Risk Management Handbook for Health Care Organizations, Student Edition.* AASHRM. San Francisco: Jossey-Bass.

Kaveler, F., and A. Spiegel. 2003. *Risk Management in Health Care Institutions: A Strategic Approach,* Second Edition. Sudbury, MA: Jones and Bartlett Publishers.

Orlikoff, J., and G. B. Landau. 1981. "Why Risk Management and Quality Assurance Should be Integrated." *Hospitals* 55 (11): 54–55.

# Part II

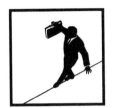

# HEALTHCARE LAW AND HIGH-RISK ADMINISTRATIVE ISSUES

The ED is the location in the hospital with a prevalence of high-risk scenarios. It is also the focus of specific legislation and legal requirements that are unbending. There is endless opportunity to run afoul of civil and criminal laws in the ED. This section is a walk through the high-liability minefields in the emergency department with answers to the most frequently asked questions and myth busting around EMTALA, HIPAA, Stark, and kickbacks. The remarkable thing about this section of the book is the sheer magnitude of misinformation circulating about these laws and their application to the ED. Even leaders who believe they are well informed may find they are carrying around erroneous beliefs about these laws.

The emergency department also has some risks that are situational, such as transfers, informed consent, and treating underage or incapacitated patients. Strategies for minimizing those risks are offered, and the law is brought to life with real-life cases. Documentation in the ED is also covered in this section, along with standardized order sets and protocols. Areas of legal risk particular to the ED are broken down and clarified, and system solutions are offered.

# CHAPTER 14

# HIPAA in the ED, Part I

**In This Chapter**

- Back to the Beginning
- The HIPAA Myth Buster
- Sharing Health Information as Necessary for Treatment
- The Much-Maligned White Board
- Dealing with Families and Loved Ones
- The Role of Executive Leadership
- Case Study
- Strategies for Healthcare Executives

## BACK TO THE BEGINNING

The Health Insurance Portability and Accountability Act (HIPAA) was passed in 1996, and many remember the significant upheavals, delays, and revisions encountered by the Privacy Rule before its compliance date, April 14, 2003. That shared experience may be where common knowledge ends. Even at the time of this writing significant misunderstandings, myths, and convoluted reasoning about HIPAA remain.

At the end of the day, the Privacy Rule was intended to provide "federal protections for personal health information held by covered entities and [to give] patients an array of rights with respect to that information. At the same time, the Privacy Rule is balanced so that it permits the disclosure of personal health information needed for patient care and other important purposes" (HHS n.d.(b)). The law was never meant to endanger patients, nor specifically to prevent physicians, nurses, hospital staff, and other providers from sharing personal health information (PHI) necessary to ensure safe and effective patient care. This is not to say that patient privacy is unimportant. Healthcare professionals have always had ethical duties related to the privacy of their patients.

> ### Reasons for Confusion About HIPAA
>
> - Delays and revisions of the original law
> - Varying state laws
> - Myths perpetuated by vendors
> - Embellishments by The Joint Commission
> - Lack of clarity in the original law

Each state had its own laws, regulations, and other enforceable rules that predated HIPAA. In fact, the federal requirements of the HIPAA Privacy Rule created a floor, not a ceiling, for laws passed by any state; states had to meet the federal requirements as a minimum standard but were free to require more stringent protections. Many states did so. In addition, various accrediting bodies (most notably The Joint Commission) also embellished the requirements required by the federal law.

Adding to the confusion around HIPAA, particularly in the beginning, were the voices of numerous vendors that had products to sell. Nothing assists in marketing better than fear, so the most aggressive penalties in the law (such as jail for criminal activity) were purposely confused with more lenient penalties for accidental disclosures by conscientious providers.

In sum, political battles, numerous revisions during the rulemaking by the US Department of Health and Human Services (HHS), differing state requirements, variety in interpretation by different agencies, and a subset of unscrupulous marketers all created a cacophony around HIPAA. That by itself is irritating; when patients are injured or their families are unnecessarily left with inadequate information in an emergency, it is tragic.


## THE HIPAA MYTH BUSTER

There are multiple commercial resources available about HIPAA, but even the best may fail to clarify what information is misleading, particularly regarding penalties and risk. It is best to rely on a definitive source that comes from the government directly.

To its credit, HHS has been trying to dispel the myths that have been circulating all these years. Through summaries, guides for the public and covered entities, and the Frequently Asked Questions (FAQ) section of its website, HHS has provided clearly worded, succinct, and easily accessible information to clarify what was intended under the HIPAA Privacy Rule.

Healthcare executives must keep in mind the possibility that state law may require more of them and must confirm the details of their own state laws through the relevant state agency, their state hospital association, their medical association, and/or their state bar association. In addition, all institutional providers must of course look to the accrediting authority for compliance with rules. More on that later in this chapter.

## SHARING HEALTH INFORMATION AS NECESSARY FOR TREATMENT

The most dangerous HIPAA myths are those that result in the nondisclosure of patient information that is necessary for patient care and safety. Particularly in an ED, physicians and other providers must have immediate access to patient information, including from private physician offices in the community. Unfortunately, and frequently, this is not the case.

Information can be shared via fax, by e-mail, or over the phone (HHS n.d.(b)). Conversations, particularly in a loud ED, may be overheard.

**Can healthcare providers engage in confidential conversations with other providers or with patients, even if there is a possibility that they could be overheard?**

Yes. The HIPAA Privacy Rule is not intended to prohibit providers from talking to each other and to their patients. Provisions of this rule requiring covered entities to implement reasonable safeguards that reflect their particular circumstances and exempting treatment disclosures from certain requirements are intended to ensure that providers' primary consideration is the appropriate treatment of their patients. The Privacy Rule recognizes that oral communications often must occur freely and quickly

(continued)

in treatment settings. Thus, covered entities are free to engage in communications as required for quick, effective, and high quality healthcare. The Privacy Rule also recognizes that overheard communications in these settings may be unavoidable and allows for these incidental disclosures.

SOURCE: HHS (2006a).

The government recognizes that in "an emergency situation, in a loud emergency room, or where a patient is hearing impaired, such precautions may not be practicable" (HHS 2006a). Information may be overheard because the sharing of patient information is more important than privacy at that time. An improper balance between privacy and patient care can often be seen in the arduous precautions espoused by numerous "experts" as compared to the level of protections actually envisioned by HIPAA.

**Does the HIPAA Privacy Rule require hospitals and doctors' offices to be retrofitted to provide private rooms and soundproof walls to avoid any possibility that a conversation is overheard?**

No, the Privacy Rule does not require these types of structural changes be made to facilities.

Covered entities must have in place appropriate administrative, technical, and physical safeguards to protect the privacy of protected health information. This standard requires that covered entities make reasonable efforts to prevent uses and disclosures not permitted by the rule. The department does not consider facility restructuring to be a requirement under this standard.

For example, the Privacy Rule does *not* require the following types of structural or systems changes:

- Private rooms
- Soundproofing of rooms
- Encryption of wireless or other emergency medical radio communications that can be intercepted by scanners
- Encryption of telephone systems

(continued)

> Covered entities must implement reasonable safeguards to limit incidental, and avoid prohibited, uses and disclosures. The Privacy Rule does not require that all risk of protected health information disclosure be eliminated.
>
> SOURCE: HHS (2006b).

## THE MUCH-MALIGNED WHITE BOARD

Given the priority placed by the government on patient care and safety—not as *opposed* to patient privacy but as *balanced* with it—why have hospitals across the country been required to take down their white boards tracking patients in the ED (Welch and Fontenot 2010)?

These boards have a specific purpose: patient safety. In a busy ED it is imperative that all hands on deck know *who* is in the ED, *where* each patient is, and can *at a glance* distinguish between the room that holds a woman in labor and the room with the severe asthmatic. These boards, similar to ones used in the OR, are a means of communicating patient information to everyone involved in patient care. They are for safety's sake, and they are not prohibited by HIPAA.

Needless to say, a similar board in a pediatrician's office—"ear check in room 3"—may not be *reasonable*, and it goes without saying that the white board is not posted in the ED waiting room. However, in the staff area of an ED, which may transiently contain members of the public, the information posted is what is necessary to facilitate care and prevent accidents.

## DEALING WITH FAMILIES AND LOVED ONES

One area where HIPAA misunderstandings have really gotten out of hand is in defining what is meant by "family." The law was meant to give patients control over their own privacy, and it would make sense that HIPAA allows a patient to choose who will have access to her private information. For example:

> We propose to require covered entities to obtain the individual's oral consent before…speaking with next of kin "or other individual involved in the individual's healthcare."
>
> SOURCE: HIPAA Privacy Rule, Final Rule §164.510.

Similarly, the FAQs on the HHS website include the following:

> If the patient is present and has the capacity to make healthcare decisions, when does HIPAA allow a healthcare provider to discuss the patient's health information with the patient's family, friends, or others involved in the patient's care or payment for care?
>
> If the patient is present and has the capacity to make healthcare decisions, a healthcare provider may discuss the patient's health information with a family member, friend, **or other person if the patient agrees** or, when given the opportunity, does not object. (HHS (2006a))

It is clear that the intention of HIPAA was that the person identified by the patient as a "loved one" could be given appropriate information. Sadly, in the midst of HIPAA confusion some providers started confusing "family" with the *legal* definition and felt they could not follow a patient's request to share information to a same-sex partner or other nonlegal "family" member (Simmons 2010). In June 2010 HHS released new regulations clarifying a patient's right to choose whom she wants as a visitor in the hospital, including a same-sex domestic partner.

Other HIPAA issues in the ED involving "family" are fairly standard and well documented in the HHS FAQs.

Does the HIPAA Privacy Rule permit a doctor to discuss a patient's health status, treatment, or payment arrangements with the patient's family and friends? Yes. Is that true even if the patient is not present or is unconscious? Yes. Specific examples provided in the FAQs include those in the two boxes that follow.

---

### Examples of Situations That Do Not Violate HIPAA

- An emergency room doctor may discuss a patient's treatment in front of the patient's friend if the patient asks that her friend come into the treatment room.
- A doctor's office may discuss a patient's bill with the patient's adult daughter who is with the patient at the patient's medical appointment and has questions about the charges.
- A doctor may discuss the drugs a patient needs to take with the patient's health aide who has accompanied the patient to a medical appointment.

(continued)

---

- A doctor may give information about a patient's mobility limitations to the patient's sister who is driving the patient home from the hospital.
- A nurse may discuss a patient's health status with the patient's brother if she informs the patient she is going to do so and the patient does not object.

SOURCE: HHS (2006a).

### Examples of Situations That Do Violate HIPAA

- A nurse may not discuss a patient's condition with the patient's brother if the patient asked that he not be given information.
- A healthcare provider may not discuss a celebrity patient's condition with the media.
- An ED staff member may not discuss a patient's case with his own family or friends if the patient asks that information not be given.

SOURCE: HHS (2006a).

HIPAA has strict guidelines around releasing information to the media. For example:

- Celebrities are to be given the same privacy as any other patient.
- Hospital directory information (the patient's name, one-word condition, and location in the hospital) may be given if an inquiry is made about the patient by name and if the patient has given permission for this disclosure.
- Media representatives and photographers should contact the hospital's designated spokesperson for assistance in obtaining interviews and photographs of patients, employees, and areas of the hospital.
- Hospital policies usually require that a hospital representative accompany news personnel any time they are on hospital grounds.
- No photographs, audio/visual recordings, or interviews of patients may be taken within the facility or on hospital property without the patient's prior written consent or the written permission of a parent or legal representative.

- Even with permission, news media representatives should use good judgment when airing images or printing photographs of patients who are ill or injured. Deceased or unconscious patients should never be photographed under any circumstance.

The following activities require a written and signed authorization that meets all HIPAA privacy standard requirements from the patient:

- Releasing a detailed statement (includes anything other than a one-word condition); the patient or her legal representative must sign the written authorization approving any detailed statement
- Taking photographs (either video or stills) of the patient
- Conducting media interviews with patients

Other FAQs address notification of clergy and responding to inquiries by visitors or callers regarding the patient's location and general condition if the patient does not object. The ability to respond to inquiries may extend to other hospitals or providers who are using information obtained from your ED, if the patient is informed and has the opportunity to restrict the disclosure. Communication with family or other loved ones is also permitted via an interpreter as necessary. Finally, and perhaps most poignantly, an ED may *initiate* contact by calling loved ones of a patient who arrives in the ED subsequent to an accident or critical health event.

## THE ROLE OF EXECUTIVE LEADERSHIP

It is essential that executive leadership clarify for the organization exactly what the basic tenets of HIPAA are and combat the tendency to over-read the law. This requires education of clinical, risk management, and information technology personnel. Patient safety should not be sacrificed due to a distorted interpretation of the law.

An emergency department with 23 beds and peak seasonal volumes of 89 patients a day is told that the ED whiteboard is a HIPAA violation, so staff remove it. A misinformed patient safety officer also advises the ED to cover patient clipboards and charts with a plastic sheet to prevent any patient information from being seen by passersby.

The ED experiences a series of sentinel events, including tests and x-rays being performed on the wrong patients, patients being administered the wrong medications, and waits and delays in patient care due to confusion of the locations of patients. Consultants and ancillary service technicians cannot readily locate patients in the department without the whiteboard. Covered patient information on the charts amplifies the problem.

An outside consulting firm called in to evaluate the performance of the emergency physician group immediately faulted the department for these lapses and instructed the emergency department to replace its whiteboard.

SOURCE: Welch and Fontenot (2010).

### Strategies for Healthcare Executives

- Take the initiative to read government resources and understand HIPAA correctly.
- Make patient privacy a cultural imperative for your organization.
- Articulate that safety comes before privacy and that the ED is a unique healthcare setting.

## Recommended Readings

A complete list of Frequently Asked Questions on privacy is available at www.hhs.gov/ocr/hipaa

Simmons, J. 2010. "Some Hospitals Falling Short of Protecting for Gay Patients." Healthleaders Media, June 8. www.healthleadersmedia.com/content/QUA-252125/Some-Hospitals-Falling-Short-of-Protecting-for-Gay-Patients.

# CHAPTER 15

# HIPAA in the ED, Part II

**In This Chapter**

- Public Health Emergencies, Law Enforcement, and National Disasters
- Penalties: The Real Scoop
- The Threat of Incarceration
- When the Inspector Says You Are Wrong
- New Sheriffs in HIPAA Enforcement Get to Work
- The Role of Executive Leadership
- Case Study
- Strategies for Healthcare Executives

## PUBLIC HEALTH EMERGENCIES, LAW ENFORCEMENT, AND NATIONAL DISASTERS

The location in any hospital that will most likely be involved in a public health emergency, a summons for law enforcement, or a national disaster is the ED. HIPAA implications for all three scenarios are addressed in the HHS Frequently Asked Questions (see box on page 142): Disclosure may be necessary and permitted to address a public health emergency and/or a threat of bioterrorism; notification of law enforcement is permitted as necessary to allow "important law enforcement functions to continue"; and waivers may be necessary to allow public authorities to deal with a national disaster.

**Is the HIPAA Privacy Rule suspended during a national or public health emergency?**

No; however, the secretary of HHS may waive certain provisions of the rule under the Project Bioshield Act of 2004 (PL 108-276) and section 1135(b)(7) of the Social Security Act.

*What provisions may be waived?*
If the president declares an emergency or disaster *and* the secretary declares a public health emergency, the secretary may waive sanctions and penalties against a covered hospital that does not comply with certain provisions of the HIPAA Privacy Rule:

1. The requirements to obtain a patient's agreement to speak with family members or friends involved in the patient's care
2. The requirement to honor a request to opt out of the facility directory
3. The requirement to distribute a notice of privacy practices
4. The patient's right to request privacy restrictions
5. The patient's right to request confidential communications

*When and to what entities does the waiver apply?*
If the secretary issues such a waiver, it only applies:

1. In the emergency area and for the emergency period identified in the public health emergency declaration
2. To hospitals that have instituted a disaster protocol. The waiver would apply to all patients at such hospitals
3. For up to 72 hours from the time the hospital implements its disaster protocol

When the presidential or secretarial declaration terminates, a hospital must then comply with all the requirements of the Privacy Rule for any patient still under its care, even if 72 hours has not elapsed since implementation of its disaster protocol. Regardless of the activation of an emergency waiver, the HIPAA Privacy Rule permits disclosures for treatment purposes and certain disclosures to disaster relief organizations. For instance, the Privacy Rule allows covered entities to share patient information with the American Red Cross so it can notify family members of the patient's location.

SOURCE: HHS (n.d.(c))

In summary, EDs should be allowed to do what they know best: respond to emergencies as presented by a particular patient, law enforcement, the community (public health disasters), or the nation (national disasters).

## PENALTIES: THE REAL SCOOP

Penalties for violations of a patient's privacy should not be discounted. Casual, willful, or malicious sharing of a patient's secrets can subject a physician or other provider to discipline by the appropriate licensing agency (e.g., medical board, board of nursing), disciplinary action by the employer, and the possibility of a suit brought by the patient or his representative.

The state statute-based liabilities associated with privacy breaches predate HIPAA and should have always controlled the inappropriate sharing of patient information, although one would hope good manners and a sense of professionalism would have been enough alone.

Even since the ascendency of HIPAA, however, it has been commonly believed and repeated that an accidental violation of a patient's privacy could result in significant fines or jail time. Let's review what the HIPAA Myth Buster would say in answer to that assertion.

### Civil Financial Penalties

The Office for Civil Rights (OCR) within HHS may impose a penalty on a covered entity for a failure to comply with a requirement of the Privacy Rule. Penalties will vary significantly depending on factors such as the date of the violation, whether the covered entity knew or should have known of the failure to comply, or whether the covered entity's failure to comply was due to willful neglect. Penalties may not exceed a calendar year cap for multiple violations of the same requirement.

|  | For violations occurring prior to 2/18/2009 | For violations occurring on or after 2/18/2009 |
|---|---|---|
| Penalty amount | Up to $100 per violation | $100 to $50,000 or more per violation |
| Calendar year cap | $25,000 | $1,500,000 |

SOURCE: HHS (2003).

The sharp increase in penalties reflects changes made under the American Recovery and Reinvestment Act (ARRA) and the Health Information Technology for Economic and Clinical Health (HITECH) Act of 2009. There is a distinction between cavalier, willful acts and breaches that occur despite the best efforts to comply with the HIPAA Privacy Rule. This line between caring, careful providers with *accidental* disclosures and the truly negligent is underscored by the following from the HHS site:

---

**No Penalty**

A penalty will **not** be imposed for violations in certain circumstances. If the failure to comply was not due to willful neglect, and was corrected during a 30-day period after the entity knew or should have known the failure to comply had occurred (unless the period is extended at the discretion of OCR), a penalty will not be imposed.

In addition, OCR may choose to reduce a penalty if the failure to comply was due to reasonable cause, and the penalty would be excessive given the nature and extent of the noncompliance.

---

This does not dismiss the potential penalties for electronic breaches affecting large numbers of patients or the prospect of being listed on the "wall of shame" of breaches by HHS under the HITECH Act, but those are not the type of penalties encountered in an ED. The HIPAA issues faced routinely in an ED are much more personal, such as posting patient information to improve coordination and ensure patient safety or comforting a family member by appropriately sharing information regarding the status of a loved one. These well-intentioned, patient-centric efforts should be encouraged, not discouraged.

## THE THREAT OF INCARCERATION

The threat of jail was a seductive element of the HIPAA Privacy Rule for some vendors. Both consultants and IT software vendors perpetuated misinformation to sell their products. The net result is that fear spread throughout the healthcare community, and the misinformation has been repeated ever since by smart, honest, and caring people (Turner 2002). But the damage was done at the beginning and has been hard to correct. Notice that there has been no mention thus far in this discussion of incarceration. That is because we have been discussing *civil* penalties, and yet the healthcare providers who are trying the hardest to get the law right seem to be the most worried about going to jail.

People can, and have, gone to jail for violating a patient's privacy under the HIPAA Privacy Rule. That is true. What is not true is that the people incarcerated did all the right things but inadvertently responded to a family member's question against a patient's request or otherwise "broke HIPAA." People who need to worry about incarceration are those who participate in conduct "committed with intent to sell, transfer, or use individually identifiable health information for commercial advantage, personal gain, or malicious harm" (42 U.S.C. 1320d–6 §177(b)(3)). If you should ever fall into that category, watch out for the US Department of Justice, the government entity responsible for criminal prosecutions under the Privacy Rule.

---

**Go Straight to Jail**

Selling, using, or transferring identifiable health information for:

- Commercial advantage
- Personal gain
- Malicious harm

---

## WHEN THE INSPECTOR SAYS YOU ARE WRONG

The prospect of being questioned by any authority about your facility's compliance is enough to cause concern for even the most stalwart administrator. At the same time, there is an emperor-wears-no-clothes quality to many of the "rules" enforced in the name of HIPAA.

Assuming you have made an appropriate effort to comply with your state law and all relevant rules from your accrediting body, what is an administrator to do when an investigator casts aspersions on measures you have taken to ensure patient safety but which could arguably present a privacy issue (such as the whiteboard in your ED)? For lack of a better description, we hope there could be an appropriate level of push-back best encapsulated in the words "prove it."

If there is a bona fide rule or regulation that can be verified, there may *still* be an appropriate argument to make in the name of patient safety, albeit one that would be more appropriate for the state agency, not the investigator in your hallway. It is our expectation that many challenges to HIPAA requirements will be met with a resounding silence. For almost a decade providers have been accepting modifications in their communication systems (Welch and Fontenot 2010), even when some of the most commonly held beliefs fly in the face of running an efficient, effective ED. From the removal of the whiteboard that conveys critical patient identifiers and location to double and triple (and time-consuming) log-ons for computer systems, misunderstandings about HIPAA have led to changes that imperil the efficient communication of critical information in the ED. We all believe in privacy, but the roughshod enforcement of unnecessary precautions must stop. If the battle is ultimately in the name of patient safety, it is a battle worth fighting.

A new and unanticipated aspect of patient privacy involves camera phones and photography in the ED. Organizations should have an institutional policy about this to protect patients and their privacy from other patients and their visitors and to protect healthcare workers from unwanted imaging. A strict policy with placards and signs prohibiting amateur photography in the ED is the best and the easiest to enforce. Photography for the health record or for educational purposes is done with hospital equipment after signed consents are obtained, and the images do not leave the hospital.

## NEW SHERIFFS IN HIPAA ENFORCEMENT GET TO WORK

The American Recovery and Reinvestment Act of 2009 (ARRA) made a number of changes to HIPAA, such as increasing financial penalties for egregious violations. As already discussed, these new penalties should not apply to well-meaning providers who make an inadvertent mistake and respond appropriately.

The most potentially intrusive change under ARRA involves the enforcement of HIPAA. After years of no real enforcement of the civil side of the law, attorneys general in every state were authorized by ARRA to enforce the federal law under their own state jurisdiction. According to Nicastro (2010), "HHS has yet to levy any civil penalties...since the HIPAA Privacy Rule was in force April 13, 2003, but now there are 50 new sheriffs in town.... Most state attorneys general are elected, and almost all of them do everything they can to get re-elected." This may mean new aggressive applications and enforcement of HIPAA.

Many people in the healthcare industry, and most in health law, anticipate that the interpretation of 50 different state offices will only add to the confusion about what HIPAA does, and does not, require for patient privacy. Time will tell; at the time of this writing only one state has taken up the challenge: In July 2010 Connecticut announced a $250,000 settlement with Health Net stemming from a breach of personal health information that involved the loss of a computer disk drive, after which the company delayed notifying consumers and law enforcement authorities for about six months from the time of the breach (Nicastro 2010).

Of course the application of state law was always the province of the attorneys general, but the addition of federal law enforcement to their docket bears watching.

## THE ROLE OF EXECUTIVE LEADERSHIP

People attracted to healthcare as a profession are overwhelmingly people of good intentions and sincere caring. Patient privacy is important to healthcare executives because they are generally good people. The same can be said for the licensed and nonlicensed professionals and personnel involved in all of the various functions of a healthcare entity. An executive does well when he confronts privacy as an individual concern and directs policy from the perspective that privacy is a shared concern for all employees.

At the same time, compliance efforts, policies, procedures, and supervision of all people in a facility are meant to discover and remove people who do not share that principled view of privacy. This no-tolerance policy must extend to employees and independent professionals equally.

A commitment to privacy must be balanced with a primary concern for patient care and safety. To deliver excellence in healthcare, patient information must be shared appropriately among everyone assisting in that patient's care. A true leader helps the team understand that sharing patient information is not only allowed under HIPAA, it is encouraged, given that reasonable protections are in place. Leadership in healthcare requires that an executive has an understanding of HIPAA, not only its components, but also how the law affects patient care and safety. At the end of the day, an educated response to patient privacy protections is the best leadership of all.

### Case Study

A nurse is cleaning the wound of a patient with multiple lacerations when his friend begins to photograph her at work with his camera phone. She is taken aback but does not have a script to follow for managing the situation. She forgets about the episode until someone informs her that her image is on YouTube with unflattering commentary.

(continued)

The whole scenario is upsetting to her, to human resources workers who feel she should have been protected from this situation, and to hospital public relations personnel.

In response the health system for which she works began crafting "Social Media Policies" to address this new phenomenon. Around the country healthcare organizations are taking different approaches. Some ban photography altogether, while others allow photographs to be taken with hospital photography equipment (and thence control of the images and their distribution) with consent forms signed.

SOURCE: Welch (2010d).

---

### Strategies for Healthcare Executives

- Make privacy and its impact on policies and procedures the domain of the highest executive level in the organization.
- Constantly police for compliance.
- Understand and help draw the line in the ED between patient safety and patient privacy.
- Address the issue of camera phones and photography in the ED.

## Recommended Readings

Alexander, B., B. M. Broccolo, K. F. Conley, A. R. Daniels, M. Dube, R. G. Hoban, C. B. Hutto, C. C. Loepere, D. E. Matyas, T. W. Mayo, J. J. Miles, R. E. Sallade, M. F. Schaff, S. O. Scheutzow, D. J. Schwartz, and E. T. Thomas. 2008. *AHLA Fundamentals of Health Law,* Fourth Edition. Washington, DC: American Health Lawyers Association.

Wing, K., and B. Gilbert. 2006. *The Law and the Public's Health,* Seventh Edition. Chicago: Health Administration Press. See Chapter 3, "Government Power and the Right to Privacy," for an excellent general discussion on the right to privacy.

# CHAPTER 16

# Stark in the ED

**In This Chapter**

- Background of "Stark"
- Stark Defined
- Penalties Under Stark
- Stark Versus Kickbacks
- The Role of Executive Leadership
- Case Study
- Strategies for Healthcare Executives

## BACKGROUND OF "STARK"

The Omnibus Reconciliation Act of 1989 (commonly known as "Stark," in honor of California Representative Pete Stark, a key force behind the law) prohibits a physician from referring a patient to a facility, such as a clinical laboratory, in which he has an ownership interest. However, Stark does have exceptions. "The law came about after a 1989 study by the Office of Inspector General (OIG) demonstrated increased utilization of services—and therefore increased cost—when a physician had an ownership stake. A study in Florida at that time demonstrated similar findings" (McDowell 1989).

The Stark rule aims to prevent the physician financial relationships that lead to overuse of services. However, additions and changes to the Stark regulations and interpretations have plagued the healthcare industry for decades. Some of these changes have been issued via Stark Final Regulations; other alterations have been passed through other federal legislation, such as the Medicare Modernization Act of 2003, the Deficit Reduction Act of 2005, and the Inpatient Prospective Payment Proposed Rule of 2008. The frequency of changes, combined with the varied location of legislative guidance, has only increased the confusion in the healthcare industry about the law.

### Reasons for Stark Confusion

- Additions and changes to the original Stark law have been peppered into other federal legislation.
- Changes occurred before the previous iteration was well understood.
- The first version was particularly complex and included sweeping changes.
- The rule had a dormant period before implementation while other legislation moved forward.
- Providers struggled with interpretation and received conflicting legal advice.

As one healthcare accounting firm put it, "How could the government possibly make matters worse for hospitals and physicians doing their best to avoid Stark violations in their everyday business transactions? Simple: just take one of the most complicated sets of regulations ever imposed, and change it up to *three times* in the course of a year!" (Johnson and Schroeder 2011). Additionally, Stark was dormant during a period when a number of other pieces of federal legislation were capturing much of the attention of the healthcare industry, such as the HIPAA Privacy Rule and Security Rule. In 2008 the American Healthcare Lawyers Association noted in its monograph about Stark Rules, "After several years of relative quiet in the Stark regulatory field, the last half of 2007 and the first half of 2008 unleashed a flurry of actual and proposed rulemaking, including some of the most sweeping and dramatic changes in a decade" (AHLA 2009).

Any evaluation of a potential Stark violation must, therefore, include analysis of multiple rules and regulations. It is also important to note that Stark analysis is fact-specific; providers cannot rely on the legal analysis of a similar situation with any level of assurance. This means that one "pass" in the industry does not translate to global permission; every provider must seek guidance from appropriate legal counsel.

Any time there is payment or any return of value in exchange for healthcare services, the specter of Stark needs to be raised.

Complicating matters, the same fact pattern will also frequently create the possibility of a kickback. Providers must understand that an activity could pass Stark analysis but still be illegal as a kickback, or vice versa.

## STARK DEFINED

The Stark law itself is succinct: Physicians are prohibited from making a referral for a designated health service to entities with which the physician (or an immediate family member) has a financial relationship, unless an exception applies.

The devil, of course, is in the details. The following are definitions of the terms within the law:

### Physician

Stark regulations apply to physicians of all kinds:

- Doctor of medicine
- Doctor of osteopathy
- Doctor of dental surgery
- Doctor of dental medicine
- Doctor of podiatric medicine
- Doctor of optometry
- Chiropractor

### Referral

As a practical matter, a referral occurs anytime a physician is not going to personally perform a service. Stark defines a referral as "a request by a physician for an item or service payable under Medicare or Medicaid (including the request by a physician for consultation with another physician and any test or procedure ordered or performed by such other physician)" (StarkLaw.org 2010). A service performed by someone under the ordering physician's supervision may be viewed for Stark analysis as if the ordering physician had performed the service herself (Burgess n.d.). Many physicians have been led to believe that an employee performing a service under orders is always permitted under Stark, but that is not true unless an exception applies, such as those pertaining to bona fide group practices.

## Designated Health Service

The list of what constitutes a designated health service has grown significantly over time, and many of the services listed are conducted in an ED, such as:

- Clinical laboratory services
- Radiology/imaging services
- Provision of outpatient prescription drugs
- Outpatient hospital services

## Immediate Family Member

Stark prohibits referral if the physician has a financial interest in that service and also if the physician's family has a financial interest. The definition of family is exceedingly broad:

- Husband or wife
- Birth or adoptive parent, child, or sibling
- Step-parent, step-child, or step-sibling
- In-laws of all kinds
- Grandparents or grandchildren
- Spouse of grandparent or grandchild

A physician may not, therefore, prescribe services that benefit her financially (or benefit her mother-in-law) *unless* an exception applies.

## Financial Relationship

Any financial benefit that results from the referral of a designated health service may result in a Stark violation. That financial benefit does not need to be money per se, but could also include ownership or investment interests or other compensation arrangements. Even a retirement plan or stock option may constitute "a compensation arrangement" and must therefore fall under a Stark exception to be permitted. In fact, retirement plans have come under increased scrutiny in recent years as they are often seen as conduits for giving physicians value in exchange for referrals. A multilevel corporate structure cannot be used to hide an incentive to a physician for referrals.

If an arrangement does not give a physician any incentive for referrals it may be permitted, but any such arrangement should be brought to appropriate counsel for analysis. Even the implication of hidden incentives may cause the physician trouble later if the arrangement is scrutinized.

## Exceptions

Stark in effect prohibits *all* self-referral by *all* physicians. This is true by design, as it is a statute of exception, which means that an entire category of behavior is prohibited, with specific exceptions. In Stark analysis of any particular business plan, any *one* exception that fits is enough to allow the referral pattern in question. If one exception can be found, the plan should survive.

There are many, many exceptions under the law. Exceptions include those that apply to certain compensation methodologies, such as specific ownership and compensation exceptions; ownership-only exceptions; compensation arrangement exceptions; exceptions for physician services or in-office ancillary services; and exceptions pertaining to academic medical centers, to name just a few.

Stark analysis continues to change over time, and common behaviors that were acceptable in the past are now subject to scrutiny; some common exceptions have been closed altogether. For example, a common reimbursement methodology known as "per-click" (in which the ordering physician was paid for every referral) was felt to include an incentive to increase orders (and therefore income) and has been closed. Similarly, "under-arrangements" (in which a physician not employed by a hospital was able to pass his charges through the hospital) have been disallowed, requiring that physician to submit his charges directly at a lower rate of reimbursement. Even the time-honored tradition of professional courtesy has come under Stark scrutiny.

ED physicians concerned with possible Stark violations need to review their practices in light of their employment status. If they are outside of hospital employment they should contact their own attorney for review of their contractual obligations to the hospital, such as renegotiating any lease or rental agreement they have for equipment or office space. This is true even if the ED physicians constitute a group practice as defined by the Stark law, as the exceptions permitted to those practices that can meet all nine conditions for classification as a group practice have been changed in recent years.

Of particular interest to the ED is recent re-evaluation of what constitutes "fair market value" for hourly reimbursement of ED physicians. As the market has ratcheted up these figures, the government has become increasingly loath to have published indices or actual market conditions determine if hourly reimbursements meet the fair-market-value requirement.

Written advisory opinions are available through the Office of Inspector General (OIG) on whether a referral relating to a designated health service is actually prohibited under the Stark law. Unfortunately, the OIG will not make specific determinations regarding whether a situation meets the fair market value standard. There are third parties available commercially to make this determination, but again these companies cannot be used as a ruse to channel additional incentives back to referring physicians.

The only safe recourse to any provider—institutional or personal—is to have all contractual relationships and compensation agreements between service providers and physicians assessed by competent legal counsel.

---

**Stark Exceptions**

- Academic centers
- Specific ownership
- In-office ancillary services
- Specific compensation methodologies
- Under-arrangements
- Group practice exemptions

---

## PENALTIES UNDER STARK

The first concern for a physician violating Stark is that she will not be paid for an illegal referral. Of far greater concern is that Stark allows for a civil penalty of up to $15,000 for *each* bill or claim submitted for a service the person knew violated the Stark regulations, plus up to three times the amount of *each* claim wrongfully submitted. An additional penalty of up to $100,000 may be incurred for each *arrangement* or scheme for inappropriate reimbursement.

As significant as these penalties are, it is the possibility of exclusion that should concern physicians most. Sanctioned providers that may not participate in any government healthcare reimbursement program rarely survive the length of the exclusion, even if it is only a year. More is said about exclusion in Chapter 37.

## STARK VERSUS KICKBACKS

In listing the penalties under Stark, it should be noted that jail is not mentioned. That is because Stark is a *civil* statute, and civil violations do not result in incarceration. This is the biggest difference between Stark and antikickback legislation, which does allow criminal penalties. The differences between Stark violations and kickbacks are listed in Exhibit 16.1.

In discussing Stark, it is important to emphasize that the same set of facts could lead to Stark *and* kickback liability. Again, analysis must consider both possibilities, as activity acceptable under one federal law may still be illegal under the other.

## THE ROLE OF EXECUTIVE LEADERSHIP

Healthcare executives are charged with knowing how they can steer their organization into partnerships, ventures, and alliances that foster growth and stability and increase patient care services *without* posing liability risks. Good leaders not only watch out for their own institutional liabilities, but for the conflicting duties of possible business partners as well. Even if the hospital does not have exposure, an executive leader must be assured that relationships entered into do not pose liabili-

**Exhibit 16.1: Stark Violations Versus Kickbacks**

| Stark Violations | Kickbacks |
| --- | --- |
| Civil | Criminal |
| No intent needed | Requires intent |
| Is limited to physician behavior | Applies to any healthcare provider |

ties for the other party. The effort, time, and expense of a partnership are wasted if the other organization must withdraw from the venture.

While it is true that Stark pertains to physician behavior and physician self-referral, this does not mean that institutional providers should be cavalier about the law. Under the determination that claims filed subject to a physician self-referral are not lawful, the following case illustrates how an institutional entity can have a False Claims Act investigation "bootstrapped" to the underlying Stark violation.

### Case Study

Real estate deals that allegedly violated the Stark law are at the heart of a Midwest hospital's $1.5 million False Claims Act settlement, which grew out of a whistle-blower lawsuit filed by the organization's former director of real estate and an orthopedic surgeon. The settlement resolves allegations that the hospital submitted false Medicare claims from 2000 to 2007 by entering into noncompliant office-space leasing arrangements with two physicians and three medical groups.

The hospital allegedly made rent and other office-space concessions to an obstetrician/gynecologist between 1997 and 2002. Similar rent and office-space concessions allegedly were bestowed by the hospital from 1999 through 2006 on "a certain internal medicine group and a certain solo practitioner obstetrician/gynecologist." Finally, between 2001 and 2007, "a certain solo practitioner obstetrician/gynecologist, a certain urology group, and a certain neurosurgery group" did not have written, fully executed leases with the hospital or pay rent in a "timely and consistent manner," the settlement alleges.

The government bootstraps Stark violations to the False Claims Act on the premise that Medicare claims are false if they stem from the referrals by physicians whose financial arrangements with the entities providing the services are not Stark-compliant. The hospital did not admit liability in the settlement. In a statement, hospital spokespeople said it cooperated fully in the investigation.

"The government found a limited number of technical violations involving a handful of doctors. The total sum of the benefits allegedly received by these doctors amounted to $547,000, about one-third of the total monetary penalty," according to the statement. "The remaining portion of the almost $1.6 million settlement includes a multiplier of damages and a separate penalty for unsigned leases."

SOURCE: *Health Business Daily* (2010).

**Strategies for Healthcare Executives**

- Legal counsel must carefully review every financial arrangement between the organization and providers.
- Conduct training sessions for medical staff to help them understand the complexities of Stark law.

## Recommended Readings

Alexander, B., B. M. Broccolo, K. F. Conley, A. R. Daniels, M. Dube, R. G. Hoban, C. B. Hutto, C. C. Loepere, D. E. Matyas, T. W. Mayo, J. J. Miles, R. E. Sallade, M. F. Schaff, S. O. Scheutzow, D. J. Schwartz, and E. T. Thomas. 2008. *AHLA Fundamentals of Health Law,* Fourth Edition. Washington, DC: American Health Lawyers Association.

*Health Business Daily.* 2010. "Report on Medicare Compliance." Atlantic Information Services, posted March 23. www.aishealth.com/Bnow/ hbd032310.html.

Matyas, D., and C. Valiant. 2006. *Legal Issues in Healthcare Fraud and Abuse: Navigating the Uncertainties,* Third Edition. Washington, DC: American Health Lawyers Association.

Oppenheim, C. B. 2008. *AHLA Stark Final Regulations: A Comprehensive Analysis of Key Issues and Practical Guide,* Fourth Edition. Washington, DC: American Health Lawyers Association.

# CHAPTER 17

# EMTALA 101: The Basics

**In This Chapter**

- EMTALA in Nine Words
- EMTALA, A Brief History: Who, What, Where, When?
- EMTALA: Risks and Penalties for Institutional Providers
- The Fundamental Flaw: Physician Participation
- The Role of Executive Leadership
- Case Study
- EMTALA: A Look to the Future
- Strategies for Healthcare Executives

## EMTALA IN NINE WORDS

There have been multiple revisions to the Emergency Medical Treatment and Active Labor Act (EMTALA) regulations over the decades since its inception, and the interpretation and rule-making by agencies behind the rule have swung from strict to more lenient and back again. The actual law, however, has remained consistent at 108 words (42 U.S.C.A. §1395 dd):

> In the case of a hospital that has an emergency department, if any individual (whether or not eligible for Medicare benefits and regardless of ability to pay) comes by him or herself or with another person to the emergency department and a request is made on the individual's behalf for examination or treatment of a medical condition by qualified medical personnel (as determined by the hospital in its rules

and regulations), the hospital must provide for an appropriate medical screening examination within the capability of the hospital's emergency department, including ancillary services routinely available to the emergency department, to determine whether or not an emergency medical condition exists. (42 U.S.C.A. §1395dd(a))

If you want to bring EMTALA down to its essential elements, you could reduce the law to this:

---

**EMTALA in a Nutshell**

- Provide a mandated medical screening examination for all persons presenting for a nonscheduled visit.
- Provide stabilizing care.
- Do not transfer unstable patients.
- Maintain an adequate on-call system.
- Provide medically appropriate transfers.
- Accept appropriate transfers to your facility.

---

We have now brought EMTALA down to 43 words, which makes it easy to memorize like a mantra. However, if you want to make EMTALA really easy, you could restate it in this manner: Treat all patients the same, without regard to reimbursement.

That's EMTALA in nine words! End of story.

If it was truly that easy, this would be a short chapter. But, as is true with all laws, to understand EMTALA it is necessary to start by defining the terms in the legislation.

## EMTALA, A BRIEF HISTORY: WHO, WHAT, WHERE, WHEN?

EMTALA first appeared as a four-page section in the Consolidated Omnibus Budget Reconciliation Act (COBRA) in 1986 following reports of egregious cases in which patients were "dumped" by one hospital on another. Many of the stories that made the news were cases involving women in active labor, often with bad outcomes. That first foray into "anti-dumping" legislation has been described as "a federally mandated social policy calling for guaranteed access to healthcare" (Frew and Giese 2008). Decades have passed since the government established EMTALA as the standard for equal access to emergency care, yet the grumbling has not abated.

This chapter will briefly review EMTALA compliance and what the law requires, but it is the failure of the medical community to embrace the goal of equal access to emergency care that has led to the problems with its enforcement (see "The Fundamental Flaw: Physician Participation" on page 166).

## Who? Which Patients

EMTALA pertains to a person who presents to an ED requiring emergency treatment regardless of whether he or a representative asks for evaluation or treatment. If he doesn't ask, the "prudent layperson" would know he needs examination or treatment for a medical condition based on his appearance or behavior.

EMTALA application is not limited to the ED and *may* be triggered in other parts of the hospital, such as the labor and delivery suite, the psychiatric unit, or the grounds surrounding the hospital. This is particularly true as, in many facilities, patients enter directly into the labor and delivery suite or the psychiatric unit. Having said that, EMTALA does not apply to inpatients (despite attempts to expand the law to inpatient wards). It should go without saying that a person cannot be processed through the ED and admitted to avoid EMTALA.

## Who? Which Provider

When EMTALA is triggered, a medical screening exam (MSE) must be performed. This exam should be done by a physician, but under some circumstances the MSE may be completed by a mid-level provider, such as an advanced practice nurse (APN) or physician assistant (PA). The designation of the provider eligible to complete the MSE is based on a review of pertinent state law and the scope of practice of that professional as determined by the relevant state licensing agency.

Assuming an MSE is within a mid-level provider's scope of practice, the following conditions must also be met to make the MSE EMTALA-compliant:

### An MSE performed by a nonphysician provider *requires*

- Board approval
- Written authority to order tests and procedures and the ability to interpret results

(continued)

- Written parameters detailing when a physician must be contacted and when a physician must come to the ED to assume patient care
- A physician on call (not the APN or PA employed by the physician/physician group) named on the on-call roster

Regardless of who performs the MSE, if a decision is made that the services of an on-call physician are necessary, it is the person with eyes on the patient in the ED—the person actually looking at and evaluating the patient—who should control what happens next.

## What? Emergency Medical Condition

It is the "prudent layperson" who sets the standard for evaluating whether a person requires emergency evaluation and potentially treatment; that decision is not to be made on the level of, for example, the highly trained cardio-thoracic vascular surgeon who *knows* over the telephone that the symptoms point to a condition that ultimately will not cause the patient any harm.

Mental health disturbances may also constitute an emergency condition under EMTALA. Suicidal gestures, self-mutilation, manic status, or any altered mental status should raise the concern that the patient is presenting with a mental health emergency. Symptoms of substance abuse, including use of alcohol and drugs, are also an emergency medical condition under EMTALA.

As the dumping of pregnant women in active labor was a primary motivating factor in the passage of EMTALA, the definition of an emergency medical condition triggering EMTALA naturally includes a definition specific to labor.

### Emergency Medical Conditions

- A medical condition manifesting itself by acute symptoms of sufficient severity (including severe pain, psychiatric disturbances, and/or symptoms of substance abuse) such that the absence of immediate medical attention could reasonably be expected to result in—

(continued)

(A) placing the health of the individual (or, with respect to a pregnant woman, the health of the woman or her unborn child) in serious jeopardy;

(B) serious impairment to bodily functions; or

(C) serious dysfunction of any bodily organ or part; or

- With respect to a pregnant woman who is having contractions—

    (A) that there is inadequate time to effect a safe transfer to another hospital before delivery; or

    (B) that transfer may pose a threat to the health or safety of the woman or the unborn child.

SOURCE: Excerpted from EMTALA (42 U.S.C.A. § 1395).

## Where? Dedicated ED Versus Other Hospital Departments or "Campus"

As noted above, EMTALA is not confined to one geographic area of a hospital; confusion around the law increases as the person requiring emergency evaluation and treatment moves beyond the confines of the ED. The confusing nature of EMTALA can be found in the rule itself. For example, in the preamble to the final rule, the Centers for Medicare & Medicaid Services (CMS 2003) reaffirms that "EMTALA does not apply elsewhere on on-campus hospital property other than a dedicated emergency department unless *emergency* services are requested" (emphasis in original).

Due to a highly publicized and inflammatory incident in Chicago in 1998, CMS revised the definition of a hospital "campus." Allegedly because of a hospital policy prohibiting personnel from leaving the grounds while on duty, emergency room personnel at Ravenswood Hospital failed to provide assistance to 15-year-old Christopher Sercye, who had been shot at a nearby school playground and whose friends had brought him to an alley just off hospital grounds. The boy died from his wounds. In 2000 and again in 2003 CMS issued rules to expand the responsibility of the emergency room to respond to any "presentation" on the hospital campus. Currently a hospital campus includes the parking lot, sidewalk, driveway, and any building within 250 yards of the main buildings of the hospital. The implication of the on-campus extension beyond the actual ED is that EMTALA protections now extend to individuals on the hospital campus for other than outpatient services (such as hospital employees or visitors) who experience what may be an emergency medical condition.

The extension of EMTALA beyond the ED has resulted in the creation of some confusing distinctions. For example, any person who comes to a hospital department for nonemergency services (such as outpatient care or diagnostic testing) and has begun to receive those services does not fall under EMTALA, even if he develops an emergency condition while receiving those services (such patients are, however, protected under the Medicare Conditions of Participation [COP]). For instance, a patient receiving outpatient physical therapy who develops chest pain is not an EMTALA patient, even if she is transferred to the ED for evaluation and treatment.

It should be noted that there are some areas or structures that are not included in the definition of "campus" for EMTALA purposes, including physician offices, rural health centers, skilled nursing facilities, or "other entities that participate separately under Medicare, or restaurants, shops or other non-medical facilities" (EMTALA.com n.d.).

## Dedicated Emergency Department

EMTALA defines a dedicated emergency department as "any department or facility of the hospital that either is licensed by the state as an emergency department; held out to the public as providing treatment for emergency medical conditions; or if one-third of the visits to the department in the preceding calendar year were unscheduled and provided treatment for emergency medical conditions on an urgent basis" (Frew and Giese 2008). Under this definition, both labor and delivery suites and psychiatric units may be included under EMTALA if care is delivered in an unscheduled and urgent manner with sufficient frequency.

## When? Response Time

The time allotted for a response by an on-call physician is set by the medical-staff bylaws of the hospital and should be given in specific minutes rather than un-enforceable, open-to-interpretation phrases such as "timely" or "adequate."

Specific time measurements are not included in EMTALA, but the commonly accepted definition as established through previous evaluation and enforcement suggest the following:

- STAT response: 30 minutes
- Routine response: 60 minutes

One consequence of this requirement is that a physician cannot be providing appropriate on-call coverage if she is more than 30 minutes from the ED at any time while on call.

## EMTALA: RISKS AND PENALTIES FOR INSTITUTIONAL PROVIDERS

Enforcement of EMTALA is the responsibility of the CMS within the US Department of Health and Human Services through that department's OIG. Information gained as part of an EMTALA investigation could be shared with other authorities, such as the Office for Civil Rights or the Internal Revenue Service (IRS) for questions regarding a hospital's tax-exempt status, which may lead to investigations of violations of other federal requirements. Patients who are treated differently for financial reasons may file a private action against a hospital, hospital employees, or any physician involved in that discriminatory decision making.

The *EMTALA Field Guide* states, "An EMTALA action may be brought in state or federal court, and is separate and distinct from any medical malpractice cause of action. The Plaintiff need not establish any deviation from the standard of care, but only need prove that they received different treatment than another patient similarly situated and that an EMTALA requirement was violated" (Frew and Giese 2008). A hospital that has violated EMTALA by providing a different level of evaluation and treatment for financial reasons will be subject to a penalty. A hospital may also be fined for inappropriate transfers or refusing to accept transfers from other hospitals due to the lack of reimbursement for the patient's care.

### EMTALA Violation Penalties

- Civil penalty (i.e., a fine but without criminal implications) of up to $50,000 per violation
- A maximum penalty of $25,000 per violation for hospitals with fewer than 100 beds
- Revocation of provider agreement
- Risk of investigation by other federal authorities, which could jeopardize a hospital's tax-exempt status
- Termination of Medicare participation

The greatest risk to any hospital facing an allegation of non-compliance with EMTALA is termination from Medicare participation. Exclusion from government reimbursement is sufficient to close down most, if not all, institutional providers and most private physician practices as well. Revocation of a provider agreement is the "Medicare Death Penalty"; the threat alone is enough to provide the biggest incentive for hospitals to be diligent in their attention to EMTALA compliance.

An investigation of a hospital for EMTALA compliance can be initiated by a complaint from a patient or from another hospital. In fact, a hospital is required to notify authorities if a patient in the facility was wrongfully denied a transfer to another hospital.

"Hospitals that fail to report possible violations committed by other hospitals may be terminated from Medicare participation in the same process as if they had committed a direct violation themselves" (Frew and Geise 2008). This requirement between hospitals to be your brother's keeper is included even in the transfer of documentation at the time of patient transfer. The transferring hospital sends to the receiving facility all medical records related to the emergency condition for which the individual has presented, available at the time of the transfer, including records related to the individual's emergency medical condition, observations of signs or symptoms, preliminary diagnosis, treatment provided, results of any tests, and the informed written consent or certification and the name and address of any on-call physician who has refused or failed to appear within a reasonable time to provide necessary stabilizing treatment (42 U.S.C.A. § 1395dd C (2)).

## THE FUNDAMENTAL FLAW: PHYSICIAN PARTICIPATION

The fundamental flaw in EMTALA is that the performance of all parties depends, in large part, on the physicians in a community. Most of those physicians do not perceive the law as *their* problem but the hospital's. This is largely because the fines and penalties and enforcement activities by the government to date have focused on the hospitals and the EDs far more than on individual physicians. However, EMTALA does include penalties specific to physicians, which could translate to more investigations and enforcement in the medical community.

### Physician Penalties

Any physician who is responsible for the examination, treatment, or transfer of an individual in a participating hospital, including a physician

(continued)

on-call for the care of such an individual, and who negligently violates a requirement of this section, including a physician who—

- signs a certification ... that the medical benefits reasonably to be expected from a transfer to another facility outweigh the risks associated with the transfer, if the physician knew or should have known that the benefits did not outweigh the risks, or
- misrepresents an individual's condition or other information, including a hospital's obligations under this section,

is subject to a civil money penalty of not more than $50,000 for each such violation and, if the violation is gross and flagrant or is repeated, to exclusion from participation in this subchapter and State health care programs. 42 U.S.C.A. § 1395dd (D)(1)(B)

SOURCE: Fosmire (2009).

Therefore, physician liability, including civil monetary penalties or exclusion, can result if a physician signs a certificate for transfer knowing that the transfer did not actually outweigh the risk of moving the patient, or by misrepresenting the condition of the patient or the ED's abilities to appropriately care for the patient.

### An Old Oath and a Good Rule of Thumb

Treating all patients equally is a principle in medicine that goes back to the Hippocratic Oath. Straying from that principle puts the professionalism of physicians in question and raises legal questions.

Treatment decisions based on anything other than the patient's best interest are likely to raise questions regarding EMTALA liability.

### Common EMTALA Complaints Involving Physician Behavior

In the world of EMTALA, the person in control of the on-call physician's actions is the person making the request from the ED, the person who has her eyes on the patient. This person is most likely to be another physician but may also be a mid-level practitioner in the emergency department. In a perfect world, physicians would respond appropriately and no one, including the physician, would be subject to an EMTALA enforcement action. Stephen A. Frew, JD, an acknowledged leader in the country on EMTALA, lists the most common EMTALA pitfalls.

### The Most Common EMTALA Pitfalls

- When asked to come in to see an ED patient, the on-call physician responds with instructions to admit or to run various tests and that he will see the patient at a later time.
- When asked to come in to see an ED patient, the physician debates with the ED physician over the necessity of coming in.
- When asked to come in to see an ED patient, the physician refuses and suggests that the patient be seen by another specialty.
- When asked to come in to see an ED patient, the physician refuses and orders the patient transferred to another facility because of severity or scope of condition.
- When asked to come in to see an ED patient, the physician declines without seeing the patient based on the premise that the patient's apparent needs exceed the physician's scope of practice.
- When asked to come in to see an ED patient, the physician declines the patient because of the payer plan status or self-pay status.
- When covering more than one hospital on call, the physician asks for the patient to be sent to the hospital where the on-call physician is currently seeing patients instead of going to the patient's location.
- When asked to come in to see an ED patient, the physician declines on the basis that the patient was previously discharged from the physician's practice for noncompliance, prior litigation, or nonpayment.
- When asked to come in to see an ED patient, the physician declines on the basis that the specialist physician is "not interested" in a case of that type.
- When asked to come in to see an ED patient or an in-house patient on an emergency consult to rule out an emergency medical condition or provide stabilizing care, the physician declines because the patient is aligned with another neurosurgeon or physician who is unavailable or declined to come in.
- When contacted by another hospital seeking transfer of a patient, the physician declines the patient because a specialist at the first hospital is not available or turned down the patient improperly.

(continued)

- The physician refuses to participate in the call list, which leads to gaps in the list, but expects to be called for her own patients and for patients of physicians for whom she is covering.
- The physician refuses to be listed individually on the call list and insists that only the group or answering service name and number be listed.
- The physician lists only a PA or NP on the call roster instead of her own name.
- The physician insists that an admitting physician must request a consult before the on-call consultant has to come in.
- The physician insists that calls must come from the ED physician or qualified medical provider when contacted by a nurse or other person on behalf of the ED physician.
- The physician fails to make a detailed record of the assessment and treatment of the patient when called in.

SOURCE: Frew and Giese (2008).

The vast majority of errors in EMTALA compliance are due to the response of the on-call physician, yet Frew and Giese (2008) reveal that *physician* penalties account for a very small number of the fines actually levied. The fundamental flaw in EMTALA, therefore, is that the law causes hospitals much time, effort, and concern, but the hospitals in most communities don't have any leverage over the primary players, the on-call physicians. At the same time, the physician community largely views EMTALA compliance and penalties as a hospital problem and does not understand their own liabilities under the law, or understands but does not have any motivating fear of the potential penalties (McDonnell 2006).

## THE ROLE OF EXECUTIVE LEADERSHIP

EMTALA presents numerous areas that demand leadership. ED staff must be well versed in EMTALA and the requirements of the law. Dispatch and triage must be sure their communications and assessments are not only appropriate but documented. Patient complaints, test results, diagnosis, treatment, and monitoring must be clearly charted. Patients (or their legal representatives) must be consulted about their rights. The request, acceptance, and certification of transfers must be fully compliant with the law.

Leadership is necessary for an ED to accept these requirements, not out of legal obligation but as actions consistent with the role of an ED to serve the emergency needs of the community.

At the same time, leadership is needed to work with physicians to deal *cooperatively* with the needs of the public presenting at the ED. The importance of EMTALA compliance, as well as the hospital's mission, must be conveyed in such a way that the medical community supports the needs of the ED by participating in on-call coverage and complying with all assessment, treatment, and documentation requirements of the law.

Regardless of what happens with efforts to reform healthcare delivery, the following maxim will continue to be the core for compliance with EMTALA: Treat all patients the same, without regard to reimbursement.

A healthcare leader who can endorse this position and enroll all parties involved in that vision will lead his institution toward excellence in care *and* compliance.

---

### Case Study

After being bitten in the lip by a stray pit bull, a 12-year-old patient was screened by emergency department staff at the University of Chicago Hospital. Part of his lip was "literally gone" according to the boy's mother. He was given antibiotics, morphine, a tetanus shot, and then was told to follow up at the county hospital within one week. The boy's mother took him immediately to another hospital where he was quickly admitted for surgery.

Failure to provide immediate treatment to the child's lip laceration did not place his health in serious jeopardy and did not result in a serious impairment to any body organ or part. He received a medical screening exam, so technically the hospital may not have violated any EMTALA laws when it evaluated the boy, provided basic treatment, and referred him to a county hospital.

However, CMS is investigating the incident as an EMTALA violation. The incident likely violates the spirit and intent of EMTALA, even if it is not a technical violation. At the time of this event, the University of Chicago Hospital had just instituted a program of triaging out nonemergency patients. This inner-city safety net hospital does not have the resources to care for all the patients who present.

This case received a lot of press attention, and the American College of Emergency Physicians released a statement criticizing the University of Chicago Hospital.

SOURCE: CitronLegal.com (2009).

# EMTALA: A LOOK TO THE FUTURE

All arguments for healthcare reform in our country, regardless of political ideology or source, focus on *access* as a fundamental component in increasing the health of our population. Given this focus, it is almost unimaginable that EMTALA will go away. The only scenario where EMTALA would become a relic would be if the United States can navigate reform all the way to universal insurance of Americans. Only then would reimbursement for care become a given and distinctions between patients based on financial status become a thing of the past. Given that universal coverage is not likely to be achieved in the foreseeable future, and in fact is not a goal for a huge component of the voting public, EMTALA will continue to be a major compliance issue in EDs across the country. It may, however, become easier for hospitals and EDs to comply.

At the time of this writing, healthcare is facing many years of rule-making because of healthcare reform legislation. Some of the federal initiatives may fail altogether, but even so, state governments, private payers, and large self-insured corporations are all picking up the mantra of changing the delivery of healthcare. Recent regulations from the IRS, Department of Labor, and Public Health Service (PHS) require healthcare plans to allow access to emergency services without pre-authorization. According to Frew and Giese (2008), "Terms like emergency medical condition, emergency services, and stabilize in the regulations generally follow EMTALA language and PHS 'prudent lay person' standards, with some variations. Linkage to the existing law could be a sign that the administration considers the EMTALA law necessary to continued access to healthcare."

Perhaps the biggest wild card for the future will be utilization rates of emergency departments. Everyone on the payer side wants to see the public channeled to primary care through accountable care organizations, medical homes, and other primary resources for healthcare (Bard and Nugent 2011). If that intention is met, there will be fewer people presenting to the ED, and those patients should be truly requiring emergency care. As patient numbers decrease, the flow of patients in an ED should become more manageable, and EMTALA compliance easier to facilitate.

### Strategies for Healthcare Executives

- Educate all employees and providers in the ED on EMTALA so all components of the team can exercise EMTALA compliance in a logical (who, what, where, and when) and comprehensive manner.
- Designate specifically who is responsible to educate patients about their rights under EMTALA, including their loved ones as appropriate.
- Dispel through education the common belief that hospital on-call coverage is the *hospital's* problem; ensure that physicians are aware of their *personal* liability under EMTALA.
- Educate ED physicians (and midlevel providers as applicable) about the importance of their role as the "eyes-on" provider, and emphasize that they should seek assistance when on-call physicians do not appropriately respond to their requests for assistance with patient care.
- Involve all sectors of the hospital community in adopting a shared commitment to providing equal access to high-quality services in the ED.
- Monitor trends in the delivery of healthcare and how the employment of physicians, particularly in large provider systems, may alleviate shortages in on-call physician coverage.

## Recommended Readings

Alexander, B., B. M. Broccolo, K. F. Conley, A. R. Daniels, M. Dube, R. G. Hoban, C. B. Hutto, C. C. Loepere, D. E. Matyas, T. W. Mayo, J. J. Miles, R. E. Sallade, M. F. Schaff, S. O. Scheutzow, D. J. Schwartz, and E. T. Thomas. 2008. *AHLA Fundamentals of Health Law,* Fourth Edition. Washington, DC: American Health Lawyers Association.

Frew, S., and K. Giese. 2008. *EMTALA Field Guide: Quick Risk and Compliance Answers,* Second Edition. Kenosha, WI: Johnson Insurance Services LLC.

# CHAPTER 18

# EMTALA: The Ins and Outs of Medical Screening Exams and Transfers

**In This Chapter**

- EMTALA: Getting to the "What"
- Documenting for EMTALA Compliance
- The Role of Executive Leadership
- Case Study
- Strategies for Healthcare Executives

## EMTALA: GETTING TO THE "WHAT"

The details about compliance with the Emergency Medical Treatment and Active Labor Act (EMTALA) were discussed in Chapter 17. The most important element, however, is what an ED is supposed to do if all those other conditions apply to any particular patient. The "what" that EMTALA is trying to ensure for all patients is a medical screening exam (MSE), appropriate stabilization prior to transfer, and transfer to another facility as warranted by the patient's condition and level of need. All of this must occur without regard to reimbursement.

### Medical Screening Exam

Any patient falling under EMTALA must have an appropriate MSE before he can be transferred or discharged from the ED. The law states, "The hospital must provide for an appropriate medical screening examination within the capability of the hospital's emergency department, including ancillary services routinely available to the emergency department, to determine whether or not an emergency medical condition exists" (2 U.S.C.A. § 1395dd).

An MSE is not simple triage as traditionally performed in EDs. Triage focuses on the presenting complaint, whereas an examination limited to the complaint (e.g., evaluating only the arm when the patient says his arm hurts) is specifically not sufficient for an MSE under EMTALA; an MSE requires a more thorough assessment.

### Medical Screening Exam Guidelines

- Must rule out emergency medical conditions
- Must be more comprehensive than complaint-based exams and standard triage
- Must be performed before preauthorization call is made
- Must include all necessary testing and on-call services
- Must be performed without regard to reimbursement
- Must be performed at the same level for all patients

In addition to a medical screening, patients presenting with symptoms of a mental health disturbance and/or substance abuse must receive a health assessment that must rule out organic, toxic, and traumatic causes for any unusual behavior (AZHHA 2008). An ED must perform a mental health assessment if warranted by the patient's behavior or complaints, regardless of whether the hospital includes a psychiatric unit. Screening particular to substance abuse or suspected substance abuse may necessitate toxicology testing, including serial toxicology to determine return to normal values. Discharging a patient who is still intoxicated may constitute an EMTALA violation; EDs should hold patients until they are no longer impaired. The time a patient is held for this purpose will not be sufficient to demonstrate compliance; determination that a patient is ready for discharge must be based on objective indicators and observations regarding behavior and resolution of intoxication. When dealing with suspected drug or alcohol toxicity, providers must always treat with the potential of withdrawal complications in mind; withdrawal from alcohol or street drugs can be an emergency medical condition.

## Stabilization

Once a medical screening exam (including mental health screening, if warranted) is completed, a patient must receive sufficient treatment to be stabilized before discharge or transfer to another facility. Under EMTALA, *stabilize* means "to provide such medical treatment of the condition as may be necessary to assure, within reasonable medical probability, that no material deterioration of the condition is likely to result from or occur during the transfer of the individual from a facility, or, with respect to a pregnant woman, delivery including the placenta" (42 U.S.C.A. §1395dd(3)(A).) The use of the term "stabilization" for EMTALA purposes is different from "stabilization" in common medical parlance. According to Frew and Giese (2008), "Patients who have not yet had their conditions completely evaluated are deemed to have an emergency medical condition until it is ruled out and their condition sufficiently resolved for movement or discharge without any risk in change of condition.... Because the average physician tends to mark or document the patient as stable using medical standards and not EMTALA standards it is recommended the determination be based on whether the patient has a potential to deteriorate from their condition or from the transfer itself during the transfer." The requisite level of stabilization must be realized before a patient may be transferred to another facility.

## Exceptions to the Stabilization Requirement

EMTALA allows for exceptions to the stabilization rule in cases where delaying transfer may be detrimental to the patient, such as when there is another facility better equipped to address the patient's condition. An exception to the stabilization requirement also exists to allow for patient-documented requests.

### Exceptions to EMTALA's Stabilization Rule

If an individual at a hospital has an emergency medical condition which has not been stabilized...the hospital may not transfer the individual unless—

- the individual (or a legally responsible person acting on the individual's behalf), after being informed of the hospital's obligations under this section and of the risk of transfer, **in writing requests** transfer to another medical facility;

(continued)

- a physician...has signed a certification that, based upon the information available at the time of transfer, **the medical benefits** reasonably expected from the provision of appropriate medical treatment at another medical facility **outweigh the increased risks** to the individual and, in the case of labor, to the unborn child from effecting the transfer; or
- if a physician is not physically present in the emergency department at the time an individual is transferred, a qualified medical person...has signed a certification...after a physician...in consultation with the person, has made the determination described in such clause, and subsequently countersigns the certification; and
- the transfer is an appropriate transfer...to that facility.

SOURCE: Excerpted from 42 U.S.C.A. § 1395dd C (1).

## Making and Accepting Transfers

The guidelines for making and accepting appropriate transfers are the final "what" of EMTALA compliance.

### Appropriate Transfers

An appropriate transfer to a medical facility is a transfer—

- in which the transferring hospital provides the medical treatment within its capacity that minimizes the risks to the individual's health and, in the case of a woman in labor, the health of the unborn child;
- in which the receiving facility—
  - has available space and qualified personnel for the treatment of the individual, and
  - has agreed to accept transfer of the individual and to provide appropriate medical treatment;
- in which the transferring hospital sends to the receiving facility all medical records (or copies thereof), related to the emergency condition for which the individual has presented, available at the time of the transfer,

(continued)

including records related to the individual's emergency medical condition, observations of signs or symptoms, preliminary diagnosis, treatment provided, results of any tests and the informed written consent or certification (or copy thereof)...and the name and address of any on-call physician...who has refused or failed to appear within a reasonable time to provide necessary stabilizing treatment;

- in which the transfer is effected through qualified personnel and transportation equipment as required, including the use of necessary and medically appropriate life support measures during the transfer; and
- which meets such other requirements as the Secretary may find necessary in the interest of the health and safety of individuals transferred.

SOURCE: Excerpted from 42 U.S.C.A. § 1395dd C.

Hospitals with specialized capabilities (such as burn units, shock-trauma units, and neonatal intensive care units) have an obligation to accept transfer of any patients requiring those services if the hospital has the capacity to treat them. Communication between the two facilities, both in requesting and accepting a pending transfer, is vital, as is the free exchange of medical information accompanying the patient on transfer.

## Transfer Decisions Made Without Regard to Reimbursement

Hospitals have a duty to accept transfers without regard to reimbursement. When one hospital, unable to deliver the standard of care the patient requires, calls another hospital with a higher level of capability, that hospital must accept the transfer if a patient with a similar condition *and* reimbursement would be accepted. Hospitals that receive transfer requests must accept unless it is literally impossible to do so. A completely full hospital or a hospital with the temporary loss of necessary equipment, such as treatment facilities under repair, might be excused for refusing a transfer, but that determination would have to be the same for *any* patient. All potential transfers must be treated the same.

## DOCUMENTING FOR EMTALA COMPLIANCE

All aspects of EMTALA compliance must be well documented to avoid any question about a hospital's performance or to defend against any subsequent EMTALA investigation. Patient care documentation must also be detailed for the benefit of the patient. The exchange of information is critical for accuracy in treatment and will assist subsequent providers involved in the patient's care. Patient care documentation should minimally include:

### Patient Screening Documentation

- Initial triage and nursing evaluation
- Evidence of ongoing monitoring (in keeping with other patients similarly situated)
- Testing performed, test results, and documented review of those results by the physician
- Assessment by the physician in a narrative addressing all complaints and abnormal findings, including the physician's impressions and plan of care
- Explanation of any mental health screening
- Test results and screening specific to substance abuse
- Response and prevention in regard to any substance-withdrawal complications
- Observations and other indicators regarding the resolution of intoxication

Documentation must also demonstrate that the patient was adequately stabilized before transfer or discharge.

### Patient Stabilization Documentation

- Condition of the patient at the time of discharge, transfer, or admission
- Pain scale assessment or evidence that is used to determine patient has been stabilized or normalized prior to discharge
- Relevant lab results, fetal monitoring, or other diagnostic information used to determine stabilization

To comply with the requirements for a transfer of a patient, it is critical to have documentation of the decision-making process. All treatment, evaluation, and assessment by the physician (or other provider) must be well reflected in the patient record. In addition, EMTALA requires that the physician sign a transfer certificate immediately prior to a patient's discharge. The certificate cannot be signed in anticipation of a transfer, but must be completed at the time the patient is leaving the hospital. The responsibility for completing the certificate rests with the doctor who ordered the transfer; delegation of care to other physicians, midlevel providers, or nursing staff does not abrogate the duty of the ordering physician.

### Patient Transfer Documentation

- The patient transfer form with certification
- The signature of the physician making the transfer, at the time of transfer
- Vital signs at the time of transfer
- Other documentation regarding the patient's status at the time of transfer
- Records pertaining to the patient's care and a listing of those records
- Patient consent form
- Physician order for level of transport care, personnel support, and specialized equipment
- Documentation of acceptance of transfer, including who gave the acceptance
- Refusal of ambulance form (if applicable)
- Documentation pertaining to the patient's initiation of transfer (if applicable)

Any inability to accept a patient transfer, such as the lack of patient bed availability or inoperative or unavailable equipment, should also be well documented.

## THE ROLE OF EXECUTIVE LEADERSHIP

The list of EMTALA elements may be long and excruciatingly detailed, but the intended result of the law is simple. Any evaluation, stabilization, treatment, transfer, or acceptance of a transfer of any patient must be determined by non-economic considerations. Reimbursement (or the lack thereof) should not play a role in administering emergency care. ED care must be administered as benefits the patient, not the bottom line. A healthcare executive who keeps that principle foremost and communicates that end result clearly and consistently will have gone a long way to ensure her facility has done all it can do to comply with the law.

---

### Case Study

AP was an 88-year-old man brought to the respondent's ED at 5:41 p.m. on December 29th, 2001, by members of his family. AP's daughter-in-law told the ED registration clerk that AP was not feeling well and that his physician had directed that he be brought to the ED. AP's complaints and possible problems were recorded on the emergency room log as being "general weakness/possible stroke." AP and his family members then went to the ED waiting area to await examination and possible treatment. His condition appeared to be deteriorating and on separate occasions his daughter-in-law and son reported at the registration window that AP's condition was getting worse and that he needed to be seen by a physician. During that three-hour period, AP's condition deteriorated steadily. He manifested signs of a life-threatening emergency medical condition. AP's family repeatedly pleaded with ED staff to take notice of and to address his problems. Their pleas were unavailing. Respondent's staff did not begin to deal with AP's problems until he had deteriorated irretrievably. Eventually, AP died. The evidence presented by the inspector general establishes that AP waited for about three hours at respondent's ED without being examined by a physician to determine the reason for his complaints and his medical signs.

Respondent acknowledges that its failure to provide AP with a screening examination during the nearly three hours he waited at its ED may have comprised a negligent failure by its staff to attend to and treat AP. Respondent avers that its failure to respond promptly to AP was triggered by a single event, the triage that classified AP's condition to be "routine." Arguably, according to respondent, that classification was a negligent diagnosis of AP's condition. But it contends that its negligence—if it was negligent—cannot be construed to be a violation of EMTALA.

EMTALA does not excuse a hospital for failing to perform a screening examination where that failure is the consequence of the hospital's staff's gross negligence. EMTALA is unequivocal. A hospital must provide a screening examination to every individual who comes to its emergency department requesting treatment. There is no "negligence" exception to the law. Respondent's failure to provide AP with a screening examination comprises a violation of EMTALA.

Determination of the Inspector General to impose a civil money penalty of $50,000 sustained.

SOURCE: HHS (2009).

## Strategies for Healthcare Executives

- Once a year, have EMTALA experts review the standardized documentation that goes with transfers.
- Set time goals for performing the MSE.
- Have clear policies and procedures about who will perform the MSE, what it will entail, and what triggers more detailed evaluation and treatment of patients (e.g., unstable vital signs, chest pain, stroke-like symptoms).
- Provide annual system-wide reviews of EMTALA and what it means for that particular unit. Articulate expectations for responses to episodes on campus.
- Review the documentation on all transfers and set 100 percent compliance as the institutional goal.
- Review documentation for simplicity, forcing functions and strategies to improve documentation.

## Recommended Readings

Alexander, B., B. M. Broccolo, K. F. Conley, A. R. Daniels, M. Dube, R. G. Hoban, C. B. Hutto, C. C. Loepere, D. E. Matyas, T. W. Mayo, J. J. Miles, R. E. Sallade, M. F. Schaff, S. O. Scheutzow, D. J. Schwartz, and E. T. Thomas. 2008. *AHLA Fundamentals of Health Law,* Fourth Edition. Washington, DC: American Health Lawyers Association.

Frew, S., and K. Giese. 2008. *EMTALA Field Guide: Quick Risk and Compliance Answers,* Second Edition. Kenosha, WI: Johnson Insurance Services LLC.

# CHAPTER 19

# EMTALA and Paying for On-Call Coverage: Risks Versus Reality

**In This Chapter**

- The EMTALA Conundrum: Physician Refusal to Participate in Call Coverage
- Paying for On-Call Coverage
- 2007 OIG Advisory Opinion Background
- The OIG Answers 2007
- OIG Warnings from the 2007 Advisory Opinion
- 2009 OIG Advisory Opinion
- OIG Warnings from the 2009 Advisory Opinion
- The Role of Executive Leadership
- Case Study
- Strategies for Healthcare Executives

## THE EMTALA CONUNDRUM: PHYSICIAN REFUSAL TO PARTICIPATE IN CALL COVERAGE

It has become increasingly common for physicians to opt out of call coverage for the ED, particularly physicians who practice in the surgical subspecialty fields (McConnell et al. 2007). This has put EDs across the country in a difficult situation. How do they maintain adequate coverage to meet the requirements of EMTALA when doctors in the community won't respond to the call?

As physicians realized the way to avoid the requirements for on-call physicians was to simply stop taking call, hospitals were faced with glaring gaps in their coverage for ED services, and emergency physicians found a dwindling number of colleagues they could call to come in and assist with a patient's care. In some hospital communities, enforcing a requirement to participate in on-call coverage was as simple as revising the medical staff bylaws. Many bylaws now require on-call participation as part of the obligations of active medical staff membership, and the debate over payment for on-call services must begin with these bylaws (AHLA 2009).

## PAYING FOR ON-CALL COVERAGE

In many communities the difficulty of maintaining on-call coverage has been resolved by creating a benefit for physicians who remain on the call roster—money. Paying physicians to maintain call has become commonplace for surgeons and surgical sub-specialists, although the practice has rarely included primary care physicians.

As discussed in Chapter 16, any time money is exchanged between a hospital and a physician, there has to be concern that the payment may be construed as a kickback. The prospect of criminal liability for both the party offering and the party accepting a kickback is significant; that risk increases as a direct correlation with the amount paid for on-call coverage. Paying for on-call coverage raises issues around EMTALA, medical staff bylaws, and the federal antikickback statute (AHLA 2009). The amount being paid for physician on-call coverage differs by community and area of physician practice, but as is true with any market where one party has almost complete leverage over the other, the cost for coverage tends to ratchet up.

## 2007 OIG ADVISORY OPINION BACKGROUND

The practice of paying for call coverage is certainly not illegal per se, but the analysis will depend on the details. Fortunately, we do have examples of reimbursement strategies that have been passed by the enforcement branch of the US Department of Health and Human Services, the Office of Inspector General (OIG). The first time the OIG weighed in on the issue of paying physicians on call occurred in September 2007. The advisory opinion was sought by a tax-exempt, not-for-profit medical center with an ED, which wanted the government to lend it guidance on whether its proposed reimbursement structure would survive government scrutiny.

The hospital in question was based in a community where nearly one in four patients visiting the ED had no form of health insurance, and approximately one in ten of the uninsured patients in the ED was subsequently admitted. The medical center was having difficulty finding physicians to provide on-call coverage and uncompensated inpatient follow-up care, which necessitated the transfer of ED patients to other medical facilities both for emergency treatment and necessary inpatient care that might have been handled more conveniently and efficiently at the medical center.

In response, an ad hoc committee at the hospital developed an arrangement to relieve the call coverage issue. All the physicians on the medical center staff within the relevant specialties were offered the opportunity to contract for two-year terms under the guidelines listed in the box below.

---

### The Arrangement

1. Physicians would participate in the call rotation.
2. Physicians would be obligated to provide inpatient care to any patient seen at the ED while on call.
3. If the patient was admitted to the medical center, participating physicians would be obligated to provide inpatient care, continuing until the patient was properly discharged.
4. Participating physicians would be required to respond to calls from the ED in a reasonable time.
5. Physicians would be required to collaborate with hospital initiatives on issues including discharge planning, utilization, and review of observation patients.
6. Participating physicians would be required to document their services in timely medical records.
7. Physicians participating in the arrangement would be paid a per diem rate for each day spent on call at the ED, except for one and one-half days that each physician must contribute *gratis* to the rotation schedule monthly.
8. The per diem rate would vary based on two factors:
   1. Physician specialty, and
   2. Whether call coverage was on a weekday or a weekend
9. The difference in per diem rates among specialties would be based on the following factors:
   1. The severity of illness typically encountered by that specialty in treating a patient presenting at the ED
   2. The likelihood of having to respond when on call at the ED
   3. The likelihood of having to respond to a request for inpatient consultative services for an uninsured patient when on call
   4. The degree of inpatient care typically required of the specialty for patients who initially present at the ED.

SOURCE: Excerpted from OIG Advisory Opinion No. 07-10 (2007).

---

Participating physicians who failed to adhere to these requirements had their payments under the arrangement suspended until they demonstrated compliance; continued noncompliance would result in termination of the physician's involvement with the arrangement. Also of note, the safe harbor for personal services and management contracts, which often applies to service arrangements between physicians and hospitals, did not apply to the arrangement because the amount of compensation could not be established in advance as the payments could vary from month to month.

In submitting this arrangement for an OIG advisory opinion, the medical center certified that the ED was running more efficiently and with fewer patient transfers since the arrangement began. Also of importance to the outcome of the opinion, the medical center certified that the per diem rates paid under the arrangement were fair market value based on a consultant's analysis (the OIG does not make determinations on fair market value in advisory opinions). The medical center also certified that the reimbursement did not consider in any way the volume or value of referrals or business generated.

## THE OIG ANSWERS 2007

This arrangement survived review by the OIG, but it is important to note that the outcome of an advisory opinion is limited to the specific case in question. However, advisory opinions are released to provide general guidance to other hospitals, so it is interesting to look at what made this arrangement acceptable to the OIG.

The circumstances noted by the OIG as legitimate reasons for the agreement included:

- Compliance with EMTALA
- The scarcity of certain specialties within the hospital's service area
- The community's access to trauma services
- The hospital certifying that payments were fair market value for actual services needed without relationship to referrals
- The per diem rate was applied uniformly within a given specialty
- The arrangement prevented cherry picking because it required physicians to treat all patients who were admitted
- The per diem payments compensated the physicians for significant, quantifiable services

In particular, the OIG noted "the hospital's legitimate and unmet need for on-call coverage (reflected in part by patient transfers) which demonstrated that the arrangement was not a means to conceal unlawful remuneration for referrals" (OIG Advisory Opinion No. 07-10). In addition, the arrangement promoted the hospital's charitable mission, and the hospital, not federal healthcare programs, absorbed all costs of the on-call compensation program.

## OIG WARNINGS FROM THE 2007 ADVISORY OPINION

Beyond the specific facts of the 2007 opinion, the greatest value for guidance to other hospitals are fairly specific warnings about remuneration for on-call physicians. The OIG made it clear that it would not accept:

♦ Arrangements that purport to compensate physicians for "lost opportunities" but in reality fail to reflect any actual lost income
♦ Arrangements that pay a physician when no service is actually provided or that could result in disproportionately high payments relative to the physician's regular medical practice income
♦ Payment structures that provide payment for services for which the physician already receives reimbursement, resulting in double payment for the same services

## 2009 OIG ADVISORY OPINION

The OIG returned to the issue of paying physicians for on-call coverage in an advisory opinion released in May 2009. This opinion reiterates many of the points and the analysis of the September 2007 opinion but also added more precautions and was far more specific about the *nominal* amount of money exchanged that was at issue.

The 2009 opinion covered the following circumstances:

♦ Participating physicians submitted claims to the hospital for payment for services rendered to certain indigent and uninsured patients.
♦ The participating physicians had to be active members of the hospital's medical staff.

- Physicians agreed to respond to the ED in a timely manner (within 30 minutes).
- Physicians agreed to provide such additional evaluation and care as deemed clinically appropriate by the physician with input from the patient's family or guardian as available.
- Emergency consultations on an eligible patient presenting to the ED resulted in a flat-fee payment of $100 to participating physicians.
- If an eligible patient required admission from the ED, the physician received a payment of $300 per admission.
- Surgical procedures or procedures performed on an eligible patient admitted from the ED resulted in a $350 flat fee for the primary surgeon of record.
- An endoscopy or other second-tier procedure performed on an eligible patient admitted from the ED resulted in a $150 flat fee.

Press reports at the time announced that paying physicians for on-call services did not violate antikickback statutes (Marsich 2009), but the OIG opinion was far from a blanket approval (OIG Advisory Opinion No. 09-05). The text pointed to the significant balancing between details and criminal liability the OIG opinions addressed.

In their analysis, and of great importance legally, the OIG noted that the hospital seeking the opinion had certified that payments were made solely on the basis of services actually needed and provided without regard to referrals or any other business generated and that the amount of the payments were at a level that constituted fair market value for the services rendered. The OIG "highlighted a number of safeguards that it believed minimized the risk of fraud and abuse [including that] the hospital's payments to doctors reflected fair-market value (per hospital certification) for the actual services they provided and were tied to tangible physician responsibilities, rather than to referrals" (Sorrel 2009).

## OIG WARNINGS FROM THE 2009 ADVISORY OPINION

One element of the 2009 OIG Advisory Opinion that must be emphasized is what appears to be growing annoyance by the OIG toward the medical community for demanding payment for on-call services. The opinion states, "In sum, the Hospital states that, whereas its physicians historically performed on-call coverage out of a sense of duty to their profession, that sentiment is no longer shared by all; rather, the physicians commonly view on-call coverage as an unwanted obligation, jeopardizing the Hospital's ability to serve patients" (OIG Advisory Opinion No. 09-05).

This comment suggests that the government may become less tolerant of on-call reimbursement in the future. As tolerance wears thin, enforcement activity will undoubtedly follow.

It is also interesting to note the amount of money that was in question in the 2009 OIG opinion, a mere pittance compared to the amounts reported being paid to on-call specialists in some parts of the country. In sum, both advisory opinions serve far more as warning shots across the bow of healthcare administration than as endorsements of reimbursement to physicians to fulfill on-call duties (Abaris Group 2011).

## THE ROLE OF EXECUTIVE LEADERSHIP

The two OIG advisory opinions provide take-home messages that should be considered by any ED paying for on-call coverage. Physicians need to be educated about the risk to themselves and the institution should they attempt to "extort" money for on-call. To many physicians, this talk of criminal liability seems to be used to ratchet down physician reimbursement. It will take strong leadership to convince physicians about the realities of on-call coverage.

Hospitals must comply with EMTALA, and physician on-call coverage and appropriate response are integral to that compliance. Hospitals should take every possible measure to make EMTALA compliance a part of their standard operating procedure, and payment, if necessary at all, should be scaled to what could be considered likely to pass an inspection by the authorities. As the nation moves from medicine as a cottage industry to large healthcare delivery systems, access to on-call services should become easier, as many physicians will presumably be employees, and on-call coverage will be required for employment.

In the meantime, it is important for executive leaders to educate the physician community about the significant legal risks inherent in on-call payment programs. EDs and the medical community must work together to maintain excellent patient care in the ED *and* avoid criminal and civil liabilities.

A level I trauma center and tertiary care facility needs an anesthesiologist on-call to remain open as a level I trauma center for the weekend. The facility is informed by the anesthesiology group that there is no one to take call, and it will have to close to trauma unless an anesthesiologist is willing to take in-house call. The hospital administrator attempts to find coverage by calling individual physicians, most of whom are out of town on this summer weekend. Finally the administrator reaches one of the anesthesiologists and begins to bargain for his services. The administrator offers increasing amounts to keep the trauma center open, eventually offering a stipend of $10,000 for one night's coverage. The anesthesiologist, who was not bound by the hospital bylaws to provide on-call coverage, declined. The administrator did not realize this attempted arrangement, which resulted in the closure of the trauma center for 24 hours, would run afoul of OIG guidelines on several fronts because there was no "arrangement" beforehand with physicians taking call and the hospital, and no one would consider this fee an example of fair market value.

SOURCE: Taylor (2010).

### Strategies for Healthcare Executives

- The OIG opinions do not constitute blanket permission for paying physicians for being on call, are fact-specific, and only apply to the two cases presented.
- Any arrangement for on-call reimbursement should be in response to a documented, legitimate community need.
- A "need" should not be an excuse for extortion by physicians.
- Reimbursement can't be a ruse for increasing physician loyalty.
- Any hospital involved in reimbursement must be able to show that the payments were within fair market value.
- As payments exceed the amount of money reviewed in the OIG opinions, the specter of illegality may grow proportionately.

## Recommended Readings

Alexander, B., B. M. Broccolo, K. F. Conley, A. R. Daniels, M. Dube, R. G. Hoban, C. B. Hutto, C. C. Loepere, D. E. Matyas, T. W. Mayo, J. J. Miles, R. E. Sallade, M. F. Schaff, S. O. Scheutzow, D. J. Schwartz, and E. T. Thomas. 2008. *AHLA Fundamentals of Health Law,* Fourth Edition. Washington, DC: American Health Lawyers Association.

Frew, S., and K. Giese. 2008. *EMTALA Field Guide: Quick Risk and Compliance Answers,* Second Edition. Kenosha, WI: Johnson Insurance Services LLC.

OIG Advisory Opinion No. 07-10. See http://oig.hhs.gov/fraud/docs/advisoryopinions/2007/AdvOpn07-10A.pdf.

OIG Advisory Opinion No. 09-05. See http://oig.hhs.gov/fraud/docs/advisoryopinions/2009/AdvOpn09-05.pdf.

# CHAPTER 20

# Documentation to Minimize Risk

**In This Chapter**

- The Functions of ED Charting
- Charting for Billing and Coding
- Charting for Communication
- Charting and Work Flow
- Charting to Limit Risk
- Scribes
- The Role of Executive Leadership
- Case Study
- Strategies for Healthcare Executives

## THE FUNCTIONS OF ED CHARTING

Jim Roberts (2011)—an emergency physician, writer, entertaining speaker, and humorist—described the medical record for an ED visit this way to a group of physicians:

> The medical record produces a permanent document that serves to memorialize all the details of a stressful encounter between a group of strangers, some of whom have to prove that they did everything possible to [ensure] the best outcome. Medicare and Medicaid and Blue Cross Blue Shield know more about charting than you do, and they make their own rules! As any lawyer knows, the ED chart certainly possesses miraculous powers to make them rich beyond their wildest dreams.

There is some truth to his observations. The medical record has four distinct functions:

1.  To document the medical encounter for billing and coding
2.  To communicate to other healthcare professionals what occurred on behalf of the patient, what decisions were made, and what diagnostic considerations were involved
3.  To allow review for quality purposes
4.  To provide a document that may be used in litigation against the physician or the organization

These four functions are often at odds with one another. In particular, charting for billing and coding takes time and attention away from a chart focused on the plan of care, documentation of conversations with specialists, and responses to therapy. Emergency medicine is a zero-sum game; time devoted to one task is time away from another. The most important consideration regarding documentation systems is how well they fit into work flow.

## CHARTING FOR BILLING AND CODING

The requirements for billing and coding have become more detailed and cumbersome with each iteration issued by CMS and subsequently by third-party payers. Evaluation and management (E&M) coding and billing are based on three core elements:

1.  The patient's medical history
2.  The physical examination
3.  The medical decision making, which includes the assessment and plan

To bill the highest levels for the sickest patients and most complex cases, comprehensive documentation is required, and the chart can only be coded to the lowest level of documentation in any of these areas.

The medical history consists of four elements:

1.  The chief complaint
2.  The history of the present illness
3.  The review of systems
4.  The patient's medical history, family history, and social history

For instance, a complicated patient (E&M Level 5 is the highest level of coding for an ED patient, short of critical-care patients, and connotes the sickest and most complex patients) requires four elements in the medical history and one item each in past medical history, family history, and social history. A systems review on a complicated patient must include ten items. The physical exam may be organized by system or by body area, and you must not mix the two. Eight items of physical exam are required on a Level 5 patient. Can you see how cumbersome and time consuming this can be?

The biggest areas of lost revenue due to charting inadequacies involve downcoding because the documentation does not support the level of care that was provided. In particular, emergency physicians lose money when a Level 5 case is downcoded to a Level 4 for lack of documentation. Often this downcoding occurs with a sick or complicated patient who requires much attention from the physician for coordination of care, diagnosis, and treatment, thus leaving insufficient time to document all the details. An emergency physician in practice in Salt Lake City told one of our authors about a patient who had suffered a cardiac arrest. The chart was flagged by the billing company for poor documentation and downcoding. The patient required lifesaving endotracheal intubation and anti-arrhythmic drugs and the coordination of efforts to get him to the cardiac catheterization laboratory. The physician had no time for the systems review or a detailed physical exam, let alone a family health history. He was saving the patient's life! The resuscitation was successful, but the physician was subsequently informed by the coders that his poor documentation resulted in the bill being downcoded to that of a minor illness.

Charting in the emergency department is an expensive proposition. Most emergency departments generate approximately $500 to $600 for each patient seen by a physician in the ED. When a physician is charting, she is not seeing a new patient. In a 1998 study Chisholm found that physicians spent between 12 and 21 percent of their time charting. If an ED physician averages 2.1 patients an hour, charting costs nearly $21 a minute. Many healthcare critics note that physician charting is the equivalent of having the highest-trained, highest-educated person on the healthcare team doing data entry (Bukata 2011).

Exhibit 20.1 and Exhibit 20.2 help illustrate the complexities and detail required in the documentation of care delivered to complex patients in the ED. It is as exhaustive as that required of a hospitalist or internist doing a new patient office note or an admission note to the ICU. An internist gives himself typically 45 minutes to see a patient for the first time and document that visit. In the ED, a physician typically sees many patients an hour and spends most of a shift managing three or more patients at a time. Using the same standard of documentation for both physicians takes the ED physician from the bedside and away from other critical tasks. It also likely yields no value to the patient (most ED notes are never read in their entirety).

**Exhibit 20.1: History Level**

| History Level | | | | |
|---|---|---|---|---|
| | **Brief 1–3** | | **Extended 4 or more** | |
| **HPI**<br>Location  Severity  Timing  Modifying factors<br>Quality  Duration  Context  Associated signs/SX | None | Pertinent to problem 1 | Extended 2–9 | Complete |
| **ROS**<br>Constitutional  Ears, nose, throat, mouth  Skin/breast  Endo<br>Hem/lymph<br>Eyes  Card/vasc  GI  Neuro  Allergy/immune<br>Resp  Musculo  GU  Psych  All others neg | None | Pertinent to problem 1 | Extended 2–9 | Complete |
| **PFSH**<br>Past medical history  Family history  Social history | None | Pertinent | | Complete |
| *Overall History Level* | Problem focused | Expanded problem focused | Detailed | Comprehensive |

History level is equal to the lowest Hx component documented in the record.

SOURCE: CMS (1997).

**Exhibit 20.2: Examination Level**

| | Examination Level | | | |
|---|---|---|---|---|
| | 0–1 | 2–4 | 5–7 | ≥ 8 |
| *Body Areas* | | | | |
| Head/face    Chest, including breasts and axillae | | | | |
| Neck    Back, spine    Each extremity | | | | |
| Genitalia, groin, buttocks    Abdomen | | | | |
| *Organ Systems* | | | | |
| Constitutional    Ears, nose, mouth, throat | | | | |
| Eyes    Resp    GI    GU | | | | |
| Cardio    Skin    Neuro    Psych | | | | |
| Hem, lymph, immune    Musculo | | | | |
| *Overall Examination Level* | Problem focused | Expanded problem focused | Detailed | Comprehensive |

SOURCE: CMS (1997).

# CHARTING FOR COMMUNICATION

Healthcare providers need efficient ways to communicate information with one another. The comprehensive electronic health record will eventually provide that, but the details will be important. Providers often complain that the amount of unimportant information contained in the record masks the important information. Many emergency physicians are looking at a model called "hybrid charting." This model combines a template, which prompts users to complete the necessary elements for full coding, with a transcribed record that focuses on the medical decision making, assessment, and plan, which are the most important elements for providers to communicate to one another during care and during hand-offs. The charting options currently available to emergency physicians and nurses in the ED include those listed below:

---

**Charting Options for the Emergency Department**

- Paper template charts
- Electronic template charts (touch screen or tablet)
- Handwritten paper charts
- Electronic charts with areas to enter free text
- Fully dictated and transcribed charts
- Hybrid charting

---

Transcription of dictated charts is considered to be the most comprehensive way of charting, but it has a number of drawbacks. It is time consuming and expensive, with a delayed turnaround time. This method does not prompt physicians to document key elements or provide clinical decision support. Outsourced transcription services run about $0.13 a line or $3 to $5 a page, with charts now running two to three pages. Templated charts are typically less than $1 a page.

Transcription can be accelerated with the creation of macros, in which a physician creates a sentence or two that are tied with a code. Macros can help speed up the documentation, especially for the systems review and the physical exam. For instance, P7 might be the code for the physical exam of the lungs. When the physician dictates "P7" the field is populated with this text: "The pulmonary excursion is adequate. Breath sounds are clear and equal bilaterally." The physician only free-texts the abnormal portions of the physical exam.

Template charting is the fastest method and has been shown to enhance billing by prompting the physician or nurse in terms of documentation items (Kanegave 2005). Typically medical staff do not like templates as they find them harder to interpret. Physicians unfamiliar with using them find that their organization and layout are not intuitive, making it hard to find the information they are looking for. Newer templates are being turned into electronically generated text. Electronic versions of the templates even have forcing functions and clinical decision support.

## CHARTING AND WORK FLOW

One of the other big issues surrounding this exhaustive requirement for real-time data entry is that it takes physicians and nurses away from patient care and interrupts work flow. Electronic charting for nurses has become cumbersome, often with many computer screens to go through to document a simple task. Physicians working in organizations with these systems can recall having to call a nurse away from the computer and charting to get help at the bedside of a critically ill patient. It can be easier to hold a nurse accountable for success or lapses in documentation than for sitting at the bedside with a patient and providing personalized care, so nurses have been pushed to be rigorous in their data entry. The patient encounter is suffering as a result (Mador 2009).

Similarly physician work flow is affected by the data-entry tasks associated with charting. In systems where discharge instructions must be created through the computer as part of the medical record, physicians too are going through countless computer screens to generate paperwork. It is conventional wisdom in EDs to note that the discharge paperwork is thrown in the trash by patients on the way out of the building. Is there any value to the patient in all of this activity?

Emergency department records, which once consisted of handwritten SOAP (subjective-objective-assessment-plan) notes written on carbon paper charts with space for discharge instructions on the bottom, have given way to dictated three-page charts by the physician and three pages of discharge instructions. At Mercy Health in Philadelphia, Jim Roberts, a senior faculty member at Drexel University College of Medicine who is intensely interested in the time physicians spend on charting, notes that their ED charting once consisted of a five-page template. That template is now 20 pages per ED visit (Roberts 2011). It is an electronic system that includes documentation and physician order entry via electronic systems. Dr. Roberts laments, "It takes four keyboard clicks and six lines of charting to order an aspirin!"

Data to accompany this observation can be found in another study that finds that physicians spent only 41 minutes out of every two-hour period at the bedside giving direct patient care (Chisholm et al. 2011). The rest of the time was spent on charting and clerical tasks. This same study found an increase in the numbers of interruptions. Prior work done ten years ago by the same researcher found ED physicians to be interrupted ten times an hour. In this new study physicians were interrupted between 10 and 16 times per hour and, even more alarming, 20 percent of the time they never got back to the task they were doing when interrupted.

---

### Goals of New Documentation Systems

- To unencumber providers and staff
- To require minimal time devoted to charting
- To generate records that are neat and legible, meet charting requirements, and provide adequate detail
- To facilitate care so that throughput is improved
- To allow subsequent providers easy access to the records
- To provide point-of-service decision support to providers

---

## CHARTING TO LIMIT RISK

Fear of litigation drives some of this busywork. Though as Rick Bukata (2011) points out, the risk of a lawsuit occurring in the emergency department is 1 in 20,000 visits. This means that all of this paper being generated is irrelevant in 19,999 cases.

Most attorneys would rather defend a comprehensive dictated chart, which of course is the most expensive and time-consuming option. The lack of documentation that costs physicians in terms of downcoded charge levels also costs in settling litigation. Physicians are not always conscientious about documenting their medical decision making and thought processes regarding a difficult case. They also often speak to consultants on behalf of patients and do not document those discussions well (Weizberg et al. 2009).

The move to a hybrid chart may help this. If the mundane portions of the chart can be managed through check boxes and templates, the physician can focus her attention on the medical decision making, assessment, and plan—the meat of the medical record.

Physicians also fail to document procedures step by step (*APS Update* 2007; Garvey 2010). Macros in the dictation or prompts in template charting can help.

Physicians are also poor at documenting times in the chart. The electronic record with time stamping will help. Some sophisticated ED tracking systems have the person completing a patient-related task in the ED indicate completion on the electronic ED tracking system. The best systems have that time stamp automatically appear in the record (e.g., 0945: The patient is returned from x-ray).

Technology can mitigate the risk of poor documentation in many ways, and technology upgrades such as ED tracking systems, charting systems, and the electronic health record should be purchased with this in mind.

## SCRIBES

One innovation gaining momentum in emergency departments in particular and healthcare at large is the idea of scribes. One of the earliest ED scribe programs began at Antelope Valley Medical Center emergency department, where the physicians individually paid to have someone work alongside them doing paperwork. Led by a physician, Mark Brown, these physicians were soon the most productive in the group; as other physicians in the department wanted their own scribes, the program was formalized. Eventually the hospital partnered with the physicians, providing benefits while the physicians paid the hourly rate. Some of the earliest scribes in the program were pre-med students who went on to become emergency physicians and came back to work for the group.

Richard Bukata of San Gabriel Valley Medical Center in San Gabriel, California, introduced scribes in his department and saw individual physician productivity rise from fewer than 2 patients an hour to 2.7 patients an hour, which more than pays for the program. He also found an unexpected benefit to his program. Because work was now less stressful and more satisfying, two older physicians who had planned to retire decided to stay and work a few more years—no small matter considering the looming physician shortage.

Consider, too, adding scribes to on-call specialists to help make their on-call work easier and more palatable.

## THE ROLE OF EXECUTIVE LEADERSHIP

Leadership can and should play a role in promoting effective documentation by all clinicians. The move toward an electronic health record will be difficult and will require sensitivity to the needs of frontline clinicians. Executive leaders must understand and require that documentation systems do not impede work flow. They can drive this message home with regular goal setting for the IT department that supports documentation strategies to improve work flow and patient flow. Leadership can also show an understanding of these often competing concerns (clinical care and the documentation of that care) by providing scribes and data-entry personnel to reduce the clerical load if the documentation system becomes cumbersome.

## Case Study

Dr. Mahmood Vahedian, an emergency physician with the Banner Health System in Arizona, wanted to improve working conditions for the physicians in his group. Struggling under staggering clerical duties during each shift, physician satisfaction was at an all-time low. Dr. Vahedian, who worked as a scribe before medical school, had an insider's view of the work. Beginning with five scribes, he launched a training program in which the scribes are paid by the 35-member physician group. He had some groundwork to lay because the job description, credentialing, and security issues had to be worked out from scratch. Since Dr. Vahedian had experience as a scribe, he was able to incorporate the necessary elements in launching his program. One clever strategy he used was to partner the scribes-in-training with the most productive physicians in his group. As most readers will intuitively understand, all emergency departments have process idiosyncrasies, and experienced, efficient physicians learn the workarounds and techniques to get workups done expeditiously. In turn, the scribes who work with the most productive physicians (and who really function as physician assistant liaisons) expose each physician in the group to the tricks of the trade they have learned from the most efficient physicians. It becomes an iterative process with benefits all around.

Dr. Vahedian tries to partner the same scribe with the same physician as much as possible so that the scribe learns the style and nuances of how that physician practices and documents. Over time the efficiency grows as the scribe and physician work as a team. Though no physician has been required to use the scribe program, the group has unanimously requested scribe services, and even the physician assistants working in the fast track want to use them. Dr. Vahedian's program now has 40 trained scribes, filling the ranks with pre-med or pre-nursing students. Many are looking for hospital experience to put on their professional school applications, and he offers them great frontline experience and a small hourly wage. The program now populates itself by referrals from other scribes, and turnover is low but expected as the students advance their education and careers.

Each scribe currently works fewer than 1,000 hours a year, which allows the physician group to pay the hourly wage but not provide benefits. Since its earliest days, Dr. Vahedian's program demonstrated an increase of $28 per chart through better documentation, along with physician and patient satisfaction gains. One physician who was slated to retire asked to stay on because he found the work environment so much less frustrating. Physicians are freed up to spend time with patients and families, and the frenetic game of chasing data and paper has been mitigated.

SOURCE: Welch (2010a).

## Professional Scribe Resources

Some professional scribe companies include:

- Emergency Medicine of Idaho
  http://emidaho.com/services6.aspx
- PhysAssist Scribes
  www.iamscribe.com
- Emergency Scribe Consultants
  http://eccpa.org/scribes/index.html
- Scribe America
  www.scribeamerica.com/
- ScribeMD
  www.scribemd.com/index.htm
- Emergency Medicine Scribe Systems
  http://emscribesystems.com
- E Square Scribe Program
  www.esstllc.com/default.htm

## Strategies for Healthcare Executives

- Understand and recognize the effect of documentation on clinical work flow.
- Understand the documentation options available and the limitations of each.
- Ensure that every documentation change and selection for the organization has a positive impact on workflow, patient flow, and staff efficiency.
- Consider some of the innovative choices for documentation, and partner with physicians to bring them about.

## Recommended Readings

Welch, S. 2010. "Beyond Scribes: A Better Idea on the Horizon." *Emergency Medicine News* 32 (1): 4.

Yu, K., and R. Green. 2009. "Critical Aspects of Emergency Department Documentation and Communication." *Emergency Medicine Clinics of North America* 27 (4): 641–54.

# CHAPTER 21

# Protocols and Standardized Order Sets

**In This Chapter**

- "Doing It the Same Way!"
- Advanced Triage Order Sets
- Legal Considerations
- Examples of Standardized Order Sets
- The Role of Executive Leadership
- Case Study
- Strategies for Healthcare Executives

## "DOING IT THE SAME WAY!"

Most of what we do in medicine is *not* evidence-based. There are not enough evidence-based data to guide the care we render, so the physician makes hundreds of decisions each day based on his experience and intuition. Brent James, one of the fathers of quality improvement in healthcare and founder of the Intermountain Institute for Health Care Delivery Research, has said, "It is more important that you do it the same than that you do it right!" (James 2006)

In other words, in terms of safety, efficiency, and quality, it is better to have standardization than not. Dr. James believes each group and each organization should craft a standardized approach to particular clinical situations. It may not be evidence-based, but the local group can develop an approach that makes sense for that medical community, based on its resources and constraints.

In 2000 the emergency physician group at LDS Hospital, the flagship hospital for Intermountain Healthcare, standardized its approach to the common chief complaints in the department. For example, pregnant patients with vaginal bleeding were often found to have an error of omission. Pregnant women who may be miscarrying and are Rh factor negative are supposed to receive a dose of Rhogam in the ED to protect future pregnancies from Rh disease. This step was typically missed because the physician forgot to send the Rh test, which would cue the need for Rhogam. By making an Rh factor test part of the standardized order set for pregnant patients with vaginal bleeding, this error was eliminated.

Dr. James advises group practices to craft standardized order sets for their group's common clinical management problems in the ED. As noted in Chapter 7, this is a safer and more efficient system, and it saves money. Examples of standardized order sets for the ED are included in this chapter on pages 209–19.

## ADVANCED TRIAGE ORDER SETS

Many innovative EDs are using locally developed and chief complaint-driven advanced triage order sets, which allow ED staff to begin diagnostic and therapeutic interventions before the physician sees the patient. These order sets are developed with patient safety, reliability, and efficiency in mind (Welch 2009b).

In the healthcare systems where such protocols are used, the orders are implemented before a physician is linked to the patient. Once a physician is linked to the patient, the physician authorizes the care retroactively by signing the medical record. This process is used widely in most inpatient settings for a host of scenarios, such as the administration of aspirin and an ECG when patients have chest pain and DVT prophylaxis for all post-op patients. Intermountain Healthcare has used advanced triage protocols in the ED of LDS Hospital for more than ten years. Other landmark studies document the advantages in nurses being allowed to institute orders at triage (Retezar 2011; Russ 2010; Wiler 2010).

## LEGAL CONSIDERATIONS

Other hospital departments improve patient care with protocols and order sets such as pre-op order sets used by anesthesia, post-op order sets for open-heart surgery, sepsis bundle order sets in the ICU, and DVT heparin prophylaxis for inpatients. These measures help prevent any local push-back to the implementation of advanced triage order sets. For reasons that are not always clear, some local nursing organizations and state health departments charge that if a nurse begins orders before a physician sees the patient, this is "practicing medicine without a license."

Though there is ample precedent for protocol-driven nurse order sets, some conservative medical communities still push back by suggesting such practices put the nurse at risk (LSU Law Center 1993):

> When nurses are working from standing orders or protocols, their authority is derived from the physician's authority, but the lines of responsibility are less obvious. Intensive care nurses may be authorized to look at a cardiac monitor and to give a bolus of lidocaine when the monitor shows premature ventricular contractions. The nurses may not realize that they are not doing this on their own judgment or responsibility. The protocols are authorized by the physician in charge of the intensive care unit. If no physician has authorized the protocols, the nurse is practicing medicine without a license.

A number of years have transpired since that quote, and nursing practice has developed as rapidly as all the other components of the healthcare system. Still, the point remains that decisions and definitions by state licensing authorities must expand to include recognition of the demands of patient care and safety in a digital world.

The American College of Emergency Physicians and the American Hospital Association have fought this battle with the Centers for Medicare & Medicaid Services, The Joint Commission, and other organizations (AHA 2008). There is nothing illegal about a nurse using guidelines to begin the care of a patient. Having nurses administer Tylenol to febrile children by protocol, ordering simple x-rays from triage, and administering aspirin to chest-pain patients on arrival are all examples of nurses treating patients by protocols or guidelines; these examples can be used to make the case for the further development and implementation of advanced triage order sets.

Protocols have a valuable role in an ED, but they must not be a barrier to independent judgment. But a physician or nurse who varies from a protocol should be able to justify that deviation; reasons for any alteration in the care process should be clearly stated in the patient record.

Protocols must also be understood—and approved—by all relevant parties. Protocols should be appropriate to the ED and the facilities available and should be evaluated from a medical, nursing, and administrative perspective to be sure they will not create unintended consequences. The process of derivation, review, and approval of a protocol should be well documented.

Finally, the protocol must be appropriately available in the patient's chart. Orders must be documented and countersigned as required under relevant state law. Any additions or deletions must also be clearly documented by the appropriate physician or other personnel as permitted under state law.

---

**Keys to the Successful Implementation of Advanced Triage Order Sets**

- The individual protocols should be developed locally or modified from other organizations and approved by the ED physician group.
- Departments should get approval of these protocols from the medical executive committee as well so that protocols become the standard of care for the organization. This step provides institutional approval and endorsement of the order sets.
- The orders may be pre-empted at the individual physician level.
- Physicians understand that they may have to explain why they deviated from a protocol, particularly if there is strong supportive evidence-based data. (For example, "Why didn't you take the patient with the acute ST-segment elevation MI to the cath lab?")
- The individual physician's signature on the medical record should authorize the protocol use.
- Protocols should be periodically reviewed and revised by the physician group based on changes in the medical literature or the needs of the department.

---

## EXAMPLES OF STANDARDIZED ORDER SETS

Exhibits 21.1, 21.2, and 21.3 are examples of advanced triage order sets from several high-performance emergency departments around the country. We recommend that these order sets be locally developed by the emergency physician group and then passed through the medical executive committee for institutional approval. These real, advanced triage protocol order sets come from the following emergency departments: Mercy Medical Center in Cedar Rapids, Iowa; Florida Hospital Fish Memorial in Orange City, Florida; and Williamsport Regional Medical Center in Williamsport, Pennsylvania.

*Adult*

*General Illness*
- If stable, insert saline lock/if unstable, initiate NS at 50ml/hour
- CBC, CMP, hold rainbow
- Obtain UA, urine HCG if female in reproductive years

*Upper Respiratory Symptoms: Sinus/Sore Throat/Cough/Fever/Body Aches*
- Obtain throat swab for sore throat
- Nasal aspirate for Influenza A/B
- Follow APAP/Ibuprofen dosing for patients with fever

*Dyspnea/Asthma/COPD (Resp. distress, severe)*
- Initiate Albuterol 2.5mg in 3 ml saline nebulizer treatment—**don't delay treatment, contact MD immediately & Notify RT**
- Obtain ABGs prior to starting oxygen therapy if patient not in extremis
- Apply cardiac monitor, pulse oximetry and initiate oxygen therapy at 2L per nasal cannula
- If stable, insert saline lock/if unstable, initiate NS at 50ml/hour
- CBC, CMP, Troponin, blood culture if fever present
- ECG
- **Do not delay oxygen if symptoms are severe**

*Overdose/Suicidal Attempt*
- Apply cardiac monitor and pulse oximetry
- If stable, insert saline lock/if unstable, initiate NS at 50ml/hour
- CBC, CMP, APAP level, ASA level, blood alcohol
- ECG

- Obtain urine for UA, drug screen, urine
- HCG, if female in reproductive years
- If patient is not with police officer, notify Security for stand by
- Notify Access Nurse

*Weakness/Generalized (General Illness)*
- Apply cardiac monitor, pulse oximetry
- If stable, insert saline lock/if unstable, initiate NS at 50ml/hour
- ECG
- CBC, CMP, Troponin
- Blood culture if fever present (ask physician for 2nd B.C. order)
- Obtain UA

*Chest Pain*
- STAT ECG
- Apply cardiac monitor, pulse oximetry
- Apply oxygen 2L per nasal cannula
- Administer four (4) baby aspirin, chewed (hold if patient has already had today, active GI bleeding, peptic ulcer disease or is allergic
- If stable, insert saline lock/if unstable, initiate NS at 50ml/hour
- CBC, CMP, PT/PTT, Troponin
- Administer sublingual Nitro 0.4mg x 3 every 5 minutes to maintain BP greater than 100 systolic (hold for patients who have had Viagra, Cialis, Levitra or any other sexual performance enhancement drugs)

*Abdominal Pain/Flank Pain/N/V/D*
- If stable, insert saline lock/if unstable, initiate NS at 50ml/hour
- CBC, CMP
- Obtain UA, urine HCG for females in reproductive years

(continued)

*Adult Continued*

- Anticipate pelvic for females in reproductive years

*Vaginal Bleeding/OB Complaints (Female GU)*
- Obtain orthostatic vitals (BP/pulse) and fetal heart tones for pregnancies 10–12 weeks or greater
- If stable, insert saline lock/if unstable, initiate NS at 50ml/hour
- CBC, Rh type, quant HCG
- Cath UA
- Anticipate pelvic exam

*Seizure*
- If stable, insert saline lock/if unstable, initiate NS at 50ml/hour
- CBC, CMP, drug level as appropriate
- Pad side rails for patient safety

*Headache, Worst Ever: Notify MD immediately*
- If stable, insert saline lock/if unstable, initiate NS at 50ml/hour
- CBC, CMP, PT/PTT
- Anticipate STAT Head CT

*AMS (CVA Symptoms/Neurological Complaints)*
- Apply cardiac monitor, pulse oximetry
- Apply $O_2$ at 2L per nasal cannula
- Glucometer check
- If stable, insert saline lock/if unstable, initiate NS at 50ml/hour
- CBC, CMP, PT/PTT
- ECG
- For Stroke Alerts: IV access X 2
- Anticipate for STAT Head CT

*Syncope/Near Syncopal Episode (General Illness Template)*
- Apply cardiac monitor, plus oximetry
- ECG

- Obtain orthostatic vitals (BP/pulse) if patient tolerates
- If stable, insert saline lock/if unstable, initiate NS at 50ml/hour
- CBC, CMP, Troponin
- Anticipate a Head CT

*Neck/Back; Facial/Head Trauma*
- Spinal immobilization as appropriate based on mechanism of injury
- Apply ice as appropriate
- Cleanse any wounds with Shur Clens and set up for laceration repair
- Update Adult DT as necessary, if no allergy
- Place neon green "pt on back board" card on chart to alert physician as appropriate

*UTI Symptoms (Female GU Template)*
- Obtain UA (hold for culture)
- If menses present, obtain Cath UA

*Alleged Assault/Abuse*
- Cleanse all wounds with Shur Clens, apply ice as appropriate
- Update Adult DT if necessary, if no allergy
- Notify police for report
- Follow Back/Neck/Extremity injury protocols as appropriate

*Defer/Suicidal/Homicidal/Clinically Intoxicated/Committals (Psych Complaints)*
- Notify Security for stand by
- Place emergency hold on patient until evaluated by physician
- Notify Access Nurse
- Call lab for draw: CBC, CMP, TSH, GGTP, RPR, Blood alcohol

*Adult Continued*

- Obtain UA, drug screen, urine HCG for females in reproductive years, if possible

*Corneal Abrasion/Foreign Body/Pain/Trauma*

- Obtain "eye kit" meds from Acudose
- Instill Tetracaine 2 drops to affected eye
- Visual acuity after Tetracaine
- If chemicals, irrigate with 1000ml of NS

*Extremity Pain/Trauma (Upper/Lower Template)*

- X-ray area of tenderness, apply ice, elevate, and splint or position for comfort
- Urine HCG for female in reproductive years
- Cleanse any abrasions/wounds with Shur Clens and set up for laceration repair
- Update adult DT as needed if no allergy
- Notify physician if patient will need multiple x-rays

*Pain, Severe (General Illness Template)*

- Initiate IV of NS at 50 ml/hour
- Draw and hold rainbow from IV start

*Trauma Alert (Major Trauma)*

- Apply cardiac monitor, pulse oximetry
- If stable, insert saline lock/if unstable, initiate NS at 50ml/hour
- Consider 2 large bore IVs
- CBC, CMP, PT/PTT, Lipase
- Type and Screen
- Hold for rainbow
- STAT ECG as appropriate
- Obtain urine for UA, urine HCG if female in reproductive years

- Notify ED physician immediately
- Anticipate x-rays and CT

*MVC*

- Spinal immobilization as appropriate
- Apply ice as appropriate
- Place neon green "pt on back board" card on chart to alert physician as appropriate

*Burns*

- Calculate BSA. For BSA greater than 20% initiate NS at 1000 ml/hour
- Draw and hold rainbow
- **Notify MD immediately**
- For minor burns, update adult DT if necessary, if no allergy

*Diabetes Out-Of-Control (General Illness Template)*

- Glucometer check
- Initiate IV of NS at 500 ml/hour (if cardiac disease check with Physician)
- CBC, CMP
- Obtain urine for UA, urine HCG for females

*Infectious Disease (General Illness Template)*

- Assess for a) Unusual wt loss/fatigue/night sweats; b) cough greater than 3 weeks/bloody sputum; c) travel outside US less than 30 days ago; d) neck pain/rigidity, fever and/or headache
- If answered "yes" to any preceding question, consider masking patient and send directly to private exam room

*Fever (General Illness Template)*

- Treat temperatures greater than or equal to 102° F rectal or 101° F oral with antipyretics (APAP 1000mg PO)

(continued)

*Adult Continued*

*Body Fluid Exposure (General Illness Template)*
- For high-risk source or suspected high-risk source, Triage Level 2. Initiate Body Fluid Exposure protocol including Source panel and Exposed panel

*Epistaxis/ENT*
- Hold pressure for 5 minutes or apply nose clips
- If systolic BP less than 90 or heart rate greater than 120, initiate IV NS at 50 ml/hour and draw CBC, PT/PTT, & hold for rainbow
- If patient on Coumadin obtain CBC, PT/PTT and hold for rainbow
- Set up room for physician exam/nasal packing procedure
- **Pediatrics - (Anticipate use of LMX Cream for IV/Lab Access)**

*Abdominal Pain (Peds Illness)*
- NPO
- Obtain UA

*Diabetes Out of Control (Peds Illness)*
- Glucometer check
- Anticipate IV access

*Extremity Trauma (Peds Trauma)*
- X-ray area of tenderness
- Apply ice, elevate, splint, position for comfort
- Notify physician if patient will need multiple x-rays

*Chemotherapy Patient (General Illness Template)*
- Patient with fever, mask in Triage
- Take to private exam room
- Access infusaport, if present; otherwise initiate IV of NS at 50 ml/hour
- CBC, CMP, Blood culture x 1 from port (ask physician for 2nd B.C. order)
- Order old medical record

*Fever (Peds Illness)*
- **Fever greater than 100.4° F rectal in infants younger than 60 days of age, Expedite chart to Physician.**
- If older than 60 days, treat temperatures greater than 102° F rectal or 101° F oral with antipyretics. (APAP per weight (15mg/kg) or Ibuprofen (10mn/kg))

*Ear/Throat Pain (Peds Illness)*
- APAP per weight chart (15mg/kg) or Ibuprofen per weight chart

**Exhibit 21.2: Florida Hospital Fish Memorial Emergency Department Protocols**

❏ *Abdominal pain and/or vomiting*
- CBC, CMP
- Amylase, Lipase, BHCG on premenopausal females of childbearing age
- Urinalysis with urine culture
- Minicath on females
- IV Saline Lock In Treatment Room
- ECG for age greater than 35
- Consult ED MD for analgesic medication, antiemetics, fluids

❏ *Chest Pain-Presumed Cardiac in Nature*
- **Expedite to Treatment Area**
- Initiate Cardiac Order Set Labs
- ECG and show to ED MD
- Send any applicable drug levels
- IV Saline Lock In Treatment Room
- $O_2$ @ 2L via N/C, Cardiac monitor, pulse oximeter
- Consult ED MD for medication administration.
- Notify physician for persistent pain
- **Goal for thrombolytics in STEMI is 30 min. from arrival Pleuritic Chest Pain**
- CSR, ECG and show to ED MD, pulse oximeter

❏ *Fever greater than 100.5F GREATER THAN 50 years of age; R/O sepsis*
- CBC, CMP, Urinalysis with culture
- Blood cultures x2, serum lactate
- BHCG on pre-menopausal females of childbearing age
- pCXR, cardiac monitor, continuous pulse oximetry
- IV saline lock, $O_2$ @ 2L via N/C
- Acetaminophen 1 gm PO or 650 mg rectally prn for temp greater than 100.5F
- Consult ED MD for administration of antibiotics
- **Goal for antibiotics in CAP is 4 hours from arrival**

❏ *Seizures - Active or subjective*
- Continuous cardiac monitoring
- Pad side rails, side rails up, bed low position
- Administer oxygen as appropriate
- IV Saline Lock or Normal Saline at KVO rate in treatment room
- Obtain CBC, CMP, any applicable drug levels, urinalysis, Notify ED MD of patient's presence
- Consult ED MD regarding CT scan of the brain
- Consult ED MD regarding anti convulsants

❏ *Mental Status*
- CBC, CMP, Urinalysis with culture
- pCXR, Blood Culture x2, cardiac enzymes
- ECG and show to ED MD
- $O_2$ @ 2L via N/C, cardiac monitor
- IV Saline Lock In Treatment Room
- Continuous pulse oximetry
- AccuChek

❏ *Dyspnea in the absence of chest pain*
- CBC, CMP, BNP
- Any applicable drug levels
- pCXR, ECG and show to ED MD
- $O_2$ as appropriate
- 2L via N/C for COPD pts
- Maintain pulse ox greater than 92% for non-COPD pts
- IV Saline Lock In Treatment Room
- Stat albuterol/atrovent neb with peak flow before and after
- Consult ED MD for administration of diuretics, steroids, and/or antibiotics
- **Goal for antibiotics in CAP is 4 hours from arrival**

(continued)

**Exhibit 21.2: Florida Hospital Fish Memorial Emergency Department Protocols (continued)**

❏ *Head Injury*
- Consult ED MD for CT head (only if loss of consciousness, on blood thinners, or with subsequent altered mental status)

❏ *Patients on Coumadin w/bleeding*
- PT/PTT
- CBC, CMP, T&S
- Pulse oximetry
- IV Saline Lock In Treatment Room
- Consult ED MD for administration of intravenous crystalloid solutions

❏ *Sickle Cell Crisis*
- Notify ED MD of patient's presence and presentation
- Initiate IV access in Treatment Room
- Obtain CBC, CMP, Reticulocyte count
- Consult ED MD for administration of IV fluids
- Administer high flow $O_2$ If febrile, also obtain blood cultures x2, urinalysis with culture, CXR, and notify ED MD for prompt antibiotic selection & administration.

❏ *Animal Bites*
- Remove jewelry from affected extremity if applicable
- Cleanse wound with Betadine or chlorhexidine
- Use sterile 4x4 gauze pad to dry wound
- Anticipate suture by MD
- Obtain tetanus immunization status
- If no allergy, administer 0.5ml Tetanus Toxoid if immunized greater than 5 yrs ago or if it is unknown.
- Complete Animal Bite Report form and fax to the number on the Animal Bite Report.

❏ *Extremity Injury*
- Assess & document pain quality and intensity on 0–10 scale.

- Determine mechanism of injury and exact location of pain. Evaluate joint and joint below the injury for tenderness. Order appropriate x-ray.
- Immobilize/Elevate injured extremity
- Apply cold compress if injury is less than 48 hrs old
- Saline lock for obviously displaced fracture in Treatment Room
- BHCG for pre-menopausal females of childbearing age
- Consult ED MD for administration of analgesic medication.

❏ *Oncology Patients with Fever/Weakness*
- CBC, CMP, PT, PTT
- Blood Cultures x2
- Urinalysis and urine culture
- pCXR
- Pulse oximetry
- Maintain patient in private room
- Consult ED MD for administration of antibiotics
- Administer acetaminophen 1 gm PO

❏ *Asthma*
- $O_2$ @ 2L via N/C
- Continuous pulse oximetry
- Stat albuterol/atrovent neb with peak flow before and after
- Notify ED MD of patient's presence and presentation
- Consult ED MD for administration of IV or PO steroids

❏ *Fever-Adult*
- 15 mg/kg of acetaminophen with a max dose of 1000 mg orally OR
- 15 mg/kg of acetaminophen with a maximum dose of 650 mg rectally
- Reassess patient's temperature within 60 minutes and document
- Notify MD for further orders if fever persists

**Exhibit 21.2: Florida Hospital Fish Memorial Emergency Department Protocols (continued)**

❑ *Fever-Pediatric*
- Obtain weight (kg)
- Obtain rectal temp for children less than 2 years of age
- Obtain rectal temp on other children who do not tolerate oral temps
- Verify and document antipyretic administration prior to arrival
- Administer Children's Motrin 10 mg/kg for temp greater than or equal to 100F
- If Motrin was administered prior to arrival, administer Tylenol 15 mg/kg orally or rectally
- Reassess and document temperature within 30–60 minutes

❑ *Lacerations*
- Cleanse wound with normal saline
- X-ray injured area if indicated to rule out foreign body or a suspected fracture
- BHCG on pre-menopausal females of childbearing age
- Document tetanus immunization status.
- If no allergy and greater than 5 years, administer 0.5ml TD IM.
- Suture set-up at bedside
- Anticipate post-suture clean up and dressing administration.

*Other Orders*
No IV's are to be started in Triage. Treatment rooms ONLY.

**Exhibit 21.3: ED Nursing Protocols, Williamsport Hospital Emergency Department**

*Underlying Principles*

1. These protocols are intended to facilitate rapid patient evaluation, testing, and treatment as well as overall patient flow by specifying appropriate testing and treatment for selected clinical situations prior to provider evaluation. It is anticipated that (1) in the majority of situations, the actions specified would have been ordered by the provider anyway, and that (2) in a small number of situations, a provider might not have ordered some actions. Furthermore, it is anticipated that the upside for patients in terms of rapid onset of care and enhanced patient flow will outweigh any downside associated with using protocols.
2. These protocols can be initiated by the triage nurse or by the nurse(s) caring for the patient in a treatment area.
3. More than one protocol can apply to any single patient.
4. All steps in protocol do not need to be carried out at the same time. When considering a specific action, nurses can use good judgment and should consider how long before the provider evaluation is likely to occur. If provider evaluation is not likely to be soon, then nurses should more strongly consider initiating *all* protocols that apply to a patient.
5. Moving patients to a treatment area should not be unreasonably delayed by these protocols.

(continued)

**Exhibit 21.3: ED Nursing Protocols, Williamsport Hospital Emergency Department (continued)**

6.  These protocols should be consistently applied regardless of the ED providers on duty, time of day, etc.
7.  If questions arise regarding the application of these protocols, a provider on duty should be consulted. Any problems should be reported to the ED manager and the ED medical director.

*Complaint-Specific Protocols*
1.  Chest Pain, Potentially Cardiac[1]
    a.  ECG (show to ED physician immediately), CBC, BMP, PT/PTT, CK-MB, Troponin, CXR(PA/Lateral preferred – discuss with provider), drug levels as appropriate
    b.  Oxygen, IV access, cardiac monitor, pulse ox
    c.  Repeat ECG if patient had significant change in pain, recurrent pain, or rhythm changes. Show to physician immediately.
2.  Respiratory Distress (adult)
    a.  Assure patent airway, assist ventilation as needed, anticipate need for BiPAP or intubation. Notify ED physician.
    b.  Oxygen, IV access, cardiac monitor, pulse ox. Consider ECG.
    c.  DuoNeb x2 if actively wheezing
3.  Respiratory Distress (pediatric)
    a.  Assess respiratory rate, work of breathing, pulse ox
    b.  Assure patent airway, assist ventilation as needed, anticipate need for intubation. Notify ED physician.
    c.  Consider IV access, cardiac monitor, ECG
    d.  Xopenex via nebulizer if actively wheezing
4.  Extremity Trauma/Injury
    a.  Initiate x-rays based on mechanism of injury and examination of extremity, especially palpating for bony tenderness.[2]
    b.  Consult ED provider if more than one contiguous study is needed, or if more than 2 non-contiguous studies are needed
    c.  Urine pregnancy test for potentially pregnant females
5.  Eye Injuries
    a.  Alcaine drops as needed
    b.  Visual acuity measurement
    c.  Saline irrigation for chemical exposures
6.  Potentially Pregnant Female
    a.  UA dip and urine pregnancy
7.  Pregnant Female With Vaginal Bleeding
    a.  Quantitative HCG, CBC, T&S
    b.  IV access and 300 cc NSS bolus if patient has abnormal vital signs or signs of shock, Notify ED physician.
8.  Significant Abdominal Pain (defined as: severe, associated with diaphoresis, tachycardia, hypotension, fever, or GI bleeding, or pregnancy-associated)
    a.  CBC, BMP, UA. Save extra tubes.

    b.  Urine pregnancy test for potentially pregnant females

    c.  Quantitative HCG if pregnant

    d.  Amylase/lipase if patient has epigastric pain and tenderness

    e.  ECG if epigastric pain in patient >30 years old[3]

    f.  IV access. 300 cc NSS bolus if patient has abnormal vital signs or signs of shock. Notify ED physician.

    g.  NPO

9.  Flank Pain – Presumed Renal Colic

    a.  IV NSS, UA, Urine pregnancy for premenopausal females. Draw blood tubes.

    b.  Palpate epigastrium for AAA[4]

    c.  Notify ED physician

    d.  If not allergic, give morphine 4 mg IV. May repeat x1 after 10 minutes

10. Febrile Infant <1 month (Rectal temp 38.0 or greater)

    a.  Rectal Temperature

    b.  Manual BP, pulse ox

    c.  CBC, BMP, cath UA, Urine C&S, CXR, blood culture x1

    d.  Notify ED physician

11. Febrile Elderly Patient

    a.  CBC, BMP, blood cultures x2, cath UA micro/C&S if indicated, CXR, drug levels as appropriate. Pulse ox.

    b.  IV access

    c.  Tylenol

12. Altered Mental Status – Hypoglycemia

    a.  Check FBS (if not done already)

    b.  Juice (or other sugar-containing food) if able to take PO

    c.  Administer 1 amp D50 IV if unable to take PO

    d.  Notify ED physician

    e.  Feed patient when mental status normalizes

    f.  Recheck FBS

13. Altered Mental Status – Normoglycemic

    a.  Cardiac monitor, pulse ox, oxygen, ECG

    b.  CBC, BMP, PT/PTT, UA micro/C&S if indicated, portable CXR, drug levels as appropriate

    c.  Hold blood cultures x2

    d.  Consider Head CT and UDS

    e.  IV access

    f.  Narcan 2mg IVP

14. GI Bleed (Significant)

    a.  CBC, BMP, PT/PTT, T&S, drug levels as appropriate

    b.  IV access. Cardiac monitor, pulse ox. Orthostatic HR/BP if able. Stool guiaic.

    c.  NSS bolus 300cc

    d.  Notify ED physician

(continued)

15. Acute Neurologic Deficit – potential TPA candidate[5]
    a. CBC, BMP, PT/PTT, ECG, CXR, Stat head CT, drug levels as appropriate
    b. Cardiac monitor, pulse ox
    c. IV access. Oxygen
    d. Notify ED physician
    e. IV access, draw blood. If hypotensive, 300 cc NSS bolus if patient has abnormal vital signs or signs of shock.
    f. Cardiac monitor, pulse ox, oxygen, ECG, FBS as needed
    g. CBC, BMP, UA micro/C&S if indicated. Drug levels as appropriate.
    h. Notify ED physician
    i. Call toxicologist for advice
16. Suspected UTI
    a. Dip urine and UA/micro, culture if indicated
    b. Urine pregnancy test for potentially pregnant females
17. Urinary Retention
    a. Place foley in obvious cases. Get bladder scan if uncertainty exists.
    b. Dip urine and UA/micro culture if indicated
18. Possible Pneumonia
    a. Patients Categories eligible for this protocol:
        i. Category 1: Patients who are elderly, have active cancer, symptomatic heart/ lung/ liver/renal/cerebrovascular disease, or are nursing home patients AND have fever (or history of recent fever), new or worsened dyspnea, new or worsened hypoxemia, new cough, or new sputum production.
        ii. Category 2: A patient not in Category 1 who looks "sick" with what could be pneumonia (i.e. fever, tachycardia, hypoxemia, tachypnea at rest, hypotension, significant dyspnea)
    b. CBC, blood cultures x2, CXR (PA/Lateral preferred). Drug levels as appropriate. Hold other tubes.
    c. Notify ED physician
19. Sore Throat
    a. Patient's chief complaint should be sore throat
    b. Rapid strep test – rub tonsils vigorously to get adequate specimen
20. Nosebleed
    a. Set up for provider evaluation: towel, emesis basin, headlamp, cotton pledgets, nasal speculum, alligator forceps, silver nitrate sticks.
    b. Mix lidocaine and epinephrine 1:1 in small cup
    c. PT/PTT (and hold CBC) if on warfarin (Coumadin)

*Other Protocols:*
1. Fever Management
    a. Tylenol[6] or Motrin PO[7]
    b. Children less than 2 years should have a rectal temperature if fever is the chief complaint or if an infectious problem is potentially present. Rectal temperatures should be done in any other patient where a reliable temperature cannot be obtained and infection is a consideration.

2. Wound Management
   a. Tetanus booster (Td or Tdap), LET, oral analgesic, ice, immobilization
   b. Wound repair preparation. Discuss with ED provider: anesthetic, cleaning/ irrigation, equipment for suturing/stapling/taping/Dermabond
   c. Cover with moist sterile gauze
   d. Give local anesthetic SC and/or irrigate as ordered by provider
3. Pain Management
   a. Tylenol/Motrin PO
   b. Tylenol with Codeine or Lortab PO
   c. Ice and immobilization as indicated
4. Urine Specimen Collection
   a. Female: Cath if patient is elderly, incontinent, obese, has vaginal bleeding or vaginal discharge, or is unable to perform the mechanics of a clean catch
   b. Male: Cath if incontinent or if unable to perform the mechanics of a clean catch
   c. Infants: If a urinary tract infection is potentially present, a cath specimen should be collected. Bag urines can be done when a UTI is not being considered, such as for monitoring urine output.
5. Patients Taking Warfarin (Coumadin)
   a. Draw and hold PT/INR if drawing blood for other purposes.
6. Behavioral Health Admissions to DPH
   a. Clean catch UA and urine drug screen
   b. EtOH level if alcohol recently ingested. Drug levels as appropriate.
   c. Urine pregnancy test for potentially pregnant females
   d. The behavioral health admission process and disposition should not be delayed by the absence of urine test results.
7. Tetanus Immunization
   a. Administer Td (or Tdap if age ≥19 and ≤64 and patient has not had Tdap) for any patient with a qualifying wound if they have not had a tetanus booster in 10 or more years. Note: Tdap is only give once. (N.B. Review CDC vaccine information statement as needed.)
8. Patient Undressing Guidelines
   a. Mild respiratory complaints – undressed from waist up
   b. Abdominal complaints, chest complaints, focal neurologic complaints, back pain – completely undressed except underpants

Footnotes:

[1] Coronary ischemia can present in a variety of nonspecific ways. Therefore, ECGs should be done liberally. The rest of the tests should be done before provider evaluation only when there is a greater suspicion of coronary ischemia.

[2] Remember the Ottawa Rules for ankle injuries.

[3] Cardiac ischemia can present with epigastric pain or "indigestion."

[4] A kidney stone is the most common diagnosis in cases of misdiagnosed abdominal aortic aneurysm (AAA).

[5] Selected relevant TPA criteria: Inclusion – age >18, symptoms <3 hours. Exclusion – Improving deficits, headache/stiff neck suggestive of SAH, pregnant/lactating female, platelets <100K, on anticoagulants, major surgery or trauma within 14 days, head trauma within 3 months, GI or GU bleeding within 3 weeks, non-compressible arterial puncture or LP within 1 week, systolic BP >185, diastolic BP >110, prior intracranial bleed, glucose <50 or >400, symptoms consistent with acute MI or post-MI pericarditis, or seizure associated with stroke onset.

[6] Compensate for under-dosing prior to patient's arrival.

[7] Avoid Motrin if patient is allergic to ibuprofen, NSAIDS, or aspirin, if age is less than 6 months, or if there is a history of GI bleed/ulcer.

# THE ROLE OF EXECUTIVE LEADERSHIP

Standardization can be a hard sell to clinicians, in particular to physicians. Physicians may be more receptive to the process if the executive leadership makes it an organizational priority. Often physicians who push back against advanced triage order sets are the same ones who complain when the nurses are not using them fully!

---

### Case Study

At Hospital Corporation of America (HCA) in Denver, Dr. Dickson Cheung is leading his system in chief complaint–driven ED protocols that streamline and standardize care. Using pilot studies and rapid cycle testing, eight Denver-area hospitals use standardized order sets implemented in triage to decrease the time it takes for labs to be received from the emergency department. In his early trials Dr. Cheung tracked the time from patient presentation to the time lab specimens were received and logged in to the laboratory. The early trials are showing improvement:

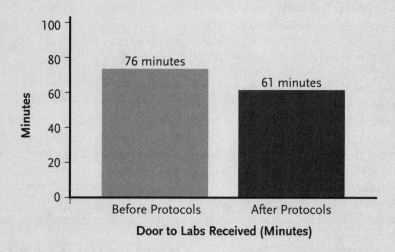

SOURCE: Cheung (2011).

---

## Strategies for Healthcare Executives

- Encourage the ED physician group to craft standardized order sets for the most common ED chief complaints.
- Pass each order set by the medical executive committee for institutional approval.
- Publicly endorse their implementation at all levels of the organization.
- Consider bringing in a respected national leader in ED quality and safety to help launch an ED standardization initiative.

## Recommended Readings

Emergency Medicine Practice Subcommittee. 2007. "Crowding and Surge Capacity Resources for EDs." Dallas, TX: American College of Emergency Physicians.

Institute for Healthcare Improvement. 2003. *Optimizing Patient Flow: Moving Patients Smoothly Through Acute Care Settings.* Boston: Institute for Healthcare Improvement.

Seay, T., and D. Fite. 2006. "Approaching Full Capacity in the Emergency Department: An Information Paper." Dallas, TX: American College of Emergency Physicians.

Wilson, M. J., B. Siegel, and M. Williams. 2005. "Perfecting Patient Flow: America's Safety Net Hospitals and Emergency Department Crowding." Washington DC: National Association of Public Hospitals and Health Systems.

# CHAPTER 22

# Consent, End of Life, and the Law

**In This Chapter**

- The Right to Consent
- What Is Incompetence?
- Implied Consent
- End-of-Life Issues in the ED
- The Role of Executive Leadership
- Case Study
- Strategies for Healthcare Executives

## THE RIGHT TO CONSENT

Every competent patient has the right to consent to care, based on an understanding of all the significant risks and benefits of that treatment, as well as the risks and benefits of any alternative treatments (including doing nothing) and other information that a reasonable person would want to know to make an informed decision. As stated by Justice Benjamin N. Cardozo (*Schloendorff v. Society of New York Hospital,* 211 N.Y. 125, 105 N.E. 92 [1914]), "Every human being of adult years and sound mind has a right to determine what shall be done with his own body; and a surgeon who performs an operation without his patient's consent commits an assault, for which he is liable in damages." Obtaining consent in an elective setting, properly done, should include a thorough review of all relevant information as well as adequate time to discuss any questions or concerns the patient (or her representative) may have. Families and other loved ones should also be considered, as is appropriate to the situation and the relevant state law. This lengthy process is often impossible in an emergency. When care is emergent, consent can be under the emergency treatment exception, which has long been recognized by the courts and state statutes. For example, in a frequently cited case from 1931, the Iowa court found a man had implied consent for the removal of his arm that had been severely damaged in a train accident, when in the physician's judgment immediate removal of the limb was necessary to save the man's life (*Jacovach vs. Yocum,* 237 N.W. 444, Iowa, 1931). The presumption of consent increases as the danger to life or loss of function becomes more immediate.

Respect for a patient's right to consent should never outweigh his safety. However physicians in an ED cannot be cavalier about consent, and whenever the patient's acuity allows, full informed consent should be obtained.


## WHAT IS INCOMPETENCE?

Incompetence in patients could be temporary (such as from a head injury, intoxication, or anesthesia) or permanent (deficiency in mental processes, dementia, or retardation). A patient is also incompetent to give consent before she reaches the age of majority, which is 18 years in most or all jurisdictions. When a patient is incompetent, who should consent to her care?

When an incompetent person is a patient in the ED, all personnel must be aware that a representative of that patient should be included in any decision making. This does not mean that necessary emergency intervention is delayed; patient safety and patient rights must be continually balanced on a case-by-case basis. The identity of the appropriate representative will be a matter subject to state law. Certainly in all states the right to consent for a child rests with a parent; the conflicting roles of divorced parents are again subject to state law, although in all jurisdictions the ultimate tool for assessing rights is the divorce decree.

Patients who have chronic issues with mental processes, such as dementia or retardation, often have a state-appointed guardian or representative. If a guardian has not been identified by the appropriate state agency, there are laws in all states that allow for loved ones to be placed in the position to grant consent on a hierarchy based on their relationship to the patient (think Terri Schiavo). Patients who come to the ED with temporary incompetence will obviously not have a court-appointed guardian. In those cases, most state laws allow loved ones to be consulted for purposes of consent.

As a practical matter, patients do not arrive in the ED with state papers pinned to their chests revealing the identities of their guardians. Children do not carry their parents' divorce decree in their backpack. In reality, in an ED there must be an awareness of the legal rights and responsibilities of the parties involved, but the critical priority is emergency intervention. Most questions involving conflicting wishes of divorced parents or which adult daughter can speak for Mom are resolved after the ED, when the patient reaches the hospital floor and time allows for more investigation. In the meantime, any attempt to determine the appropriate representative, or any effort to locate a parent, should be documented in the ED record.

## IMPLIED CONSENT

**Implied consent** is an important legal principle in two scenarios: the most innocent gesture and the most critical intervention. Innocent gestures refer to actions patients take every day that constitute implied consent. Turning an arm to give access for a shot, holding out an extended elbow for a blood draw, lifting a shirt for inspection of a rash on the abdomen—these are all examples of an action that implies consent. Even silence, or failure to object, may constitute implied consent.

> **Implied consent:** Signs, actions, or facts, or an inaction or silence, that raise a presumption that consent has been given.

On the other hand, in the most critical emergencies implied consent can come to bear because it is implied that the patient would consent to treatment necessary to save his life. In a true emergency the priority must always be placed on *treatment*.

## END-OF-LIFE ISSUES IN THE ED

People obviously die in emergency departments. Even with the best care, not everyone can be saved. In these cases the proper notification of loved ones and temporary storage of the body pending funeral home removal are all subject to various state laws and should be well represented in the ED policies and procedures.

The patient who is brain dead presents another kind of end-of-life issue in the ED. The prospect of a body still supported in breathing and circulation with no brain activity was not possible until advancements in medical technology in the second half of the last century. A person with no brain activity (as determined in most states by the Harvard Brain Death Criteria) is legally dead under state statutes that were all amended to deal with this situation. If the patient is brain dead, regardless of family wishes, all life supports must be terminated.

Problems arise in cases in which a patient is not legally dead but is receiving life-supporting care that is futile. These cases often result in agonizing, and often prolonged, discussions that must occur with the physicians, hospital, family, and other loved ones. These cases must take into account any advanced directive left by the patient, which should be controlling and must consider state law as well as potential legal claims by loved ones.

Cases involving brain death or the termination of life supports should not be dealt with in the ED. Declaration of death in the ED must be made by a physician or other state-recognized person such as a medical examiner or coroner. However, cases where death cannot be declared should be dealt with in a far more subdued, reflective environment. Every hospital has social workers or chaplains who are well versed in dealing with these difficult issues; also, any case involving the termination of life supports should always include the hospital attorney. Even determination of brain death should take time beyond what is appropriate for a patient to be held in the ED.

From the perspective of the ED, what is important is to treat. If it turns out the intervention saved a patient's life but results in a permanent vegetative state, that must be dealt with at another time in a different part of the hospital by people with different training and skill sets.

## THE ROLE OF EXECUTIVE LEADERSHIP

The protection of patient rights is a fundamental responsibility of a healthcare executive. Of those rights, few are more important than the right of informed consent. As the leader of a healthcare entity, an executive must be vigilant in ensuring that all employees of the facility, as well as all providers delivering patient care under hospital privileges, respect and protect a patient's right to consent.

At the same time, in the ED there will be many cases where the need for treatment is too emergent to allow for the informed consent process, or the patient will be unable to consent and no representative will be available. At all times the right to consent must be protected but never at the risk of patient care and safety.

On December 26, 1982, Susan Kozup was admitted to the High Risk Obstetrical Unit of Georgetown University Hospital when it appeared that delivery of her child would involve complications. On January 9, 1983, Kozup went into labor. Matthew was born on January 10, and shortly thereafter, Georgetown began giving Matthew blood transfusions for hypovolemia, a condition associated with premature birth. Over the course of two days, Matthew received three transfusions contaminated with HIV.

The American Red Cross (ARC) supplied the contaminated blood to Georgetown. According to ARC records, the blood had been donated in October 1982 by an individual who subsequently developed AIDS and died from opportunistic infections associated with the disease. At the time of his donation, however, the donor was in good health. Kozup alleged that as a result of the transfusions Matthew received in the days immediately following his birth, he was infected with AIDS. On July 10, 1986, Matthew died, allegedly from complications related to infection with the AIDS virus.

The Kozups sued Georgetown and ARC for $15 million under nine separate counts, alleging negligence, breach of implied warranty, strict liability, lack of informed consent, violation of the District of Columbia Consumer Protection Act, and battery.

The District Court found that Georgetown failed to obtain any consent from the parents for Matthew's transfusions. The general rule in the District of Columbia states, "A surgeon who performs an operation without his patient's consent commits an assault for which he is liable in damages." In the case of a minor patient, the relevant consent is that of the parents, with certain exceptions: in situations where there is a bona fide medical emergency; when the patient is a "mature minor"; when the parents are not readily accessible; or when the parents have given their implied consent. Georgetown argued and the District Court held that the implied consent exception applied in this case. As the District Court put it: "The transfusions were absolutely necessary to save his [Matthew's] life. Confronted with a decision whether to permit this treatment or to decline it...no reasonable person in the Kozups' position would have declined."

That may well be true, but it is not the standard. Despite the ruling for summary judgment (in which the court can dismiss a claim without a full trial), the Appeals Court ruled that determining credibility, weighing evidence, and drawing legitimate inferences from the facts are jury functions, not those of a judge. The court said a summary judgment was improper, and the family should have an opportunity to plead its case to a jury. The Kozups offered some evidence relating to other possible courses of treatment, and Georgetown's evidence did not exclude those possibilities with the certainty required at the summary judgment level.

(continued)

The message of the Kozup case is that the question of consent will not necessarily be dismissed by a court under the traditional principle of implied consent. Healthcare executives must be aware of the importance of informed consent to the courts, and how courts have weighed the right to consent more heavily in recent years. Each institution will be subject to the precedent and priorities of its own court system, but the Kozup case stands as a cautionary tale for all. Even if treatment is lifesaving and reasonable, it does not mean the courts will deny the plaintiffs from presenting their complaint to a jury. Consent must be obtained, unless that process itself would prevent necessary emergency treatment.

SOURCE: *Stephen Kozup, et al., Appellant, v. Georgetown University* (1988).

## Strategies for Healthcare Executives

- On-call support should be provided for ED staff for difficult consent issues. This support may come from legal counsel, risk management staff, or an administrator.
- Leadership should support an imperative that treats urgent matters first and clarifies consent issues later.
- The organization should provide regular training sessions for staff delineating the rights of patients and the responsibilities of caregivers, in particular when consent is unclear or unreliable.

## Recommended Readings

Alexander, B., B. M. Broccolo, K. F. Conley, A. R. Daniels, M. Dube, R. G. Hoban, C. B. Hutto, C. C. Loepere, D. E. Matyas, T. W. Mayo, J. J. Miles, R. E. Sallade, M. F. Schaff, S. O. Scheutzow, D. J. Schwartz, and E. T. Thomas. 2008. *AHLA Fundamentals of Health Law* Fourth Edition. Washington, DC: American Health Lawyers Association.

Miller, R. 2006. "Decision-Making Concerning Individuals." In *Problems in Health Care Law,* Ninth Edition. Sudbury, MA: Jones and Bartlett Learning. This chapter is an excellent, thorough review of all elements concerning informed consent.

# Part III

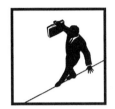

# RISK MANAGEMENT STRATEGIES FOR HIGH-RISK CLINICAL ENTITIES

Risk cannot be solely managed by the clinicians and front-line workers—it will take executive leadership to bring about real change. Dr. Welch and Dr. Klauer have more than 37 years' experience in emergency medicine between them and almost as many years as physician leaders and consultants. They believe physicians and nurses in the trenches will need help from healthcare leadership to "Move Your Dot" (IHI 2003) in risk management and patient safety. Both have observed that clinicians appreciate the help in improving quality and safety in the ED, and executive leadership always drives change.

The healthcare executive is typically not a practicing clinician. But the authors believe that the healthcare executive and leader can help the front-line clinician to succeed by providing the resources necessary to manage high-risk clinical entities and by standardizing the approach to the riskiest of them. Part III identifies the eleven clinical entities, diagnoses and scenarios that account for the overwhelming majority of lawsuits in emergency medicine. Each disease, injury, illness, or process flaw is approached in layman's terms with statistics about its incidence and prevalence and how it is often misdiagnosed. Then each entity is approached with a "Strategy for

Success," explaining the standardized management of these dangerous clinical scenarios with cases from the medical literature or from the clinicians' practices peppered into the chapters to bring the topics to life.

# CHAPTER 23

# Medication Errors

## In This Chapter

- The Magnitude of the Problem
- Challenges in the Emergency Department: The Unique Environment
- Strategies for Success: Communication
- Deadly Drug Categories
- The Ten Troublemakers of Medication Administration
- Effective Strategies to Reduce Medication Errors in the ED
- The Role of Executive Leadership
- Case Study
- Strategies for Healthcare Executives

## THE MAGNITUDE OF THE PROBLEM

Adverse events occur in 4 percent of hospitalized patients, which accounts for an estimated 180,000 deaths and 1 million injuries each year in the United States (Leape 1994). Almost 20 percent of adverse events are **medication errors**, leading to almost 100 deaths a day! One study has shown medication errors occur in 15 percent of ED visits and with higher frequency on the night shift (Vila-de-Muga 2011). This is astoundingly high in contrast to the 1.4 medication errors recorded per hospital admission (Leape 1994). Though only 2.4 percent of medication errors result in serious

> **Medication error:** Any preventable event that may cause or lead to inappropriate medication use or patient harm while the medication is in the control of the healthcare professional, patient, or consumer.

injury, that they are occurring on our watch and by our hands is a compelling enough reason to want to remedy the problem.

**Adverse drug event (ADE):** An injury associated with administration of a medication, which may include a drug reaction, drug–disease interaction, drug–drug interaction, allergic reactions or medication side effects.

**Injuries Associated with Adverse Drug Events in the ED**

- Short-term morbidity: anaphylaxis, respiratory failure, GI bleed
- Long-term morbidity: renal failure, anoxia, deafness
- Death

**Adverse drug events** have been reported in 1.7 percent of all ED encounters (Leape 1994). Ninety percent go unrecognized; the data on medication errors have only come to light when pharmacists have been placed in emergency departments to observe and monitor for errors. It is believed 70 percent of adverse drug events are preventable (Hays 2007).

Three percent of malpractice claims involve adverse drug reactions, and the average award comes close to six figures (Welch 2010e)

**Most Frequent Medication Error Allegations**

- Allergic reaction
- Excessive dosage
- Incorrect drug given
- Contraindicated medication
- Adverse drug reaction

# CHALLENGES IN THE EMERGENCY DEPARTMENT: THE UNIQUE ENVIRONMENT

Unlike other clinical specialties, the practice of emergency medicine places no limits on the number of patients that can present for care at a given time. Because of EMTALA regulations the doors can never close, even with patients arriving in surges that overwhelm the resources of the department. Multitasking and interruptions are common to this setting, and several studies have shown that the intensity of the clinical work is greater than in other office or clinic environments (Chisholm et al. 2011; Chisholm 2001, 2000). As mentioned in Chapter 1, the ED has been referred to as a "laboratory for error," where time-pressured work is performed in an environment of uncertainty. In fact, some suggest that you could not design an environment better suited for making medical errors! To devise strategies to improve safety and minimize risk in the emergency department, a thorough understanding of its unique features and elements is required.

---

**Contributors to Medication Errors**

- Distractions
- Multiple caregivers
- Handoffs
- Sound-alike drugs
- Lack of standardization
- Unfamiliarity with medications

---

## STRATEGIES FOR SUCCESS: COMMUNICATION

One of our biggest challenges will also be our best hope for reducing medical error: communication. Clinicians in the emergency department use a communication style and technique that is informal, on the fly, and rife with opportunity for medical error. Part of this may be due to the rapid changes in the specialty. This casual verbal-orders style may have been appropriate and even effective when an emergency department was seeing a mere 50 patients a day in the 1980s. Fast forward 30 years, and most departments see more than twice that. Patients arrive in surges on the evening shift and need much care that is on the clock and more technical. It is not unusual for staff to refer to patients by room number or by chief complaint: "Can you give my kidney stone more morphine?" "Dr. Welch, can I give Room 3 some more Zofran?"

Tightening this casual communication style with repeat-backs and call-backs would help the current chaotic environment of the emergency department become safer. The Institute for Healthcare Improvement uses a comparative audio recording of two cardiac arrests when teaching physicians, nurses, and healthcare leaders about communication. In the first, a civilian hospital's staff conducts a typical cardiac resuscitation in the emergency department, and it sounds like most of the codes you have witnessed. There is no clear chain of command. Orders are barked into the air at no one in particular, and it is hard to tell if anyone has acted on them.

Many people are talking at once. Then the audio switches to a cardiac arrest at a military hospital. Though there might be some soft background communication going on, there is clearly one voice in charge:

"Nurse, I would like one amp of bicarb IV push Stat!"

"Doctor, that is one amp of bicarb IV push Stat!"

"That is correct."

"I am giving one amp of bicarbonate IV push at 1815."

By using a clear chain of command, repeatbacks, and callbacks, there is no doubt in anyone's mind what has been ordered and given. The chaos is minimized, and the communication is about as tight as it can be. It follows a precise script, and it is clear who is giving orders to whom. The verbal clarity makes it easy for a charting nurse or tech to record what has been given. Medication administration, both in cardiac arrest situations and in the general practice of emergency medicine, would benefit greatly from such rigor in communication. Training in this type of communication as part of med teams training has been effective in ORs, trauma suites, and labor and delivery and is reported increasingly in the literature (Cooper et al. 2011; Hull 2011; Capella 2010).

## DEADLY DRUG CATEGORIES

In the Center for Emergency Medical Education's "High Risk Emergency Medicine" course, doctors are taught there are 11 categories of medication that account for the overwhelming majority of adverse drug events in healthcare (Exhibit 23.1) These

**Exhibit 23.1: Deadly Drug Categories**

| Cardiac medications | Psychiatric medications | Antibiotics | Immunosuppressants |
|---|---|---|---|
| Anticoagulants | Anticonvulsants | | Narcotics |
| Antihypertensives | Diabetes medications | NSAIDs | Benzodiazepines |

SOURCE: CEME (2010).

drugs have a narrow therapeutic window (the difference between a therapeutic dose and a toxic dose is small) and have the capacity for dangerous interactions with other drugs.

## THE TEN TROUBLEMAKERS OF MEDICATION ADMINISTRATION

Within the 11 categories, ten "superstar" drugs and drug categories are most likely to result in medication errors or adverse drug events.

1. *Potassium chloride (KCL).* There have been at least ten deaths from KCL in the clinical setting. Eight occurred because it was given IV push, and in six cases it was mistaken for another drug. Potassium chloride is the chemical used in lethal injections and is wildly dangerous. Standardization would prevent mixing of the solutions on clinical floors (where mistakes can be made). All potassium drips should be prepared in the pharmacy and always infused with a pump.

2. *Opiates.* While opiates are used frequently in the ED and have a remarkable potential for alleviating pain, they often cause respiratory depression or even failure and can also cause hypotension. Standardization for safety should include double checking every narcotic order by a second nurse and placing patients on pulse oximetry and telemetry whenever IV narcotics are administered. Also a standardized order for stat IV Narcan (which reverses narcotics) should be ordered whenever a nurse is worried that a patient is becoming unstable because of the narcotics.

3. *Insulin.* Low blood sugar from overdoses of insulin is a frequent occurrence and can cause coma or seizures. Standardizations such as those described for opiates might also make sense when IV insulin is being used in the ED. In addition, bedside blood sugar determinations should be part of the standardization.

4. *Heparin.* Heparin is dispensed in two concentrations: One is for therapeutic doses, and the other is for flushing IVs. Baxter, the manufacturer, has done much to change the bottles, which were once identical with slightly different-colored blue labels. Therapeutic heparin and the IV flush should be stored in distinctly different locations. This may be another medication that would benefit from a second-nurse double check.

5. *Aspirin.* Yes, that medication in your medicine cabinet—and given to every patient presenting to the ED with chest pain or stroke symptoms by well-accepted protocols—is dangerous! It increasingly accounts for GI bleeds, and aspirin allergy has been associated with asthma and other adverse events. Elderly patients and patients on steroids or other non-steroidal anti-inflammatory agents are at particular risk.

6. *NSAIDS.* Though most clinicians think of these drugs as safer than narcotic pain medicines, in fact they are the number-one cause of adverse events—typically a GI bleed. Having the pharmacist alert the high-risk patient (such as the elderly or patients taking prednisone or Coumadin) might prevent some of these adverse events.

7. *Psychotropics.* Although we do not see the serious arrhythmias associated with tricyclic antidepressants that we saw in the 1980s, there are still possible side effects associated with the SSRI classes and the newer antidepressants. Having pharmacist oversight when drugs—even antibiotics—are mixed with psychotropics is one way to combat this risk.

8. *Coumadin.* Coumadin is by far the most dangerous drug prescribed by physicians. The narrow therapeutic range, the difficulty in regulating the medication, the effects of other drugs and antibiotics on its efficacy, and the fact that it is often prescribed for frail individuals at risk of falling all contribute to a dangerous milieu. Standardization should include the automatic INR (testing for Coumadin efficacy and overdose) on each patient who lists Coumadin as a medication. Pharmacists should provide oversight for any medication to be added to Coumadin.

9. *Combinations.* When a patient is on two or more medications, he has a 13 percent chance of having an adverse drug interaction. When the seventh drug is added to the patient's regimen, that risk shoots up to almost 90 percent (Runciman 2003; Bates 1996). Nearly half of ED patients leave with a new medication. All of this means that we are likely to see more and more adverse drug interactions as the population ages and the complexity of care given increases. Pharmacist oversight is essential.

10. *Pediatrics.* Pediatric patients have a 20 times greater chance of a medication error than adults. When you mix two medications that have the potential for sedation, the risk for an adverse drug interaction is immediately 90 percent (Hughes 2005). One of the most common root causes in pediatric medication errors involves pediatric weights. All pediatric medications are administered based on weight in kilograms. If the dose is calculated on pounds, the patient will effectively get double the necessary dose. Most EDs have a scale that goes back and forth between pounds and kilograms, and

parents often want to know the weight of the child in pounds. The nurse who is trying to hurriedly triage a handful of waiting patients may not note that the scale has been switched to pounds. You could remedy this today by having engineering disable the ability to weigh in pounds or by purchasing a pediatric scale that weighs only in kilograms. Additionally, all pediatric medications should have a repeatback with the physician and a second nurse to double check the dosing calculations.

## EFFECTIVE STRATEGIES TO REDUCE MEDICATION ERRORS IN THE ED

Culture is still one of the biggest impediments to preventing medication errors. Far too many organizations still respond in a punitive way to medication errors and employ a name, blame, and shame strategy. When an adverse event occurs, the last person to touch the situation is blamed 80 percent of the time, even though analysis shows that individual is clearly responsible less than 25 percent of the time (Liang 2002).

Most organizations still respond to medication errors with the incident report approach, which carries implicit blame. Few organizations have a robust process in place to capture information and get upstream of near misses in medication errors. Most still retrain individuals when a serious medication error has occurred. In our view, if this error occurred with Dr. A and Nurse B, it can occur tomorrow with Dr. B and Nurse A. The processes and systems need to be fixed.

## THE ROLE OF EXECUTIVE LEADERSHIP

Leadership can and should play a role in promoting safety and preventing medication errors. By careful implementation of standardized protocols the most dangerous scenarios can be avoided. The biggest challenge will be to change the culture to better capture these errors and craft system-level solutions. This culture change will have to start with executive leadership and may at first be at odds with certain departments, such as risk management. But without putting an end to the old blame-and-shame culture, success in this area will be limited.

Actor Dennis Quaid's wife gave birth to twins prematurely, and the babies started their lives in the neonatal intensive care unit. They had IVs because of concern over sepsis, and they were getting prophylactic antibiotics. Both babies as well as a third in the unit had mistakenly been given full-strength heparin instead of heparin flush (a more dilute solution used to keep tiny IVs from clotting off).

All three babies were given the antidote to heparin after the error was discovered, and none suffered any adverse drug event.

These babies were cared for in the Cedars Sinai Medical Center in Los Angeles, which had a robust system of checks and balances in place even before this high-profile, high-publicity case occurred:

- Double check at pharmacy by technician
- Double check on pediatrics floor by technician
- Nurse check before administration

Baxter Pharmaceuticals had already changed the bottles of the two concentrations of heparin. Previously the bottles had been the same size and shape and had only different shades of blue lettering to distinguish one from the other. In response to reports of errors Baxter had already changed the size, shape, and color of the bottles to distinguish them and had a red warning label on the dangerous full-concentration compound.

In spite of all of these safety initiatives this medication error still occurred. Is there any doubt we need to always be on guard for the possibility of human error in the administration of medicines?

SOURCE: Landro (2008).

## Strategies for Healthcare Executives

- Make recognizing, tracking, preventing, and mitigating against medication errors an organizational priority.
- Involve the board in these initiatives.
- Consider placing a pharmacist in the ED.
- Craft standardizations for the high-risk categories, medications, and situations in the ED.
- Reward healthcare workers who identify medication errors before they occur or who find solutions that fix systems.
- Track and monitor medication errors and celebrate improvements.

## Recommended Readings

Croskerry, P. 2009. "Medication Safety in the Emergency Department." *Patient Safety in Emergency Medicine*, Chapter 21, 144–48. Philadelphia: Lippincott Williams & Wilkins.

Leonard, M., A. Frankel, and T. Simmonds, with K. Vega. 2004. *Achieving Safe and Reliable Healthcare*. Chicago: Health Administration Press.

Spath, P. 2000. *Error Reduction in Healthcare: A Systems Approach to Improving Patient Safety*. Chicago: Health Forum Inc.

# CHAPTER 24

# Appendicitis

**In This Chapter**

- The Magnitude of the Problem
- Strategies for Success: History and Physical Examination
- Strategies for Success: Laboratory
- Strategies for Success: Imaging
- Patient Care Options
- The Role of Executive Leadership
- Case Study
- Strategies for Healthcare Executives

## THE MAGNITUDE OF THE PROBLEM

Appendicitis is common, occurring in 1.1 per 1,000 individuals annually (Søreide 1984). Although it occurs less frequently in children and the elderly, it can occur in any age group. Unfortunately, appendicitis is also misdiagnosed at a rate of 9 percent in males and 23.2 percent in females (Naoum et al. 2002). Female patients are more likely to be misdiagnosed because of the greater number of diagnostic entities possible, potentially explaining the source of pain as an ovarian cyst, urinary tract infection, or pelvic inflammatory disease.

When diagnostic errors occur, patients are often discharged. Generally, if appendicitis is not diagnosed within 24 hours, it will result in complications such as rupture, sepsis, and even death.

## STRATEGIES FOR SUCCESS: HISTORY AND PHYSICAL EXAMINATION

The classic presentation of fever, right lower-quadrant pain, and anorexia (loss of appetite) is often not seen until late in the disease. Until then, the patient may experience many different symptoms and may present in a variety of ways. Patients may complain of pain in the upper abdomen, bladder, lower back, or left lower quadrant. Changes in bowel habits are common; however, patients are no more likely to experience diarrhea than constipation. Errors are frequently made attributing abdominal tenderness to constipation. Diarrhea is often assumed to be secondary to a viral infection. Thus, many cases of appendicitis are misdiagnosed as gastroenteritis. Fever is commonly described as a classic feature of appendicitis, but it is just as likely to be absent. History and physical examinations, particularly early in the course of this disease, reveal varied symptoms and nonspecific physical findings. Thus, the best plan is to consider an appendicitis diagnosis in any patient with undifferentiated abdominal pain.

## STRATEGIES FOR SUCCESS: LABORATORY

Laboratory diagnostics often discussed with appendicitis are the white blood cell count (WBC), erythrocyte sedimentation rate (ESR), and the c-reactive protein (CRP), all of which are tests for inflammatory mediators. As with all inflammatory mediators, they are sensitive but nonspecific. In other words, these levels can be elevated with appendicitis but may not be. Many patients with appendicitis have normal tests. WBC, ESR, and CRP may be factored into the diagnostic picture, but they should not be used to rule out appendicitis. Occasionally, the inflamed appendix will lie near the bladder or one of the ureters, which may even result in **pyuria** (WBCs in the urine). Pyuria, in the absence of other signs suggesting urinary tract infection, should prompt further concern about appendicitis.

> **Pyuria:** Pus cells in the urine.

## STRATEGIES FOR SUCCESS: IMAGING

Plain radiographs, such as an acute abdominal series, are not very useful in diagnosing appendicitis. One exception is the rare finding of an appendicolith (calcification within the appendix), which in the context of abdominal pain is diagnostic for appendicitis. Ultrasound may be useful but depends on the expertise of individual technologists and radiologists. In women, ultrasound is often a reasonable diagnostic option, as it can also assess gynecological disorders. However, if the appendix cannot be adequately evaluated via ultrasound, and appendicitis is in the differential diagnosis, use caution in relying on the results. For instance, in a female patient with right lower quadrant pain, in whom the appendix has not been seen on the scan, the discovery of an ovarian cyst on the ultrasound may be incidental. Such incidental findings are often the source of medical error and misdiagnosis because the physician may erroneously conclude that the patient's pain is from a cyst and not appendicitis.

Computed tomography (CT) is the most commonly used tool for the investigation of appendicitis. Although a positive CT for appendicitis is useful, a negative CT does not rule out the possibility, particularly if the appendix is not well visualized. CT may also miss early appendicitis. Patients who present soon after symptom onset may be best served by observation without CT. If a patient is observed at home, returns for scheduled ED re-evaluation, and is not improved, a CT scan can be performed at that time, avoiding the expense and radiation exposure of a second study. This may be particularly important in pediatric patients.

CT scans may also delay surgical treatment for appendicitis because many surgeons refuse to evaluate an ED patient for appendicitis unless a CT scan has been performed. Certainly, in some cases, early surgical evaluation is warranted and must be supported. CT rates for appendicitis evaluations have increased from 12.3 percent in 1998 to 88.4 percent in 2004 (Frei et al. 2008). This trend of ordering more CT scans has increased the average time to surgical intervention from 250 minutes to 426 minutes. Although there are no definitive data on patient outcomes, these delays may negatively affect patient care.

In addition, leaders should consider how CT scans are performed. Many radiologists prefer that oral and intravenous contrast be administered prior to obtaining a CT of the abdomen and pelvis. Such preparations take anywhere from one to three hours to complete and have been deemed largely unnecessary in the investigation of most abdominal processes (Ganguli et al. 2006). Especially with newer CT scanners, the routine use of contrast is not warranted. Ordering an imaging study that takes one to three hours functionally reduces the patient capacity of the emergency department. Some may argue that the appendix may not be visualized without the contrast, but this is debatable. In those patients, it is also likely that the appendix would not be visualized if contrast had been given. Further, in cases where the appendix is not visualized and no inflammatory changes are noted in the right lower quadrant, the incidence of appendicitis is much lower than in cases that did not involve a CT scan. In other words, there is negative predictive value in performing a CT that does not visualize the appendix.

## PATIENT CARE OPTIONS

The diagnosis of appendicitis should be included in the differential diagnosis in any patient with abdominal pain, no matter how atypical the presentation may seem. One study reports that 30 to 45 percent of patients will present with atypical symptoms (Frei et al. 2008). Every patient in the emergency department should be advised of the consideration of appendicitis and of the signs and symptoms to watch for if discharge is being considered. In patients with equivocal evaluations, observations over 12 to 24 hours should always be considered. The clinical circumstances will dictate the appropriateness of inpatient versus outpatient observation. In cases of outpatient observation, scheduled follow up in the ED should be considered as a patient safety and risk management tool. Reassessing these patients should occur as early as eight hours later, but no later than 24 hours.

---

### Solutions for Success: Appendicitis

- Provide appropriate analgesics to the patient, which will facilitate the ability to perform an abdominal examination.
- Understand the substantial limitations to diagnostic studies and discuss them with each patient.
- Order CT scans judiciously and without the routine use of contrast.
- Perform immediate surgical evaluation for patients with a clinical presentation consistent with appendicitis.
- In patients with equivocal evaluations, observation over time—no more than 24 hours—should be used to further assess the patient.

---

Even if a CT scan is performed and a normal appendix is visualized, the patient should not be told, "You cannot have appendicitis." It is appropriate to advise the patient that it is less likely that appendicitis is the cause of her symptoms. However, due to the natural history of appendicitis, the diagnosis is still possible; emphasize appropriate follow-up.

# THE ROLE OF EXECUTIVE LEADERSHIP

The executive leadership team should be involved with setting protocols for performing CT scans to investigate the possibility of appendicitis, acknowledging that the routine use of contrast can be unnecessary and inefficient. Share with the medical staff your expectation that when a surgical consult is requested, prior to CT, the surgeons will not refuse to evaluate the patient. Further, it may be helpful to approach primary care medical staff members about admitting select patients who require inpatient observation but do not clearly need a surgeon at the time of admission.

---

### Case Study

A 19-year-old male presents with eight hours of right lower quadrant pain. Though he has a low-grade fever he has not had nausea, and in fact he reports just eating a "tall stack" of pancakes without vomiting.

The emergency physician is concerned about the young man's clinical exam. The patient has signs of peritonitis. The physician calls the surgeon, but the surgeon will not see the patient without a CT scan. A CT scan is ordered without oral contrast, which has been the protocol for some time, but the radiologist is new and demands that the patient drink oral contrast first. The patient is now feeling sicker and is having a hard time drinking the contrast, despite the administration of antinausea medications. He finishes the contrast but then promptly vomits all of the contrast material up. The ED physician orders a nasogastric tube to administer the contrast. But the CT technician refuses to do the CT scan until the contrast has been in the gut for 45 minutes, because that is the protocol.

The patient has been in the ED more than four hours when the CT report comes back positive for appendicitis with likely perforation.

SOURCE: Welch, risk management case review.

---

## Strategies for Healthcare Executives

- Recognize the limitations of laboratory testing in diagnosing appendicitis.
- Recognize the complexity of the diagnosis of appendicitis and the complexity of diagnostic evaluation of abdominal pain patients.
- Avoid delays using oral contrast protocols.
- Establish a protocol of surgical evaluation when requested by the emergency physician.
- Employ the strategy of scheduled ED follow-up in equivocal cases
- Include discussions about the possibility of appendicitis in the discharge instructions of all patients presenting with a complaint of abdominal pain.

## Recommended Readings

Ege, G., H. Akman, A. Sahin, D. Bugra, and K. Kuzucu. 2002. "Diagnostic Value of Unenhanced Helical CT in Adult Patients with Suspected Acute Appendicitis." *British Journal of Radiology* 75 (897): 721–25

Frei, S. P., W. F. Bond, R. K. Bazuro, D. M. Richardson, G. M. Sierzega, and J. F. Reed. 2008. "Appendicitis Outcomes with Increasing Computed Tomographic Scanning." *American Journal of Emergency Medicine* 26 (1): 39–44.

Keyzer, C., P. Cullus, D. Tack, V. De Maertelaer, P. Bohy, and P. Gevenois. 2009. "AMDCT for Suspected Acute Appendicitis in Adults: Impact of Oral and IV Contrast Media at Standard-dose and Simulated Low-Dose Techniques." *American Journal of Roentgenology* 193 (5): 1272–81.

# CHAPTER 25

# Ectopic Pregnancy

**In This Chapter**

- The Magnitude of the Problem
- Strategies for Success: Lab Testing
- Strategies for Success: Imaging
- Added Risk: Methotrexate in the ED
- The Role of Executive Leadership
- Case Study
- Strategies for Healthcare Executives

## THE MAGNITUDE OF THE PROBLEM

Ectopic pregnancy is a pregnancy outside of the uterus, usually in one of the fallopian tubes. Most ectopic pregnancies occur in women between the ages of 25 and 34 and are responsible for 10 percent of maternal deaths. If an ectopic pregnancy goes undetected, it will likely rupture, with a mortality rate of 1 in every 1,000 ectopic pregnancies.

Ectopic pregnancies are not considered viable under any circumstances. The primary objective is to protect the mother from a complication secondary to rupture. Ectopic pregnancies are common, occurring in between 1 in 40 and 1 in 160 pregnancies, but can be difficult to detect when they present. Data suggest that the diagnosis of ectopic is often delayed, and even when detected, errors may occur, resulting in treatment decisions that do not meet the standard of care (Tayal, Cohen, and Norton 2004). Fertility drugs increase the likelihood of ectopic pregnancies.

In a patient who is not on fertility drugs, an ultrasound showing an intrauterine pregnancy would reduce the likelihood of ectopic pregnancy to a very low level. Thus, in most cases, no further investigation is necessary. However, if the patient is on fertility drugs, a twin ectopic gestation must be considered. In fertility patients who have symptoms suggesting ectopic pregnancy, the presence of an intrauterine pregnancy should not dissuade the prudent physician from pursuing the diagnosis of ectopic pregnancy.

## STRATEGIES FOR SUCCESS: LAB TESTING

Timely access to diagnostic information is critical. The National Quality Forum has endorsed performing a pregnancy test on any female patient of childbearing age who is capable of becoming pregnant and is presenting with abdominal pain. Urinary pregnancy tests are sensitive at seven days post-conception. However, dilute urine (specific gravity < 1.015 g/dl) may produce false negative results due to the dilutional effect on human chorionic gonadotropin hormone (HCG) levels. Serum qualitative tests may be ordered as an alternative. When the specific gravity of the urine is not dilute, the sensitivity of the two tests is the same, and the bedside urine test is much more efficient.

Ideally every emergency department should have a standing order for a urine pregnancy test on all childbearing-aged females with abdominal pain or vaginal bleeding. The decision to order this test need not be left to the individual physician. A standardized order is more appropriate and effective.

Quantitative HCG sampling provides an actual pregnancy hormone level. Through research, physicians have tried to identify a "discriminatory zone," a hormone level at which an intrauterine pregnancy would most likely be detected. Discriminatory zones were not designed, and should not be used, to determine when an ultrasound should be performed to investigate concern for ectopic pregnancy. New research increasingly shows they are unreliable at predicting outcomes (Wang et al. 2011). Any woman with abdominal pain and a positive pregnancy test should have an ultrasound.

# STRATEGIES FOR SUCCESS: IMAGING

Ultrasound access is an issue in many hospitals. If the service is available during the normal service hours, limited studies for life-threatening diagnoses such as ectopic pregnancy should be available after hours as well. If your institution does not have such resources available, transfer agreements should be in place for the emergent evaluation of patients with suspected ectopic pregnancy.

Another alternative is the endorsement and support of emergency department bedside ultrasound. Investing in bedside ultrasound units may be capital dollars well spent to provide this service, generate revenue, and reduce risk. Though bedside ultrasound is still found in only a minority of community hospital emergency departments, it is becoming more prevalent.

Even with ultrasound, the diagnosis of ectopic pregnancy can be challenging. If a gestational sac is seen in the uterus, the diagnosis has been effectively excluded. But in many cases it can be too early to see the sac. In particular it can be virtually impossible to differentiate an early pregnancy in the uterus from an ectopic pregnancy before eight weeks. Remember, the ultrasound cannot tell blood from fluid in the abdomen. Many women with a ruptured ovarian cyst will have fluid visible on pelvic ultrasound, and many physicians consider small amounts of fluid to be normal. But any free fluid seen on an ultrasound to diagnose ectopic pregnancy can be blood and should be considered an indication of ruptured ectopic until proven otherwise.

When the diagnosis of ectopic pregnancy is suspected but has not been excluded or confirmed, patient management and disposition issues will bedevil the emergency physician. The early ectopic pregnancy may require time and repeat labs and imaging to confirm. Who will manage the patient and assume the risk in this gray interval?

---

### Patient Care Options: Ectopic Pregnancies

- For stable patients with normal ultrasound, contact the ob/gyn on call to arrange follow-up and discharge the patient.
- For patients with free fluid in the pelvis, no intrauterine gestational sac, and ongoing pain, arrange a bedside consultation with the on-call ob/gyn
- For all unstable patients, admit for observation.

---

Discharge with close follow-up is appropriate only after phone consultation to confirm the plan and availability of the ob/gyn consultant to see the patient and

**Exhibit 25.1: Diagnostic and Process Error Related to Ectopic Pregnancy**

| | | | |
|---|---|---|---|
| *Diagnostic access* | No point-of-care testing for urinary HCG in the ED | No quantitative HCG (measured hormone level) | No pelvic ultrasound available 24/7 |
| *Misapplication of data* | Dilute urine produces false negatives | Discriminatory zones used to determine when and if an ultrasound should be performed | Concluding that an empty uterus does not exclude ectopic pregnancy; free fluid implies a ruptured ectopic |
| *Medical staff accountability* | No ob/gyn on call and available 24/7 | No next-day follow-up available | No ob/gyn available for bedside consultation when requested |

only in the most stable patients. This disposition should be limited to patients with a normal ultrasound. Discharge after bedside consultation should be reserved for stable patients with equivocal findings on ultrasound. Deference should be given to the consultant to decide if admission or outpatient follow-up is appropriate, provided the patient is stable. Patients who are not appropriate for discharge may be admitted to the floor to await evaluation of the consultant.

Perhaps the easiest management decisions will surround the patient who has a proven ectopic and who is unstable. We believe such patients should not go to the floor for any interval, but rather they should go from the ED to the OR. Finally, stable patients with confirmed ectopics need ob/gyn consultation immediately.

On a final note, ectopic pregnancies often result in bad outcomes, including death. The time to intervene is often prior to the definitive diagnosis being made.

## ADDED RISK: METHOTREXATE IN THE ED

Methotrexate is an antimetabolite that inhibits rapid cell division and pregnancy implantation. In the past, ectopic pregnancy was considered a gynecologic surgical emergency and patients were taken almost immediately to the operating room. Our ability to diagnose pregnancy at an early stage and the added technology of ultrasound have taken the urgency out of the diagnosis. In addition there is now a nonsurgical approach to the treatment of early ectopic pregnancy—methotrexate—which is a widely accepted treatment for ectopic pregnancies. However, there is risk that ectopics treated with methotrexate may result in rupture, just as other ectopic pregnancies do. If methotrexate is to be used, patient, provider, and hospital risk must be managed by strictly adhering to recommended treatment guidelines. Methotrexate cannot be used after rupture, in hemodynamically unstable patients, or if fetal cardiac activity is detected.

Although opinions vary about the exact parameters of optimal serum HCG levels, gestational age, and size of **adnexal mass**, the consensus is that the smaller and the younger the gestation, the less the risk of rupture. Following is a list of accepted standards for the administration of methotrexate that will minimize risk.

> **Adnexal mass:** A mass in the space in and around the fallopian tube or ovary that is suggestive of an ectopic pregnancy. It may also be a malignancy, a complex ovarian cyst, or an infectious process.

## Guidelines for Methotrexate Use

- No evidence of rupture or hemoperitoneum
- Hemodynamically stable
- Less than eight weeks' gestation
- Serum HCG less than 5,000
- Adnexal mass less than 4 cm
- No fetal cardiac activity
- Confirmed ectopic, not requiring surgical confirmation

SOURCE: Jazayeri (2008).

The nuanced and risky decision to treat an ectopic pregnancy patient with methotrexate instead of surgery belongs in the hands of the ob/gyn, not the ED. In addition, the administration of methotrexate, a highly toxic drug, should not be done in an uncontrolled environment such as the ED. Organizations such as Intermountain Healthcare require that all orders for methotrexate to treat ectopic pregnancy be given by an ob/gyn and all infusions be given by an infusion nurse (with special credentials and certifications) in an infusion center. Remember this drug has another life as a chemotherapy agent. Although methotrexate is an acceptable treatment for some ectopic pregnancies, the fact remains that this is a surgical disease. We recommend the careful crafting of policies and procedures that recognize the dangers and possible side effects of this treatment and offer the safest options, taking into account the resources of the facility.

There is no room for the "art of medicine" when there is irrefutable evidence for a best practice in a given clinical situation. Thus, individual physician decision making in such circumstances is not only risky but also inappropriate and inefficient.

## Standardization and Policies to Reduce Missed Ectopic Pregnancies and Minimize Risk

- Pregnancy test on all childbearing age females with abdominal pain or vaginal bleeding, preferably in triage before the physician encounter
- Ultrasound on all females with positive pregnancy test and abdominal pain or vaginal bleeding
- Bedside ob/gyn consultation if the ultrasound is abnormal and ectopic is suspected or the patient has shown signs of instability. Continued pain should be considered a potential sign of ruptured ectopic or raise suspicion for increased risk for rupture
- Timely and guaranteed ob/gyn follow-up if ultrasound is normal and ectopic is suspected (stable patients)
- ED protocols in place for "gray zone" patients who are stable and have normal ultrasounds
- Bedside ob/gyn consultation for confirmed ectopic, even if the patient is stable
- Unstable patients with confirmed ectopic are resuscitated in the ED until they go to the OR or to the ICU to await surgery
- All methotrexate decisions made by ob/gyn, and all methotrexate orders given by ob/gyn
- Standardize when, where, and who administers methotrexate in your institution

## THE ROLE OF EXECUTIVE LEADERSHIP

The role of the hospital executive in reducing risk with ectopic pregnancies is to ensure access to appropriate diagnostics. The essential diagnostics are urinary pregnancy test (preferably in triage), qualitative serum HCG, serum quantitative HCG, and most important, access to pelvic ultrasound. In addition, providing a call schedule that includes ob/gyn coverage is essential. For those without obstetric services, this need can be filled by those practicing gynecology alone. By providing the consultants with the hospital's expectations regarding response and availability, the treatment of patients with suspected or confirmed ectopic pregnancy can be much safer. Leadership must articulate these expectations to the medical staff at large and to the ob/gyn practitioners in particular. Discussing the bad outcomes or near misses with the ED and the ob/gyn department can help make the case to the clinicians. Celebrating the good outcomes once the policies are initiated can increase staff support for the initiatives.

### Case Study

EMP (Emergency Medicine Physicians) is a large staffing and management group composed of more than 700 emergency physicians. EMP is physician-owned and -operated and has a robust and comprehensive quality improvement program. Among the standardizations recommended at its more than 60 locations is a pregnancy test as a standing order for women of childbearing age with abdominal pain.

EMP is self-insured and fastidiously tracks closed claims data to improve patient safety and to inform their providers about malpractice risks and trends, so standardizing this evaluation was a primary objective. (The National Quality Forum has endorsed performing a pregnancy test on all women with abdominal pain presenting to the ED, and this performance measure has been sent to CMS for consideration.) By enacting this recommendation along with other protocols and guidelines for the management of patients who may have an ectopic pregnancy, EMP has a near-zero miss rate for ectopic pregnancies.

SOURCE: Nipomnick (2009).

### Strategies for Healthcare Executives

- Provide laboratory diagnostic resources.
- Ensure 24/7 availability of pelvic ultrasound.
- Ensure access to ob/gyn consultation and patient follow-up.
- Avoid delegating the methotrexate treatment decision to the emergency physician.
- Craft an institutional plan for methotrexate administration.

## Recommended Readings

Dart, R. G., B. Kaplan, and C. Cox. 1997. "Transvaginal Ultrasound in Patients with Low Beta-Human Chorionic Gonadotropin Values: How Often Is the Study Diagnostic?" *Annals of Emergency Medicine* 30 (2): 206–9.

Jazayeri, A. 2008. "Surgical Management of Ectopic Pregnancy." http://emedicine.medscape.com/article/267384-overview, posted January 7.

Rabischong, B., X. Tran, A. A. Sleiman, D. Larraín, P. Jaffeux, B. Aublet-Cuvelier, J. L. Pouly, and H. Fernandez. 2010. "Predictive Factors of Failure in Management of Ectopic Pregnancy with Single-Dose Methotrexate: A General Population-Based Analysis from the Auvergne Register, France." *Fertility and Sterility* 95 (1): 401–4.

Stein, J. C., R. Wang, N. Adler, J. Boscardin, V. L. Jacoby, G. Won, R. Goldstein, and M. A. Kohn. 2010. "Emergency Physician Ultrasonography for Evaluating Patients at Risk for Ectopic Pregnancy: A Meta-Analysis." *Annals of Emergency Medicine* 56 (6): 674–83.

# CHAPTER 26

# Aortic Aneurysm and Dissection

**In This Chapter**

- The Magnitude of the Problem
- Strategies for Success: History and Physical Examination
- Strategies for Success: Imaging
- Patient Care Options
- The Role of Executive Leadership
- Case Study
- Strategies for Healthcare Executives

## THE MAGNITUDE OF THE PROBLEM

Aortic aneurysms and aortic dissections are both potential vascular catastrophes. Although many healthcare providers use these terms interchangeably, each represents a distinct pathological entity with unique characteristics. An **aortic aneurysm** is a dilation of the aortic width by 50 percent of the normal artery. This can occur in the thoracic or abdominal aorta. However, it is most commonly reported in the abdomen. Abdominal aortic dissection (AAA) is called the "triple-A" in ER jargon. In the abdomen, a minimal dilation of 3 cm is necessary to meet the definition. Aneurysmal dilation may result in weakening of the arterial wall, resulting in a leak or rupture.

An **aortic dissection** is a separation of the layers of the arterial wall. This may occur in conjunction with arterial degradation and aneurysm formation. Aortic dissection does not imply the presence of an aneurysm. Aortic dissections typically occur in the chest. Aortic aneurysms may also have associated dissection. However, a ruptured or leaking aneurysm does not imply associated dissection.

**Aortic dissection:**
A separation of the layers of the arterial wall. This may occur in conjunction with aneurysm formation. This typically occurs in the chest, in the thoracic aorta.

**Aortic aneurysm:** A ballooning or widening of the main artery (the aorta) as it courses down through the body. The aneurysm weakens the wall of the aorta and can end in the aorta rupturing with catastrophic consequences. These are typically found in the abdomen.

In contrast to aortic aneurysms, the prevalence of aortic dissection is difficult to assess, as it is often diagnosed during autopsy. The incidence is estimated to be 5 to 30 cases per million lives annually. Dissections are noted in 1 in 10,000 hospital admissions, and 2,000 cases are reported annually. Dissections occur primarily in African-American males between the ages of 40 and 70 years, with the peak incidence between ages 50 to 65 years. Despite this peak age group, it is important to recognize that this disease has a bimodal age distribution, with another spike in younger patients in their 20s to 40s who have other diseases such as Marfan's syndrome, which predisposes to dissection. Aortic dissection is three times more likely in men than in women. The mortality rate is 1 to 2 percent every hour for the first 24 to 48 hours of a dissection.

The prevalence rate for AAA is 0.5 to 3.2 percent. Rupture occurs in 4.4 cases per 100,000. The disease is seen most often in white males aged 50 or older (peak incidence at age 70) and occurs five times more often in men than women. Ruptured AAA is the 13th most common cause of death in the United States. Most are asymptomatic prior to rupture, and the rate of rupture is 5 to 10 percent at 5 to 6 cm and greater than 20 percent with aneurysms greater than 7 cm. Some patients experience abdominal pain and back pain as warning symptoms as the aneurysm begins to leak. Twenty-five percent of patients with leaking from an abdominal aortic aneurysm die prior to arrival at the hospital, and 51 percent die if rupture occurs prior to operative intervention (Isselbacher 2005).

Misdiagnosis of either a leaking or ruptured aneurysm or of a dissection will result in delays in definitive management and increased morbidity and mortality.

## STRATEGIES FOR SUCCESS: HISTORY AND PHYSICAL EXAMINATION

Aortic aneurysms are misdiagnosed in approximately 30 percent of cases and given a variety of diagnoses. Exhibit 26.1 lists the most common misdiagnoses given to patients with AAA.

**Exhibit 26.1: Misdiagnosis of Ruptured Aortic Aneurysms**

| Diagnosis | Rate |
| --- | --- |
| Renal colic | 24% |
| Diverticulitis | 13% |
| Gastrointestinal bleed | 13% |
| Acute myocardial infarction | 9% |
| Back pain | 9% |

SOURCE: CEME (2010).

Correct diagnosis of aortic dissection may be challenging. The classic presentation is described as a "ripping" or "tearing" chest pain radiating to the back. Unfortunately, up to 30 percent of patients never experience chest pain. In addition, the presentations are variable, contributing to the 39 percent misdiagnosis rate reported by Hansen and colleagues in 2007. As the thoracic aorta dissects, the blood supply to multiple organs becomes involved, producing a wide array of symptoms. Furthermore, these symptoms are often dynamic in presentation. For instance, a patient may experience chest pain as a dissection begins. As the dissection extends, pain may radiate into the upper back, abdomen, and lower back. Stroke symptoms or headache may develop if the dissection includes the internal carotid artery. Upper extremity pulses may be absent or decreased if the dissection affects the subclavian and/or brachiocephalic arteries. Renal failure may develop if the renal arteries are involved, and of course, if the dissection includes the coronary ostia, an injury pattern may be evident on the patient's ECG. As many of these symptoms are also associated with other diagnoses, these complex presentations can easily pull the most astute physician away from the diagnosis of aortic dissection.

**Pulsatile abdominal mass:** A characteristic of an abdominal aneurysm. The mass can be felt because the aorta has ballooned out and pulses with arterial blood.

The most common misdiagnosis given to patients with AAA is renal colic. More contemporary data has confirmed that this error continues, despite attempts to educate the medical community about this diagnostic error (Acheson et al. 1998). The correct diagnosis can be difficult to make. Physicians are taught to expect the classic triad of **pulsatile abdominal mass**, abdominal pain, and hypotension. However, this triad is only seen in 25 to 50 percent of those presenting with AAA.

# STRATEGIES FOR SUCCESS: IMAGING

Imaging for AAA is reliable and diagnostic. However, the decision to order the imaging studies, in particular CT of the abdomen and pelvis, is frequently in error. Although CT is an excellent test for the detection of aneurysms and an associated leak or rupture, ordering such a study in lieu of emergency surgical evaluation increases the time to diagnosis and to definitive management. There is a linear relationship between the number of tests ordered and the mortality rate. As more diagnostics are ordered, more delays are incurred, which results in a higher likelihood of **decompensation** and bad outcomes. In short, if the patient is hypotensive or has a history suggesting hypotension prior to arrival at the hospital (such as fainting), emergency surgical consultation is the right test, not CT. However, if a patient is stable, without any signs of hemodynamic instability, obtaining a CT scan may be a reasonable choice. When in doubt, surgical consultation should be sought early.

> **Decompensation:** A catastrophic disruption of an organ system with progression to organ system failure.

Ultrasound, particularly bedside ultrasound, is an excellent tool to determine whether an aneurysm exists. However, it will not detect a leak or rupture. Bedside ultrasound may be helpful when surgical consultation seems warranted but the surgeon requests preliminary confirmation of the presence of an aneurysm. In such cases, ultrasound should be performed while awaiting the surgeon's arrival and should not be allowed to cause delays in definitive surgical evaluation and management.

CT scans with intravenous contrast are excellent for detection of dissections. However, if the clinician has not considered dissection, she is not likely to order a CT. Although dissection is a more difficult clinical diagnosis to make, surgery should be consulted early, as soon as this diagnosis is strongly suspected.

Reliance on chest x-rays to rule out thoracic aortic dissection is a frequent error. Although the chest x-ray will be abnormal in 90 percent of dissection cases, there may be nonspecific findings. Therefore, the abnormalities cannot be attributed to dissection alone. Any time aortic dissection is being considered, a CT of the chest with intravenous contrast should be performed.

Transesophageal echocardiogram (TEE) in the ED is an excellent diagnostic modality for detecting dissection. In some cases, the diagnosis may be suspected, but the patient is too unstable to leave the department for a CT scan, and the surgeon may be reluctant to take him to the OR without confirmation of the diagnosis. In such cases, TEE done in the ED can be a valuable adjunct to the diagnosis.

## PATIENT CARE OPTIONS

The most important step in detecting thoracic aortic dissection and AAA is to consider the diagnosis. Creating awareness of the difficulty in making these diagnoses is critical. Unstable patients suspected of having either diagnosis should receive emergent surgical evaluation. In stable patients, CT may be performed. Chest radiographs should not be relied on; although they are often ordered as an initial screening test, they perform poorly in this context. TEE may be useful in unstable patients requiring definitive confirmation prior to surgery. In older patients with a new onset of suspected renal colic, a CT scan should be performed to rule out AAA. Any patient with hemodynamic instability should receive an emergent surgical consultation. In addition, any patient with abnormal physical findings or symptoms suggesting multiple organ involvement should prompt serious consideration of aortic dissection.

## THE ROLE OF EXECUTIVE LEADERSHIP

The executive leader should implement training programs to raise awareness of the complexity of the presentations and the likelihood of misdiagnosis in aortic aneurysms and dissections. Adequate resources should be provided to ensure 24/7 access to CT and possibly TEE. Also, the administration should consider supporting bedside ultrasound so that brief confirmation studies can be performed. Arrangements for emergency vascular surgery coverage and blood availability must be mapped out in advance.

### Case Study

In September 2003, actor John Ritter presented to an emergency department in Burbank, California. He complained of chest pain, nausea, and vomiting. Suspecting an acute myocardial infarction, the ED staff contacted a cardiologist.

Ritter died of an aortic dissection. His family sued the hospital and individual physicians for $67 million in damages. The suit criticized the cardiologist for not ordering a chest radiograph. The cardiologist argued that when someone is having a heart attack, which is what Ritter appeared to be having, treatment should not be delayed to wait for a chest x-ray. Ritter undoubtedly looked very ill upon arrival and had chest pain, nausea, and vomiting. Thus, this diagnosis was difficult to make, as is the case with most aortic dissections. The jury ruled in favor of the defendants. Aortic dissection, with its deceptive presentations, caused Ritter's death, not the physicians who cared for him.

SOURCE: Celizic (2008).

## Recommended Readings

Assar, A. N., and C. K. Zarins. 2009. "Ruptured Abdominal Aortic Aneurysm: A Surgical Emergency with Many Clinical Presentations." *Postgraduate Medical Journal* 85 (1003): 268–73.

Hansen, M. S., G. J. Nogareda, and S. J. Hutchison. 2007. "Frequency of and Inappropriate Treatment of Misdiagnosis of Acute Aortic Dissection." *American Journal of Cardiology* 99 (6): 852–56.

Von Kodolitsch, Y., C. Nienaber, C. Dieckmann, A. Schwartz, T. Hofmann, C. Brekenfeld, V. Nicolas, J. Berger, and T. Meinertz. 2004. "Chest Radiography for the Diagnosis of Acute Aortic Syndrome." *American Journal of Medicine* 116 (2): 73–77.

# CHAPTER 27

# Wounds and Fractures

**In This Chapter**

- The Magnitude of the Problem
- Strategies for Success: Foreign Bodies
- Strategies for Success: Fractures and Dislocations
- Strategies for Success: Radiology Follow-Up
- The Role of Executive Leadership
- Case Study
- Strategies for Healthcare Executives

## THE MAGNITUDE OF THE PROBLEM

Wounds and lacerations are among the most frequent chief complaints that present to the emergency department; one in ten ED visits is for wound care. Five percent of wounds treated in the emergency department become infected. Though these bad outcomes involve smaller dollar amounts individually than other high-risk situations, the aggregate numbers mean that wounds and their complications account for 28 percent of malpractice cases and are one of the top eight causes for malpractice suits.

Common wound management problems include failure to get x-rays, failure to seek consultation, inadequate discharge instructions, inadequate documentation, and inadequate follow-up arrangements. A complete chart for a wound should include elements of the patient's medical history that would put her at increased risk of infection.

## Risk Factors for Infection

- Asplenia
- Diabetes
- Peripheral vascular disease
- Use of steroids or immunosuppressive drugs
- Delay in seeking care
- Crush or contamination
- Bites, especially human

The time of the injury and the mechanism are also critical elements of the history and should appear in the medical record. Old wounds and wounds associated with a crush injury or contamination are at increased risk. The medical record should suggest that the injury increased the risk for infection and was not the result of poor care. Charting systems that encourage the physician to document these important elements of the history—such as templates or electronic health records with built-in prompts—should be an imperative.

The physical examination should also document that the patient had intact neurologic function and pulses (indicating no nerve or artery damage) and that the wound was explored for foreign bodies or tendon injury. A low threshold for x-rays to look for hidden fractures or foreign bodies should also be the standard of care for the department, and standardized order sets can help.

## STRATEGIES FOR SUCCESS: FOREIGN BODIES

Retained foreign bodies are the fifth leading cause of lawsuits, and glass is the culprit in half of these cases. Contrary to popular belief, it is usually possible to see glass on plain x-rays. Other imaging modalities include ultrasound or CT scan. Even if the foreign body is missed on imaging (which can happen), defending a bad outcome is far easier when there has been an effort to look for a foreign body. Increasingly, because of concern over costs, the authors have witnessed an increase in patients refusing to have imaging done. Two strategies to reduce risk associated with foreign bodies:

1. Standardized order sets for imaging if the mechanism of injury involved the possibility of a foreign body

2. A charting macro that states, "Despite being warned of the risk of foreign body, the patient is convinced that there is none and chooses to decline the recommended x-ray"

## STRATEGIES FOR SUCCESS: FRACTURES AND DISLOCATIONS

Eight tricky limb injuries have been identified (CEME 2011). Most clinicians have been educated about these commonly missed diagnoses. While it is ultimately the responsibility of the physician to consider these difficult diagnoses, and the clinical details are more than executive leadership needs to know, system adaptations can reduce the likelihood of these diagnoses being missed. A sample of such guidelines follows:

1. *Scaphoid/navicular fractures.* This fracture, caused by a fall on an out-stretched hand, is the most commonly missed because it frequently does not show up on the first x-ray. Delayed diagnosis often results in complications and fractures that don't heal. Standardization would include a navicular view x-ray on all patients with the mechanism of injury and splinting with a thumb spica splint (a special splint) even if the first x-ray is negative.
2. *Salter-Harris growth plate fractures.* Salter-Harris fractures affect children who are still growing. Serious fractures can result in the limb growing too fast or two slow and can result in legs of different lengths. Standardization would include temporary splinting of all children with open growth plates and automatic referral to the orthopedist for follow-up.
3. *Lisfranc fractures.* This midfoot fracture is a difficult x-ray diagnosis. Standardization would require that any trauma to the forefoot or midfoot be x-rayed, put in a temporary splint, and referred automatically to the orthopedist.
4. *Occult elbow fractures (radial head and supracondylar fractures).* There are several fractures that can easily be missed around the elbow, and some of them require surgical intervention. Automatic x-rays of the elbow and temporary splinting and referral to an orthopedist would be safest.
5. *Femoral neck fractures.* Some negative hip x-rays can be unreliable. Any elderly patient with trauma who claims she can't walk due to pain in the hip should be considered for alternative imaging. Standardization: If the hip

x-ray is negative and the patient still can't walk, automatically CT scan the hip and refer her to an orthopedist regardless of the results.

6. *Posterior shoulder dislocation.* This is another difficult x-ray reading and is frequently missed because the diagnosis is not considered. The patient's history is often critical to the diagnosis. A patient who had a seizure and woke up with shoulder pain and an athlete involved in kayaking or similar sports should be carefully evaluated for this injury. Standardization would include historical data that trigger the ordering of shoulder films with special views.

7. *Compartment syndrome.* The extremities contain compartments that hold nerves, tendons, and blood vessels. Trauma to the compartment with or without fracture can lead to bleeding into the closed space. The resulting high pressure in the compartment can destroy nerves and tendons with profound consequences. The hand and the calf are two particularly vulnerable compartments. The injury must be considered by mechanism (crush injuries) and if the patient is on Coumadin. Early orthopedic consultation is critical. These cases yield among the highest malpractice awards because of disfigurement and disability. Standardization would include automatic elevation of the limb to reduce swelling, documentation of pulses (using Doppler if necessary), and the early alert to the physician of the possibility for compartment syndrome. If the institution does not have orthopedic coverage, agreements will need to be worked out with neighboring facilities for the early transfer of such patients. Compartment syndrome is a true orthopedic emergency.

8. *Missed hand-tendon injuries.* Because tendons may be 90 percent severed and still demonstrate no loss of function, tendon injuries are easy to miss. For deep hand lacerations with possible tendon injury, standardization would include automatic immobilization and referral to a hand surgeon. The executive leadership can help by crafting plans for hand-surgery coverage for the ED because this is one area where physician shortages have a huge impact on outcome.

## STRATEGIES FOR SUCCESS: RADIOLOGY FOLLOW-UP

Emergency radiology is flawed in most institutions, which increases risk. Even when there is real-time radiology with readings made quickly available to the ED, most films are double-read, and the final reading can be different from the preliminary reading. The ED often has to act upon the preliminary reading and treat the patient accordingly. Later radiology may place in the medical record a discrepant reading that may suggest an entirely different management plan. Should the patient have a bad outcome, this system problem lays the entire institution, the emergency department, and radiology open to litigation. The same thing can occur if the ED physician does a "wet read" from the emergency department that differs from the final official radiologist's reading.

Emergency physicians have an excellent track record reading plain x-rays in the ED (wet reads). A number of studies show that the emergency physician's readings agree with the radiologist's reading 97 to 99 percent of the time (Petinaux et al. 2011; Williams et al. 2000; Robinson, Culpan, and Wiggins 1999). Further studies show that the discrepancies are clinically relevant only 0.6 percent of the time.

In an ED seeing 50,000 visits a year, those numbers translate to approximately 100 x-rays taken each day. With three x-ray misreads or discrepancies, and 0.6 percent needing a change in management, one patient will need to be contacted every two days, and the management will be changed. This means 15 to 30 cases per month that require an airtight process to capture, track, document, and manage.

Executive leadership may need to require contractually that radiologists work with emergency physicians and staff to develop and implement a process to remedy this system. Typically radiology groups will not become engaged in the management of x-ray discrepancies, which leaves the institution at risk.

## THE ROLE OF EXECUTIVE LEADERSHIP

Though administrators have not traditionally assumed a role in the clinical particulars of patient care, this area is ripe for the involvement of leadership and management because it leaves the organization vulnerable on several fronts. With the help of physicians and other clinicians, executives can set up processes and systems that maintain quality and safety for patients and reduce organizational risk. Support for a wound-check clinic in the ED is also a good risk management strategy.

### Case Study

A 34-year-old man is fleeing police when he jumps six feet to the ground and rolls over in pain. The police apprehend him and bring him to the emergency department for evaluation of foot and ankle pain. By protocol the nurse orders both an ankle and a foot x-ray because he has pain in both areas. The real-time radiology reading of both films is negative. The physician evaluates the patient quickly in

(continued)

view of the negative films and the police officers' desire to make the booking, She orders an ace wrap and discharges the patient with instructions appropriate for an ankle sprain and a foot contusion.

The patient is instructed to follow up with an orthopedist if he has not recovered in one week. The patient, who was briefly incarcerated, seeks care from a podiatrist two weeks later when his pain has persisted. A repeat x-ray shows a Lisfranc fracture.

Meanwhile, back at the hospital, the day after the initial real-time radiology reading had been rendered by a physician using teleradiography, the hospital radiologist overreads the original reading and diagnoses a Lisfranc fracture. The new official reading is transcribed and is part of the medical record, though no alert is sent to the emergency department and the patient is never informed.

The first the emergency physician and the hospital hear of this discrepancy is from an attorney when the patient files a lawsuit against the emergency physician, the radiology group, and the hospital.

SOURCE: CEME (2011). Reprinted with permission.

### Strategies for Healthcare Executives

- Understand that these "minor" injuries hold the biggest risk to the provider and the institution.
- Work with ED physicians and radiology to reduce discrepancies and medical errors.
- Provide support to manage the tasks and clerical work associated with x-ray discrepancies.
- Institute a wound-check clinic for the ED and the hospital as a strategy to minimize the risk of wound complications.

## Recommended Readings

Kahn, J. H. 2009. "Emergency Medicine Clinics of North America: High-Risk Presentations in Emergency." *Risk Management* (November): 747–65.

Pines, J. M. 2007. *Evidence Based Emergency Care.* West Sussex, UK: Wiley & Sons.

Weinstock, M. B. 2007. *Bouncebacks! Emergency Department Cases: ED Returns.* Columbus, OH: Anadem Publishing.

# CHAPTER 28

# Acute Coronary Syndrome

**In This Chapter**

- The Magnitude of the Problem
- Strategies for Success: Electrocardiograms
- Strategies for Success: Lab Testing
- Strategies for Success: Imaging
- Strategies for Success: Response to Treatment
- Patient Care Options
- The Role of Executive Leadership
- Case Study
- Strategies for Healthcare Executives

## THE MAGNITUDE OF THE PROBLEM

Six million patients each year come to emergency departments complaining of chest pain. This equates to 5.3 percent of all ED visits. Only 15 to 25 percent of these patients are diagnosed with acute coronary syndrome (ACS), while 2 to 8 percent of ACS patients are discharged without proper diagnosis from the emergency department. These undiagnosed patients have a 25 percent mortality rate. The American Heart Association reported in 2010 that 785,000 new "coronary attacks" occur per year, and 470,000 patients will have recurrent attacks. Also, of particular importance is that 21 percent of acute myocardial infarctions (AMIs) will

> **Silent myocardial infarction:** Heart attack that presents with vague or atypical complaints, such as sweating, nausea, or jaw pain, instead of the typical chest pains.

be **silent**, presenting no chest pain symptoms (George and Dangas 2010). This is particularly true of patients with diabetes. The frequency of the complaint, the complexity of the decision making, and the potential for bad outcomes with misdiagnosis make chest pain evaluations risky. A thorough risk management program will include strategies to address common errors in diagnosis and management of ACS. ACS is a continuum of disease, ranging from unstable angina to AMI, all of which result in morbidity and mortality if misdiagnosed or mismanaged. Undiagnosed or misdiagnosed heart attacks are the leading reason for malpractice dollars paid out from the ED.

## STRATEGIES FOR SUCCESS: ELECTROCARDIOGRAMS

The diagnostic categories for ACS are electrocardiograms (ECG), cardiac biomarkers, and imaging. ECGs are the standard. However, as a stand-alone test, they are poor screening tests for ACS. In a series of nearly 400,000 AMI patients, the initial ECG was diagnostic for AMI in only 57 percent of the cases (Welch et al. 2001). In addition, 35.1 percent had nonspecific changes and 7.9 percent were totally normal. These data are humbling when considering the reliance placed on ECGs to detect ACS. One strategy to improve the sensitivity of ECGs for patients at risk for ACS is to do a second ECG 30 to 60 minutes after the first. The American College of Emergency Physicians (2006) developed and released an evidence-based clinical guideline in 2006 reporting this standard, among others. For all patients in whom a nondiagnostic ECG is performed to investigate the possibility of ACS, a second should be automatically performed within this time frame. If this action is left to the discretion of the physician, the risk of missed ACS will likely increase. An additional strategy is to compare every ECG obtained with a previous ECG. Again, this should be a forced function, as opposed to a discretionary function. When a new ECG is performed, the physician should be handed the most recent previous one as well. This comparison may identify subtle changes and also forces the physician to take a closer look at the new ECG, again reducing the likelihood of misdiagnosis. Finally, it is an accepted standard that in all patients with a left bundle branch block (LBBB) pattern on the ECG (a nonspecific but common pattern read on ECGs), a **STEMI** (ST segment elevation myocardial infarction) be strongly considered. There can be STEMI changes (those at-a-glance changes that suggest an MI on the ECG and are easiest to read and interpret), buried or hidden by the bundle branch block.

> **STEMI (ST segment elevation myocardial infarction):** These heart attacks are more easily diagnosed because findings are readily visible on the ECG. The evidence is clearest on how to manage these patients.

Therefore a good clinical rule is for all patients with suspicion for ACS who have new LBBB should be presumed to have acute coronary syndrome, with the possibility of a STEMI.

## STRATEGIES FOR SUCCESS: LAB TESTING

The laboratory diagnostics we have to aid us are primarily the following biomarker assays: myoglobin, creatine phosphokinase (CPK), CPK-MB fraction, and troponin. The theory behind biomarkers is that they will rise above normal serum levels in the face of myocardial injury (infarction). To varying degrees, each may have false positives and false negatives, consequently overdiagnosing and underdiagnosing myocardial injury. Myoglobin is sensitive for myocardial injury, but it is nonspecific as its elevations can be due to injury of any muscle type. Although some have reported benefit from using this biomarker, within one to two hours post-injury the number of false positives results in too many unnecessary admissions and evaluations. CPK, in isolation, also has little value in today's diagnostic evaluation because it is not specific enough for myocardial injury to be used effectively in the decision-making process. Nonetheless, it is often sampled in hospital ordering sets. CPK-MB is relatively specific for myocardial muscle and is more useful than either myoglobin or total CPK. However, it takes three to four hours to rise, peaks at 12 to 24 hours, and returns to normal within two days. Although CPK-MB has been used for decades, it has largely been replaced by troponin, which has similar onset of elevation post-injury and time to peak concentrations. However, it stays elevated for seven days, allowing the provider to more accurately identify subacute myocardial injury (see Exhibit 28.1). Finally, troponin is more sensitive than CPK-MB. In one study, 30 percent of patients thought to have unstable angina due to having a negative CPK-MB actually had a positive troponin (Sabatine et al. 2002). Therefore, these patients actually had NSTEMIs and not unstable angina. Thus, it is cost effective, efficient, and supported by the literature to sample troponin only.

**Exhibit 28.1: Characteristics of the Three Cardiac Markers**

|  | Onset of Rise | Peak | Normalization |
|---|---|---|---|
| Myoglobin | 2 hours | 4–6 hours | 24 hours |
| CPK-MB | 3–4 hours | 12–24 hours | 1–2 days |
| Troponin | 3–6 hours | 12–24 hours | 7 days |

How many sets of troponins would be necessary prior to discharging a patient from the ED? This is the wrong question and one that will lead to error. Hypothetically, one may rely on a single negative troponin to rule out myocardial infarction. However, that single troponin would have to be six hours or more from the time the infarct began. Unfortunately, we have no reliable means to determine when an infarct actually begins. The most important question is often overlooked: "What have we ruled out with a negative troponin?" Although we can rule out myocardial injury, we can never rule out the entire spectrum of disease with cardiac markers. Unstable angina does not result in a rise in cardiac biomarkers as there is no heart damage, yet. Emphasizing "yet," a decision to discharge a patient should never be based on the negative blood tests, if the suspicion is high.

## STRATEGIES FOR SUCCESS: IMAGING

Imaging is often ordered as part of the diagnostic evaluation in the emergency department. The options are often limited to provocative testing, such as standard exercise treadmill testing, nuclear medicine stress testing, or myocardial perfusion imaging (sestamibi or thallium) and CT coronary angiogram.

Standard exercise treadmill testing has minimal value, particularly in application to ED patients with acute chest pain presentations. The sensitivity of standard exercise treadmill tests is only slightly greater than 50 percent for coronary artery disease (Giannarosi 1989). The sensitivity of myocardial perfusion imaging has been reported as high as 97 to 100 percent for AMIs, but much lower (89 percent) for acute coronary **ischemia** (Kim 2001). However, these tests function best when patients are actively having pain. Unfortunately, it is not reasonable or safe to send a patient with chest pain to have a stress test outside of the ED. Stressing patients with active coronary ischemia may result in decompensation. And once patients are stabilized and pain free, the sensitivity of these tests is much lower. CT coronary angiography, which scans the heart vessels, is an interesting modality. It is appealing at first blush because it is noninvasive and can be done with resources readily available in the ED. It is fast and safe. However, the current data strongly suggest that it is not ready for ED application yet. An early review of its reliability and efficacy has found it to be less sensitive and specific than stress perfusion studies (Hollander and Litt 2006). Much of the research is limited by referral bias, from use of an inappropriate standard, and from low sample sizes. Stress testing may be factored into the decision to discharge. However, this should only be performed once the patient has had acute injury ruled out.

> **Ischemia:** Inadequate blood flow to tissues or organs.

## STRATEGIES FOR SUCCESS: RESPONSE TO TREATMENT

Frequently, yet inappropriately, physicians make a disposition decision based on the chest pain patient's response to certain treatments: gastrointestinal (GI) preparations (e.g., antacids) and nitroglycerin (NTG). Responses to treatment should not be factored into the decision to admit or discharge the patient. In the past it was thought that a positive response to NTG was predictive that the chest pain was cardiac in nature. A number of studies have now proved that premise to be wrong (Henrikson et al. 2003; Steele et al. 2006; Diercks et al. 2005). Similarly, it was also once believed by clinicians that a positive response to antacids indicated that the chest pain was GI in nature. This has also been proved wrong (Mattu and Goyal 2007). Although it may be appropriate to use GI preparations in certain patients with chest pain, it is not appropriate to make disposition decisions based on their response. Also, the response to nitroglycerin does not confirm or rule out coronary ischemia.

## PATIENT CARE OPTIONS

Patients with chest pain frequently present to the ED, and many are high risk. Patients with low or ultra low risk (under the age of 40 without cardiac risk factors) may be discharged with close outpatient follow up to complete their workup. However, patients with moderate or high risk must be admitted. Patients in low-risk categories must be made aware that their risk is not zero and that there is some risk with an outpatient evaluation. Any concern expressed by the patient should prompt consideration for admission. Discharge planning should be performed with phone consultation with the referral physician. The quality of the patient's symptoms can be misleading and can prompt faulty decision making, particularly in women, who are more likely to present atypically for ACS. For instance, chest pain that is reproducible when the patient's chest wall is palpated reduces the likelihood for a cardiac etiology but not to an extent that should influence final disposition decision making. Many patients have been discharged with reproducible chest pain, presumed to be musculoskeletal, only to die later from undiagnosed ACS.

It is also worth noting that women are more likely to be misdiagnosed. Women with ACS are more likely to be older and to seek treatment later. Women with ACS are more likely to have hypertension and less likely to have had stress testing or angioplasty. Women describe pain that often does not sound cardiac: It is depicted as sharp, stabbing, or transient and more likely to radiate to the shoulder, right arm, neck, or back. Women presenting with an acute MI are more likely to have GI symptoms such as nausea, heartburn, and vomiting, and they are more likely to have nonspecific symptoms such as fainting, dizziness, fatigue, and loss of appetite. Finally, women are three times more likely to have a diagnosis of psychological chest pain rather than cardiac chest pain (Woo 2009). It is important to have a documented strategy for managing nondiagnostic chest pain. If patients are discharged, follow up and further testing should be hardwired into the system.

## THE ROLE OF EXECUTIVE LEADERSHIP

The executive leadership should understand the high-risk nature of all chest-pain presentations. To avoid risk, erring on the side of caution and admission is recommended. The medical staff need to be made aware of the administration's expectations, avoiding adversarial interactions with the ED staff when admissions for chest pain are sought. For low-risk patients, the hospital should provide resources for expedited outpatient evaluations (such as next-day myocardial perfusion imaging). Providing a chest-pain unit or an observation status with a diagnostic protocol for all chest-pain admissions will help expedite evaluations while avoiding unsafe discharges.

### Case Study

A 43-year-old male with chest pain and epigastric abdominal pain presents to the ED. He is comfortable and has a normal physical examination. His only medical history is type II diabetes mellitus. An ECG is obtained, followed automatically by another ECG 30 minutes later. The first is normal. However, the second shows an acute inferolateral wall myocardial infarction. The patient did not experience any change in symptoms despite the dramatic change on the ECG. The patient was taken to the cath lab and met the 90-minute door-to-balloon goal. He was found to have occlusions and received angioplasty and stenting with a good outcome and recovery.

(continued)

ECG 1: This is essentially a normal ECG with a slightly fast heart rate.

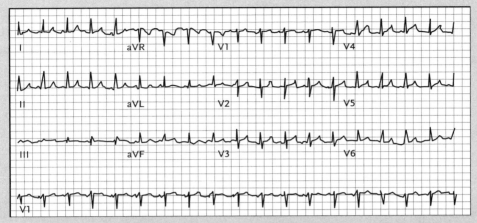

ECG 2: After 30 minutes, the ECG shows a classic STEMI in the inferolateral heads

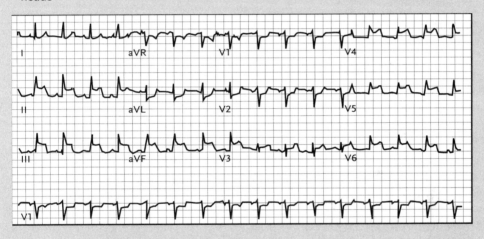

SOURCE: Klauer, quality assurance review. Used with permission.

## Strategies for Healthcare Executives

- Provide rapid turnaround on troponin results.
- Ensure repeat ECGs within 30 to 60 minutes.
- Draft a policy providing a comparison ECG automatically.
- Recognize the lack of decision-making benefit from serial cardiac enzymes, responses to treatments, and provocative testing of ED chest-pain patients.
- Define a culture encouraging short-term observation evaluation of patients with moderate or high risk for ACS.
- Articulate a chest-pain care process model for the ED and hardwire it into the system.

## Recommended Readings

American Heart Association, Statistics Committee and Stroke Statistics Subcommittee. 2009. *Heart Disease and Stroke Statistics—2009 Update.* Dallas, TX: American Heart Association.

Høilund-Carlsen, P. F., A. Johansen, H. W. Christensen, L. T. Pedersen, I. K. Jøhnk, W. Vach, and T. Haghfelt. 2005. "Usefulness of the Exercise Electrocardiogram in Diagnosing Ischemic or Coronary Heart Disease in Patients with Chest Pain." *American Journal of Cardiology* (95): 96–99.

Welch, R. D., R. J. Zalenski, P. D. Frederick, J. A. Malmgren, S. Compton, M. Grzybowski, S. Thomas, T. Kowalenko, and N. R. Every. 2001. "Prognostic Value of a Normal or Nonspecific Initial Electrocardiogram in Acute Myocardial Infarction." *Journal of the American Medical Association* 286 (16): 1977–84.

# CHAPTER 29

# Sick Babies: Sepsis and Infants

## In This Chapter

- The Magnitude of the Problem
- Strategies for Success: History and Physical Examination
- Strategies for Success: Diagnostics
- The Role of Executive Leadership
- Case Study
- Strategies for Healthcare Executives

## THE MAGNITUDE OF THE PROBLEM

**Sepsis**, particularly in **neonates**, is perhaps the greatest threat to an infant's life. Sepsis occurs in 2 of every 1,000 live births. Neonatal meningitis occurs in 2 to 4 of every 10,000 live births and accounts for 4 percent of all neonatal deaths. The mortality rate for sepsis is 50 percent if left untreated (Anderson-Berry 2010). In lawsuits involving pediatrics, the emergency department is the most commonly listed area where claims arise, accounting for 58 percent of lawsuits (Najaf-Zadeh et al. 2008). Pediatric lawsuits are always difficult, as they frequently involve death of a very young and defenseless patient, completely dependent on others for care. Despite the fact that negligence may not have occurred, pediatric cases engender a great deal of sympathy for the plaintiffs, usually the parents.

> **Sepsis:** The presence of bacteria or other infectious organisms or their toxins in the blood stream or in other tissues of the body. Sepsis can be life threatening, requiring urgent and comprehensive care.

> **Neonate:** An infant in the first 28 days of life.

The most difficult aspect of preventing neonatal sepsis lies in identifying those at risk. Many physicians inappropriately feel that assessing the physical appearance of the infant is sufficient to rule out serious bacterial infections. This is not the case. Vaccines reduce the risk of flu and pneumonia, but neonates and many older infants may not have received their immunizations. They are at great risk for serious bacterial infections, including meningitis, pneumonia, and urinary tract infections.

## STRATEGIES FOR SUCCESS: HISTORY AND PHYSICAL EXAMINATION

History and physical examination are important in detection of sepsis. Infants delivered without prenatal care and those born prematurely or at low birth weight are at greater risk. Subtle changes in behavior—such as changes in feeding patterns—are often the only indication of sepsis or meningitis. Parents may also report changes in respiratory status and irritability. A parent describing a change in respiratory pattern, even if not noted at the time of evaluation, is a red flag that cannot be ignored. For instance, any child reported to have had apnea or a change in color or muscle tone (usually floppiness) is considered to have an "apparent life-threatening event" or ALTE. Serious bacterial infection should be strongly considered in infants with ALTEs, and admission is recommended as a conservative step to reduce risk.

Of course the patient in these cases cannot provide any meaningful verbal communication, and examinations, particularly before 28 days, can be unreliable. Thus the information provided by parents is critical. Listening is the one of the most important diagnostic skills in the detection of those at risk for sepsis.

The current recommendation is to perform a complete septic evaluation, including intravenous antibiotics and admission for all neonates with a temperature of 100.4 degrees F or greater. This is the standard of care, and substantial data support this recommendation (Claudius 2010; Bonsu 2003; Caspe 1983). If this rule is not followed, serious bacterial infections will be missed and the exposure to liability is great.

As infants age, the physical assessment may become more reliable. Many providers begin to deviate from the accepted practice guideline and substitute clinical judgment to determine which infants are ill and which are not. This is a dangerous practice, in particular in the youngest infants. Caution is advised up to 90 days. Beyond 90 days, the consensus is that enough development has occurred that an experienced clinician can appropriately distinguish the sick from the nonsick and use diagnostics more selectively. However, any ill-appearing infant, regardless of age, should have a full septic evaluation performed.

In the 28- to 90-day period, physicians should consider two subsets of patients: those with a known source of fever and those without. Infants with a clear source of fever who are older than 28 days do not necessarily require a full septic evaluation. However, those with historical or physical findings suggesting systemic illness may have a serious bacterial infection. It is advised to err on the side of performing the septic workup if there is any such suspicion.

Even without a source of fever identified, some authors have reported that it may be possible to determine, based on physical assessment, which patients between 29 and 90 days old are at risk for sepsis or serious bacterial infection (Wasserman and White 1990; King, Berman, and Wright 1987; Crain and Shelov 1982). However, the most current literature reports that the most conservative physician will perform a full septic evaluation in patients up to 90 days old without a source of fever (Garra 2005; Crain and Gershel 1988). From a risk management perspective, the most conservative route is recommended, and the experience level of the physician should be incorporated into the discussion. If a particular emergency department sees few pediatric patients, providers in that ED may be less able to identify subtle physical findings than providers who see many pediatric patients. Although experience should be a consideration, it should not be viewed as a certification to avoid diagnostic evaluations. Hsiao, Chen, and Baker (2006) reported that 10 percent of infants from 57 to 180 days old with serious bacterial infections were deemed "non–ill-appearing" by experienced clinicians.

## STRATEGIES FOR SUCCESS: DIAGNOSTICS

A complete septic evaluation should include CBC with differential, catheterized urinalysis with culture, chest radiograph, and a lumbar puncture (spinal tap). This is the standard of care in febrile neonates and in any infant who appears ill or in whom sepsis is suspected.

In the 29- to 90-day age group, those without a source of fever are at greatest risk for misdiagnosis. The most conservative approach would be to perform a septic evaluation on all infants up to 90 days without a source of fever. However, some clinicians, particularly with infants older than 60 days, may begin to use some selectivity in diagnostics, guided by their assessment. Although this is an acceptable medical approach, from a risk management perspective caution is advised, especially in facilities with few pediatric visits.

Errors commonly occur in determining the source of fever. Viral upper respiratory symptoms are not adequate sources. Even when positive viral swabs for influenza or respiratory syncytial virus are obtained, there is still a significant likelihood that a serious bacterial infection will also be present. In 4.9 percent of infants with positive viral swabs, serious bacterial infections were also present.

Lumbar puncture (LP) is often the sticking point with clinicians. They are fine with checking boxes on the chart to obtain blood work, urine, and a chest radiograph. However, there is some resistance to performing the lumbar puncture. This may be attributed to the time it takes, unfamiliarity with the procedure, and concerns about complications. In experienced hands, an LP can take just a matter of minutes. Emergency physicians should be skilled in performing this procedure. LP is often more easily performed in infants than in adults because it is easier to identify landmarks. Contrary to some people's beliefs LP is a safe procedure. One complication, the "bloody tap," may obscure results but would rarely result in harm to the patient. The rare complication of the subsequent development of an epidermoid tumor (from the introduction of skin into the spinal canal by the spinal needle during the procedure) is completely avoided by the use of a needle with a stylet.

The most common serious bacterial infections in infants are urinary tract infections, or pyelonephritis. Obtaining a urine sample is critical in the sepsis evaluation. Many emergency departments use bagged specimens to avoid urinary catheterization of children. However, bagged specimens often result in false positives from perineal contamination. One pediatric study reported a contamination rate of 62.8 percent in bagged specimens, compared to 9.1 percent for catheterized specimens (Al-Orifi et al. 2000). Bagged specimens are less invasive and are convenient, but the contamination rate is far too high to warrant their use.

In the past, the white blood cell count (WBC) and differential were used to help identify infants who needed a septic evaluation from those who did not. In 1996 the Centers for Disease Control and Prevention recommended a CBC be drawn on all neonates at risk for sepsis, and the sensitivity and specificity were unacceptably low. Despite the data initially suggesting the CBC's utility, such guidelines were often not used in practice. Subsequent studies have led to a different perspective, and the current data are fairly definitive in showing no benefit in differentiating bacterial from viral illnesses using the WBC and differential (Brown, Shaw, and Wittlake 2005). That said, many pediatric medical centers, such as the Cincinnati Children's Medical Center, still include a CBC in the evaluation of infants with fever, and this has been adopted at the local level in many emergency departments (Cincinnati Children's Medical Center 2010).

# THE ROLE OF EXECUTIVE LEADERSHIP

The executive leadership should establish policies ensuring the most appropriate care for febrile infants, including performing a sepsis evaluation, administering intravenous antibiotics, and admitting all febrile neonates. The hospital and emergency department need not reinvent the wheel. The premier pediatric hospitals around the country have devised protocols for the management of febrile infants. The practitioners should be encouraged to adopt one and standardize the approach of the physicians in the department.

Practice patterns should be assessed for risky behavior. If overreliance on the appearance of febrile infants is noted, education should be provided and performance monitored. Lumbar puncture should be encouraged in the appropriate cases, and catheterized urine samples should be established as the standard.

---

### Case Study

A 26-day-old infant presented to the emergency department with her parents. The patient had a fever of 101.6. The diagnostic evaluation included a chest radiograph, urinalysis, and blood work. The patient was discharged. The diagnosis provided was "neonatal febrile illness." The urine culture grew E. coli, a common urinary pathogen. The patient developed sepsis, experienced seizures and permanent brain injury, and died. The physician did not perform a lumbar puncture, administer antibiotics, or admit the patient, all standard practices in a case of neonatal fever.

SOURCE: Courtesy Kevin Klauer, case illustration from peer review.

---

### Strategies for Healthcare Executives

- Recognize the seriousness of misdiagnosis of the febrile infant.
- Establish guidelines for the appropriate care of febrile infants.
- Ensure access to pediatric consultation is available when needed.
- Establish transfer agreements with pediatric facilities for cases outside the facility's scope of practice.
- Establish close follow-up procedures (the next day, preferably) for all febrile infants discharged from the emergency department.

## Recommended Readings

Al-Orifi, F., D. McGillivray, S. Tange, and M. S. Kramer. 2000. "Urine Culture from Bag Specimens in Young Children: Are the Risks Too High?" *Journal of Pediatrics* 200 (137): 221–26.

Baxter, A. L., R. G. Fisher, B. L. Burke, S. S. Goldblatt, D. J. Isaacman, and M. L. Lawson. 2006. "Local Anesthetic and Stylet Styles: Factors Associated with Resident Lumbar Puncture Success." *Pediatrics* 117 (3): 876–81.

Brown, L., T. Shaw, and W. A. Wittlake. 2005. "Does Leucocytosis Identify Bacterial Infections in Febrile Neonates Presenting to the Emergency Department?" *Emergency Medical Journal* 22 (4): 256–59.

Hsiao, A. L., L. Chen, and M. D. Baker. 2006. "Incidence and Predictors of Serious Bacterial Infections Among 57- to 180-Day-Old Infants." *Pediatrics* 117 (5): 1695–1701.

Najaf-Zadeh A., F. Dubos, M. Aurel, and A. Martinot. 2008. "Epidemiology of Malpractice Lawsuits in Paediatrics." *Acta Pædiatrica* 97 (11): 1486–91.

# CHAPTER 30

# Acute Cerebrovascular Syndrome, Stroke, and TIA

**In This Chapter**

- The Magnitude of the Problem
- Strategies for Success: History, Physical Examination, and the Disposition Decision
- Strategies for Success: t-PA Administration
- Patient Care Options
- The Role of Executive Leadership
- Case Study
- Strategies for Healthcare Executives

## THE MAGNITUDE OF THE PROBLEM

Acute cerebrovascular syndrome (ACVS) encompasses the entire spectrum of cerebrovascular disease, including stroke and **transient ischemic attacks (TIA)**. The incidence of stroke is high, estimated at 750,000 annually in the United States (Williams 2001, 1999). Among adults aged 20 or older, the estimated prevalence of stroke in 2006 was 6,400,000 (about 2,500,000 males and 3,900,000 females). One-third of strokes result in death; stroke is the third-leading cause of death in the United States (American Heart Association 2010). An additional 200,000 patients each

> **Transient ischemic attack (TIA):** A neurological event that shares the signs and symptoms of a stroke but is reversible. Also called a mini-stroke, TIAs typically last 2 to 30 minutes and can produce problems with vision, dizziness, weakness, or speaking. If not treated, there is a high risk of having a major stroke in the near future.

year are disabled by stroke. The combination of life-threatening pathology and high frequency should cause EDs to give ACVS substantial focus.

---

### Acute Cerebrovascular Syndrome Risk

- A stroke in evolution is not recognized.
- A transient ischemic attack (TIA) is undermanaged.
- Thrombolytic care is not considered.
- Thrombolytic care results in complications.

---

Stroke has always been challenging to diagnose and manage. However, litigation in stroke cases has skyrocketed, based on a false standard of care professed by many plaintiffs' attorneys (Liang 2008). Despite a lack of consensus in the medical community regarding the use of **thrombolytic therapy** (t-PA) clot-busting drugs in stroke, many physicians are sued for not giving this drug, and many are sued for the complications created once they have.

**Thrombolytic therapy (t-PA):** Any of the "clot-busting" drugs administered in cardiovascular and cerebrovascular disease.

An additional issue is the lack of recognition of TIA as the equivalent of "unstable angina of the brain." Conventional wisdom is that many cases of TIA that were previously diagnosed are actually strokes in their early stages. Many patients with subtle neurological symptoms are discharged and ultimately experience a stroke. The lack of appropriate intervention at the time of initial presentation is generating a substantial amount of risk.

## STRATEGIES FOR SUCCESS: HISTORY, PHYSICAL EXAMINATION, AND THE DISPOSITION DECISION

Stroke syndromes are often complex and difficult to attribute to a specific vascular cause, making misdiagnosis likely. Clinicians should realize the complexity of these syndromes and the variability in which they may present from patient to patient. It is all too common and easy to explain away an unusual set of symptoms, when in fact they may be associated with an evolving stroke. Some clinicians are reluctant to attribute minor-sounding symptoms to ACVS, in part because it would require further investigation and admission. However, it is these subtle presentations that are often early manifestations of stroke syndromes and are most amenable to treatment. When there is no explanation for a patient's symptoms and they could have a neurological cause, the clinician should consider ACVS. In such cases, either admission or neurology consultation is recommended.

TIAs (mini-strokes that go away) are often wrongly interpreted as benign events. Many events previously considered TIAs are now diagnosed as strokes in progress by identifying an ischemic pattern on MRI when the CT was negative. Therefore, unless the symptoms in question have completely resolved, the diagnosis of TIA cannot be given. In other words, if the patient has symptoms that appear to be due to cerebral ischemia, stroke in evolution must be the diagnosis until proven otherwise and discharge would be out of the question. Most TIA patients' symptoms will completely resolve prior to arrival in the ED, as the average duration is 5 to 10 minutes. Despite the short duration and complete resolution of symptoms, discharge is not appropriate for most of these patients. We would not consider sending a patient home with a diagnosis of unstable angina. A landmark article (Johnston et al. 2000) tracked ED patients with a discharge diagnosis of TIA. Ten percent returned to the ED with a stroke within 90 days. However, 50 percent returned within the first 48 hours with a worsening condition. Closed claims data also confirm that the decision to discharge patients with a new-onset TIA is problematic and is associated with poor patient outcomes and increased risk (Klauer 2011).

In some settings, expedited outpatient pathways are available, allowing for a full diagnostic evaluation to be performed within 24 to 48 hours. Such protocols are the local standard, and all TIA patients are handled this way. In such environments, admission may not be necessary. However, caution should be given to deferring an outpatient evaluation to a nonspecific provider and/or unspecified plan. Without a well-defined and well-established outpatient pathway in place, inpatient management is best in most cases to ensure that a timely and complete evaluation is performed.

The standard of care has changed dramatically in the past 25 years. In the 1980s, TIA patients were admitted. Then the recommendations were to discharge. Now a more aggressive approach to the workup is recommended.

## STRATEGIES FOR SUCCESS: T-PA ADMINISTRATION

Most controversy and litigation surrounding stroke management has to do with the administration of t-PA. Although only 1 percent of stroke patients receive it, the delivery of t-PA has driven the stroke care agenda for the past several years. The data from early trials with thrombolytic therapy were conflicting, with controversy within the specialty over whether the benefits from administering t-PA in stroke truly outweighed the risk. Emergency physicians could be faulted for giving t-PA when complications occurred (usually a catastrophic hemorrhage in the head or the GI tract), but they could also be sued if the decision was judiciously made not to administer t-PA.

Certainly, t-PA has brought focus and attention to stroke management. Furthermore, outcomes in stroke centers are better than in non-stroke centers. However, these outcomes have nothing to do with whether the patients receive t-PA or not. The improvement in outcomes has been attributed to the focus on stroke care that such institutions have, including necessary ancillary services such as speech therapy and pulmonary hygiene.

Despite the claims by many plaintiffs' attorneys that t-PA is the standard of care in ischemic stroke management, there is still no medical consensus nor irrefutable data on this topic. Where there is a lack of consensus, no standard can emerge. There are a variety of studies on t-PA for stroke (Thomalla 2007; Higashida 2003; ACEP 2002; Wardlaw 1997).

Two strategies to mitigate risk in the administration of t-PA in the ED are as follows:

1. Informed consent
2. Stroke policies

The provider offering and ordering t-PA must carry out the informed consent process. Although the task of signing a consent form may be delegated to another staff member on the team, the treating physician solely owns the act of having the informed discussion and obtaining the patient's consent. For consent to be valid, the patient must have the capacity to consent and refuse and must be advised of all risks and benefits associated with the treatment. Although the patient must be advised of the risks and benefits of administration of t-PA, the information provided is specific to that physician's interpretation of the data. That is why one physician may provide a more positive view and another a somewhat negative one. Neither is wrong, provided that a reasonable and balanced overview is provided.

It is wise to have a discussion about t-PA with every stroke patient, including those not eligible for t-PA. Documenting these discussions in the medical record protects the physician should a claim be filed.

Stroke policies are essential for every institution. Even those facilities not administering t-PA should have a policy outlining how stroke patients are managed at their institution. Providers should be educated about and adhere to the policy. Although any licensed physician could order t-PA, it is wise to have the neurologist make this decision and order the drug, thus taking responsibility for this decision. Often, the emergency physician is asked to make the decision or to order the medication following telephone or telemedicine consultation. Rarely are such consults documented in the medical record. If there is a bad outcome, there is no documentation reflecting the decision making of the consultant or her recommendations. Frequently, the consultant may have a different recollection of the encounter. This results in "finger pointing" among defendants. Once this occurs, the plaintiffs have all but won their case, as the defendants appear to be admitting each other's fault.

## PATIENT CARE OPTIONS

All patients suspected of having a stroke should receive priority triage, an expedited CT scan, and a neurology consult as soon as possible. Unless otherwise contraindicated, 325 mg of aspirin should be administered. t-PA should be discussed and offered in all applicable cases, and an informed discussion must take place about t-PA in all stroke patients.

Patients experiencing a new-onset TIA should be admitted for urgent diagnostic evaluation. However, if a previously defined local mechanism is in place for expedited outpatient workup, and the standard is for all similar patients to follow this outpatient mechanism, admission may be avoided.

## THE ROLE OF EXECUTIVE LEADERSHIP

The role of executive leadership is to provide clear guidance on the institution's expectations. Stroke policies should be drafted to outline these expectations. If the hospital is a stroke center and advocates for t-PA administration, this should be reflected in hospital policy, and the providers should be made aware. If all stroke patients will be transferred, transfer agreements with stroke centers should be drafted. The expectation for new-onset TIA patients should also be relayed to the medical staff, and barriers to admission of such patients should be removed. The aging population means that standardized stroke and TIA care are more important than ever.

## Case Study

A 20-year-old male patient presented to an ED complaining of headache, difficulty understanding, difficulty moving, and aphasia. His symptoms resolved prior to arrival. A CT and LP were performed, and both were negative. Phone consultation with a neurologist was conducted. The neurologist concluded this was an atypical migraine. The patient was discharged to follow up with his primary care physician, whom he saw two days later. Three days after the ED presentation, he suffered a massive stroke. His TIA symptoms were due to an undetected carotid dissection. A $1 million judgment was handed down against the neurologist and the primary care physician.

SOURCE: JuryVerdictReview.com (n.d.).

### Strategies for Healthcare Executives

- Establish a stroke policy, including whether or not t-PA will be used and who will administer it.
- Ensure the availability of immediate CT in all patients suspected of having a stroke.
- Consider admission of all patients with new-onset TIAs, or consider expedited outpatient TIA workups (within 24 hours).
- Educate providers about the complexity of stroke syndromes.
- Establish transfer agreements with stroke centers if the management of stroke patients is outside the scope of the facility.

## Recommended Readings

Bateman, B. T., H. C. Schumacher, B. Boden-Albala, M. F. Berman, J. P. Mohr, R. L. Sacco, and J. Pile-Spellman. 2006. "Factors Associated with In-Hospital Mortality After Administration of Thrombolysis in Acute Ischemic Stroke Patients: An Analysis of the Nationwide Inpatient Sample 1999 to 2002." *Stroke* 37: 440.

Deng, Y. Z., M. J. Reeves, B. S. Jacobs, G. L. Birbeck, R. U. Kothari, S. L. Hickenbottom, A. J. Mullard, S. Wehner, K. Maddox, and A. Majid. 2006. "IV Tissue Plasminogen Activator Use in Acute Stroke: Experience from a Statewide Registry." *Neurology* 66 (3): 297.

Hacke, W., M. Kaste, E. Bluhmki, M. Brozman, A. Dávalos, D. Guidetti, V. Larrue, K. R. Lees, Z. Medeghri, T. Machnig, D. Schneider, R. von Kummer, N. Wahlgren, and D. Toni. 2008. "Thrombolysis with Alteplase 3 to 4.5 Hours After Acute Ischemic Stroke." *New England Journal of Medicine* 359 (13): 1317–29.

Johnston, S. C., D. R. Gress, W. S. Browner, and S. Sidney. 2000. "Short-Term Prognosis After Emergency Department Diagnosis of TIA." *Journal of the American Medical Association* 284 (22): 2901–06.

Katzan, I. L., A. J. Furlan, L. E. Lloyd, J. I. Frank, D. L. Harper, J. A. Hinchey, J. P. Hammel, A. Qu, and C. A. Sila. 2000. "Use of Tissue-Type Plasminogen Activator for Acute Ischemic Stroke: The Cleveland Area Experience." *Journal of the American Medical Association* 283 (19): 1151–58.

The National Institute of Neurological Disorders and Stroke r-tPA Stroke Study Group. 1995. "Tissue Plasminogen Activator for Acute Ischemic Stroke." *New England Journal of Medicine* 333 (24): 1581–87.

Uchiyama, S. 2009. "Transient Ischemic Attack, a Medical Emergency." *Brain Nerve* 61 (9): 1013–22.

# CHAPTER 31

# Testicular Torsion

**In This Chapter**

- The Magnitude of the Problem
- Strategies for Success: Avoiding the Common Misdiagnosis
- Strategies for Success: Making the Diagnosis
- Strategies for Success: Imaging
- Management of Testicular Torsion
- The Role of Executive Leadership
- Case Study
- Strategies for Healthcare Executives

## THE MAGNITUDE OF THE PROBLEM

Testicular torsion results from the twisting of the spermatic cord, attached to the testicle. When torsion occurs, the blood supply is either completely or intermittently disrupted. Testicular torsion is a time-sensitive diagnosis. A torsed testicle has a salvage rate of 90 to 100 percent if action is taken within six hours. After 12 hours, the rate drops to 50 percent and less than 10 percent after 24 hours (Barada, Weingarten, and Cromie 1989). Early surgical intervention is the standard. Although it is important to recognize that torsion can occur at any age, it is most common in patients aged 25 or younger, with an incidence of 1 in 4,000.

Patients usually present with scrotal pain. However, particularly in pediatric patients, the only complaint may be of abdominal pain (until testicular tenderness is discovered on physical examination). The onset of pain may be associated with trauma or lifting a heavy object, which may mislead the physician into considering inguinal hernia as a more likely cause of the patient's pain. However, epididymitis is the most common misdiagnosis given to those with testicular torsion.

## STRATEGIES FOR SUCCESS: AVOIDING THE COMMON MISDIAGNOSIS

**Epididymitis** is an infection and/or inflammation of the epididymis. The epididymis is a tightly coiled tubular structure connecting the testicle to the vas deferens. As with testicular torsion, epididymitis may occur at any age. However, it is most common between the ages of 19 and 40 years. The incidence is approximately 1 in 1,000 males per year.

These facts make the misdiagnosis of testicular torsion fairly common: A study of closed claims cases from Beth Israel Hospital in New York shed much light on this high-risk clinical entity (Matteson 2001). Thirty-nine cases consisting of 58 individual claims were reviewed. Indemnity payments were made in 26 cases (67 percent), of which 25 (96 percent) were settlements, and 13 cases (33 percent) ended in favor of the physicians. Five cases went to trial, with only one verdict in favor of the plaintiff. The median indemnity payment was $45,000. Urologists were named most frequently (48 percent), and a misdiagnosis of epididymitis was most commonly cited (61 percent).

> **Epididymitis:** Inflammation or infection of the epididymis, the long coiled tube attached to the upper part of each testicle.

The mean patient age was 24.3 years. Atypical initial complaints were common (46 percent). Late presentation (greater than eight hours) did not affect the medicolegal outcome. The major liabilities for paid claims were an error in diagnosis (74 percent), a delay in or lack of referral (48 percent), lack of radiologic examination (19 percent), failure to explore (13 percent), error in surgical technique or judgment (13 percent), and falsified records (10 percent).

Perhaps the leading factor contributing to the misdiagnosis is that many physicians—particularly those trained in the 1980s, before imaging of the testes was widespread to aid in this diagnosis—are under the misconception that the two diagnoses can be differentiated based on clinical grounds alone without the aid of ultrasound. This simply is not the case. Regardless of the amount of experience with this examination, the physical findings are just too similar. In addition, some physicians are swayed toward the diagnosis of epididymitis by the presence of white blood cells on a urinalysis. White blood cells may be a nonspecific marker for inflammation. However, they are by no means confirmation that epididymitis exists and torsion does not.

## STRATEGIES FOR SUCCESS: MAKING THE DIAGNOSIS

Mistakes in diagnosing testicular torsion can occur at any time during the ED visit, especially in infants and in the absence of scrotal pain. Infants who are inconsolable should have the diaper removed and an examination of the scrotum performed. In addition every male patient with abdominal pain needs a cursory scrotal exam to look for tenderness. Performing an adequate scrotal ultrasound, with Doppler flow studies to verify blood supply, is the next essential step. Scrotal ultrasound is the standard and should be ordered in all cases of suspected torsion, and all male patients with acute testicular pain and tenderness should be considered to have testicular torsion until proven otherwise. Timely urological consultation must be available to manage these cases. The only exception to the standard ultrasound rule is for those cases in which the clinical suspicion is high enough to consult the urologist prior to performing the ultrasound, and the urologist elects to surgically explore the scrotum without performing an ultrasound. This is the preferred approach by many in treating infants with suspected torsion, as they are much less likely to have epididymitis.

---

**Root Causes of Misdiagnosis of Testicular Torsion**

- Failure to consider the diagnosis
- Inadequate physical examination
- Failure to image
- Failure to consult a urologist

---

## STRATEGIES FOR SUCCESS: IMAGING

Ultrasound, with color flow Doppler, is an excellent tool, but it is not without its limitations. The primary issue is not sensitivity or a failure to detect the disease. It is in misapplication of the test results. Ultrasound can be useful in differentiating between torsion and epididymitis. Classic torsion has no blood flow, whereas classic epididymitis has increased blood flow due to inflammation. However, reduced blood flow in torsion may be variable, dependent on the degree of torsion. If the testicle is not torsed 360 degrees, some blood flow may still be preserved. Conversely, epididymitis will never have reduced blood flow and will rarely have anything other than enhanced or hyperemic blood flow.

Therefore, it will be flawed logic to diagnose epididymitis with low, or in some cases, "normal" blood flow and may result in a dead testicle and litigation. Patients with testicular pain and anything other than hyperemic blood flow should be presumed to have torsion and require an emergency urological consult.

Ultrasound is recommended even in patients whose pain has resolved prior to or soon after arriving at the ED. These patients may have experienced intermittent torsion and detorsed spontaneously. A high percentage of these patients will suffer another torsion in the future. Thus, verifying normal blood flow at the time of their visit to the ED is essential in reducing medical malpractice risk. Such patients should receive prompt, but not necessarily emergent, urological follow up.

The importance of ultrasound in this time-sensitive diagnosis underscores the need for 24/7-ultrasound availability. If ultrasound cannot be made available, transfer agreements should be in place to expedite the transfer and performance of ultrasound. It should be emphasized that there is only one standard of care regarding ultrasound and torsion, and it is not dependent on the time of day or resource availability. All torsion patients deserve the same standard of care.

## MANAGEMENT OF TESTICULAR TORSION

Urological consultation is the final step in cases that are definitively determined to be torsion and in those in which torsion has not been ruled out. If the emergency physician strongly suspects torsion, the urologist should be contacted prior to ultrasound to reduce delays in surgical exploration. The ultrasound may still be ordered while the urologist is on her way into the hospital. However, the decision to evaluate the patient at the bedside should not be delayed waiting for the result. In the vast majority of cases, the diagnosis is unclear. The urologist can be contacted following the ultrasound if positive or suspicious for torsion, emphasizing that any case with high clinical suspicion should prompt an immediate call to the urologist. All cases of confirmed torsion and those that are indeterminate, following ultrasound, should be promptly explored in the operating room by the urologist. Noting that an unknown percentage of the equivocal cases will actually be torsions, they must all be treated presumptively to avoid delays in management that could result in a necrotic (dying) testicle.

# THE ROLE OF EXECUTIVE LEADERSHIP

The primary role of leadership is to ensure the availability of the necessary resources to appropriately care for the patients who present to the ED with symptoms of torsion. Ultrasound must be available; however, if ultrasound is not available at all or is only available at certain times of the day, transfer agreements should be made with other institutions to ensure that the appropriate diagnostic evaluation is performed in a timely manner. If these arrangements are not made, the provider may treat the patient differently than he normally would, resulting in treatment that does not meet the standard of care. The final required resource is the on-call urologist. If urologists are on the medical staff, they should participate in the on-call schedule. The urologists should be made aware of the institutional expectations for consultation in such cases.

## Case Study

A 17-year-old male presented to the ED with a 24-hour history of intermittent testicular pain without any urinary symptoms. The testis was mildly tender with no swelling and felt normal in size, shape, and position. A diagnosis of possible orchitis was made, but the patient was discharged home with a urology referral for further assessment. Surgical exploration found an engorged testis, confirming a diagnosis of intermittent torsion.

SOURCE: Somani, Watson, and Townell (2010).

## Strategies for Healthcare Executives

- Ensure that providers understand that torsion and epididymitis cannot be distinguished by physical exam findings alone.
- Provide 24/7 availability of testicular ultrasound with Doppler flow studies through an on-call arrangement with technicians.
- Work out agreements with area organizations to share the burden of on-call for technicians (and urologists as needed). One model put Hospital A on for even days of the month and Hospital B on for odd days.
- Ensure timely access to urological consultation.

## Recommended Readings

Cassar, S., S. Bhatt, H. J. Paltiel, and V. S. Dogra. 2008. "Role of Spectral Doppler Sonography in the Evaluation of Partial Testicular Torsion." *Journal of Ultrasound in Medicine* 27 (11): 1629–38.

Murár, E., P. Omaník, M. Funáková, I. Béder, and F. Horn. 2008. "Acute Scrotum Is a Condition Requiring Surgical Intervention." *Rozhledy v Chirurgii* 87 (10): 517–20.

Schmitz, D., and S. Safranek. 2009. "Clinical Inquiries. How Useful Is a Physical Exam in Diagnosing Testicular Torsion?" *Journal of Family Practitioners* 58 (8): 433–34.

Yagil, Y., I. Naroditsky, J. Milhem, R. Leiba, M. Leiderman, S. Badaan, and D. Gaitini. 2010. "Role of Doppler Ultrasonography in the Triage of Acute Scrotum in the Emergency Department." *Journal of Ultrasound in Medicine* 29 (1): 11–21.

# CHAPTER 32

# Brain and Spinal Cord Injuries

## In This Chapter

- The Magnitude of the Problem
- Strategies for Success: History and Physical Examination
- Strategies for Success: Imaging
- Patient Care Options
- The Role of Executive Leadership
- Case Study
- Strategies for Healthcare Executives

## THE MAGNITUDE OF THE PROBLEM

The incidence of traumatic brain injury in the United States is estimated to be 180 to 250 persons per 100,000 annually. When traumatic brain injury is misdiagnosed or the diagnosis is delayed, the outcomes may be devastating. The average mortality rate is 19 per 100,000, and **case fatality** rate is 17 per 100 (Cadotte, Vachhrajani, and Pirouzmand 2011). Mortality is one concern; however, many brain-injured patients face long-term morbidity. From a risk perspective, brain-injured patients are often young and require lifelong convalescent care. Special damage awards—those compensating for quantifiable monetary losses—can easily reach seven figures.

Much like traumatic brain injury, spinal cord injuries most often occur in the young, and advancements in medical care have improved the initial survival and long-term prognosis of such patients. In 2009, the National Spinal Cord Injury

Database reported life expectancies from 1.8 years to 52.6 years, dependent on many factors (Spinal Cord Injury Information Network 2009). The average lifetime cost of care for a patient with quadriplegia (also referred to as tetraplegia) from a C1-C4 injury at age 25 was more than $3.1 million. The organization also reported that 12,000 new cases are reported annually. However, no overall incidence studies have been conducted since the 1970s, so the actual incidence is not known. The mean age at time of injury is 37.7 years old. There is a four-to-one ratio of males to females, and most patients are white (66.1 percent). Motor vehicle crashes account for 45.6 percent of spinal cord injuries, while falls and violence represent 19.6 percent and 17.8 percent, respectively (Spinal Cord Injury Info Pages 2010, BrainAndSpinalCord.org 2011).

> **Case fatality:** The ratio of deaths within a designated population of people with a particular condition over a certain period of time. An example of a fatality rate would be 9 deaths per 10,000 people at risk per year. This means that within a given year, out of 10,000 people formally diagnosed with a disease, 9 died.

Not surprisingly, there is a significant incidence of concomitant head injury with spinal cord injury. The Archives of Physical Medicine and Rehabilitation reported concomitant injury to be 60 percent (Macchiocchi et al. 2008). The presence of concomitant head and spinal cord injury underscores the importance of appropriate management of such patients and avoidance of misdiagnosis.

## STRATEGIES FOR SUCCESS: HISTORY AND PHYSICAL EXAMINATION

Emergency department physicians must focus on those patients with minor head injury. Although "minor head injury" suggests that these injuries may result in minor pathology or risk, this term refers only to the mechanism of injury and the initial presentation. Many patients with minor head injury may actually suffer serious traumatic brain injury, including life-threatening intracranial injuries. Illustrating this point, Dr. Ian Stiell (2001) published data in *Lancet* in showing that small reductions in Glasgow coma scale (GCS) scores are associated with staggering increases in risk for traumatic brain injury (Exhibit 32.1).

These data confirm that subtle changes in physical examination may equate to traumatic brain injury substantially out of proportion to those findings. A detailed history and examination are critical to identifying those patients at risk. Furthermore, a seemingly minor mechanism may produce significant injuries.

The primary question with head injuries is who should receive a CT and who should not. If this question is answered appropriately, no patients with traumatic brain injury will be overlooked. Any head-injured patient with a GCS of less than

**Exhibit 32.1: Glascow Coma Scale**

| Glascow Coma Scale Score | Prevalence of CT Abnormalities |
|---|---|
| 15 | 3.5% |
| 14 | 16% |
| 13 | 79% |

| Glascow Coma Scale | | Modified GCS for Children <2 Years Old | |
|---|---|---|---|
| Sign | Score | Sign | Score |
| Eye Opening | | Eye Opening | |
| Spontaneous | 4 | Spontaneous | 4 |
| To speech | 3 | To speech | 3 |
| To pain | 2 | To pain | 2 |
| No response | 1 | No response | 1 |
| | | | |
| Motor Response | | Motor Response | |
| Obeys verbal command | 6 | Normal spontaneous movement | 6 |
| Localizes | 5 | Withdraws to touch | 5 |
| Withdraws to pain | 4 | Withdraws to pain | 4 |
| Flexes to pain | 3 | Flexes to pain | 3 |
| Extends to pain | 2 | Extends to pain | 2 |
| No response | 1 | No response | 1 |
| | | | |
| Verbal Response | | Verbal Response | |
| Oriented | 5 | Smiles, listens, follows objects | 5 |
| Confused | 4 | Irritable but consolable | 4 |
| Inappropriate words | 3 | Inappropriate, inconsolable cry | 3 |
| Nonspecific sounds | 2 | Agitated restless | 2 |
| No response | 1 | No response | 1 |

SOURCE: Stiell (2001).

the perfect score of 15 should be studied. However, up to 3.5 percent of patients with a normal GCS will have intracranial injuries on CT. Out of 3,121 patients with minor head injury, 8 percent had clinically significant intracranial injuries and 1 percent required neurosurgical intervention (Stiell 2001).

Infants and the elderly with minor head injury are at greatest risk for serious traumatic brain injury with few indications on physical exam. Forty-three percent of infants with traumatic brain injury are clinically asymptomatic (Greenes and

Schutzman 1999). As we age, cerebral atrophy occurs. This atrophy causes stretching of the dural vessels, resulting in a greater likelihood that shearing forces from head injury will injure one of those vessels, resulting in a **subdural hematoma**.

Because many elderly patients take blood thinners such as aspirin, Plavix, or Coumadin, the likelihood for significant brain injury is substantial.

> **Subdural hematoma:** A collection of blood on the surface of the brain that may cause pressure on the cerebral cortex.

Spinal cord injuries are a bit easier to detect on examination. Patients with neurological deficits and patients who present reporting intermittent **paresis**, paralysis, or **paresthesia** should be considered to have spinal cord injury until proven otherwise. In patients with neck injuries, excellent clinical guidelines have been established and should be adhered to as the standard of care (Exhibits 32.2 through 32.5). With spinal injuries, the type of imaging to perform (plain radiographs, CT, MRI) adds additional complexity to the decision-making process. In head injury, the only modality is CT; skull radiographs are obsolete.

> **Paresis:** Weakness or loss of strength.

> **Paresthesia:** Decrease or loss of sensation.

## STRATEGIES FOR SUCCESS: IMAGING

As noted, the single most important question with head or cervical spinal injury is which patients to image. In patients with a low risk of traumatic brain injury, close outpatient observation with a responsible party is a reasonable alternative to CT. Although the decision to perform a cranial CT must be weighed with the concern of radiation exposure to the brain, any head-injured patient with significant risk should have imaging performed. For patients over the age of 50 years, the risk of radiation exposure is negated by the fact that the time to develop leukemia or a solid organ tumor from such an exposure would remove the risk for this occurring during their remaining lifespan (Fazel 2009). However, in children, not only is there the risk of radiation-induced cancers, we don't know how the developing brain is affected by the ionizing radiation. Particularly in infants, whose skulls are not fully developed, the radiation exposure is substantial, similar to that experienced by those survivors standing thousands of yards from ground zero in Hiroshima, Japan. The decision to perform a CT in a pediatric patient, especially in head-injured infants, should be made carefully with the patient's parents or guardians.

As a general guide, the Canadian CT Head Rule (Exhibit 32.2) provides valuable insight into which patients may benefit from head CT and which may not.

The Canadian CT Head Rule is reasonable with one caveat: The researchers reported an additional 4 percent of patients that had "clinically insignificant inju-

**Exhibit 32.2: The Canadian CT Head Rule**

*High-Risk Factors*
- GCS of less than 15 within two hours post-injury
- Suspected open skull fracture
- Any sign of basilar skull fracture
- More than two episodes of vomiting
- Age > 65 years

*Medium-Risk Factors*
- Retrograde amnesia > 30 minutes
- Dangerous mechanism of injury

SOURCE: Stiell (2001).

ries." The implication is that these injuries could be missed without any associated bad outcomes. However, in the US medicolegal system, caution should be exercised in applying this principle, as such misses may result in significant liability exposure. It is important to note that the Canadian CT Head Rule may result in a reduction in the use of head CT by 46 percent.

Children have the greatest risk for bad outcomes and for the potential negative effects of ionizing radiation. If there is true concern for intracranial injury in any child, the clinician should err on the side of imaging. However, Kuppermann and colleagues (2009) validated the use of a decision tool that seems reliable and worth incorporating into operational and clinical practice (Exhibit 32.3). These guidelines distinguish between children younger than and older than 2 years. Each of these tools reports a negative predictive value of 100 percent: if the patient meets the parameters of the rule, a CT can be avoided, as it would be very unlikely an intracranial injury would be missed. The added benefit is reducing utilization of head CT.

The American College of Emergency Physicians in 2008 published an evidence-based clinical policy addressing the complexity of the decision to use neuroimaging in head trauma (Exhibit 32.4). Patients with high-risk factors should be imaged.

Clear-cut guidelines are in place that are regarded as the standard of care in cervical spinal evaluation: the NEXUS criteria (Exhibit 32.5) and the Canadian C-Spine Rules. When a patient presents with a cervical spinal injury, following either of these guidelines will ensure identifying those that require cervical spinal imaging. We recommend using both and documenting their use in the medical record.

NEXUS, the National Emergency X-ray Utilization Study, uses five low-risk criteria. If a patient's history and exam are negative for all five, radiographic evaluation is not necessary. NEXUS evaluated more than 34,000 patients and was 99 percent sensitive for cervical spinal injuries (Hoffman et al. 2000).

**Exhibit 32.3: Low-Risk Criteria for Head CT in Children**

*< 2 Years of Age*
Normal mental status
No scalp hematoma (except for frontal)
No loss of consciousness (or less than 5 seconds)
Nonsevere injury mechanism
No palpable skull fracture
Acting normally per the parents

*> 2 Years of Age*
Normal mental status
No loss of consciousness
No vomiting
Nonsevere injury mechanism
No signs of basilar skull fracture
No severe headache

SOURCE: Data from Kuppermann et al. (2009).

The Canadian cervical spine rule study evaluated 8,924 patients (CCC Study Group 2002). The rule was 100 percent sensitive for all "clinically important" cervical spinal injuries. The rule addresses three critical questions:

1. Are there any high-risk factors that should mandate radiographic evaluation (e.g., mechanism of injury, patient older than 65 years, paresthesis in the upper extremities)?
2. Are there any low-risk criteria that will allow range-of-motion testing (e.g., sitting position in the ED, delayed onset of symptoms, absence of midline neck tenderness, simple rear-end impact, ambulatory at any time following the accident)?
3. Can the patient rotate his head 45 degrees to the right and to the left? If there are low-risk criteria present, in the absence of the high-risk criteria, this final rotation test can be performed.

It is important to note that the plain x-ray sensitivity for cervical spinal injury is poor. Diaz and colleagues (2003) reported in the *Journal of Trauma* that plain radiographs failed to identify 52.3 percent of the fractures in the series. Other studies have found similar results (Holmes and Akkinepalli 2005). If there is significant concern, CT scan should be performed instead. Furthermore, if the patient will require a head CT and the cervical spine is to be imaged, CT is the modality of choice for the spine. It is not rational to have the patient in the CT scanner to scan

**Exhibit 32.4: High-Risk Factors for Head Trauma**

| High-Risk Factors | Odds Ratio (Confidence Interval) |
|---|---|
| Neurological deficit | 19 (13–28) |
| Signs of basilar skull fracture | 14 (8–22) |
| Loss of consciousness | 7 (4–11) |
| Severe headache | 3 (2–6) |
| Vomiting | 5 (3–8) |
| Post-traumatic seizure | 3 (2–5) |
| Anticoagulation | 8 (3–9) |
| GCS of 14 | 19 (14–26) |
| Age ≥ 65 years | 2 (1–3) |
| Dangerous mechanism | 3 (2–4) |

SOURCE: ACEP (2008).

the head and take him out to get a plain x-ray of the cervical spine, which is an inferior study.

Patients under the influence of alcohol are at risk for head and neck injuries masked by the effects of alcohol. Allowing the patient to regain sobriety and re-evaluating is a good strategy.

## PATIENT CARE OPTIONS

ED physicians have many patient care options for head and cervical spinal injuries. However, there are some specific rules that will help identify those with significant injuries and avoid testing those not likely to have such injuries. In both head injury and cervical spinal injury, one should err on the side of diagnostic imaging. Regarding head CTs in adults, apply the known high-risk criteria for intracranial injury. For pediatrics, the Kuppermann rules are excellent tools to employ. However, in every pediatric case, use informed consent for obtaining a head CT. This does not imply that a consent form must be completed on each of these cases. What is important is that the conversation takes place and is documented in the medical record.

For cervical spinal injuries, either NEXUS or the Canadian cervical spine rules will work for clinical clearance. Any patient with significant risk should have a CT performed as the initial diagnostic, not plain radiographs.

## Exhibit 32.5: NEXUS Criteria

No posterior midline neck tenderness
No intoxication
No distracting injuries
Normal level of consciousness
No focal neurological deficits

SOURCE: Hoffman et al. (2000).

# THE ROLE OF EXECUTIVE LEADERSHIP

The executive leadership should implement standard practices and guidelines for addressing imaging for patients with head injuries and potential cervical spinal injuries. Access to CT should be provided 24/7, and CTs should be encouraged over plain radiographs in appropriate cases. Also, implementing an informed consent and refusal process for CT scan evaluation of pediatric patients is worth consideration.

### Case Study

A 68-year-old intoxicated male patient presented to the ED via EMS. The patient was well known to the staff. He had struck his head, suffered a scalp laceration, and injured his shoulder. The laceration was repaired, a head CT was performed and was negative, and radiographs of the shoulder were negative for fracture. The patient was to be discharged when nursing noted he could not move his right side well. The physician reexamined him, felt he may have had a stroke, and admitted him. The patient had cervical spinal radiographs performed 48 hours later, which identified a C-7 fracture. The patient subsequently died from his spinal injury. Despite not meeting NEXUS or the Canadian Cervical Spine Rules, which would have allowed him to be safely evaluated clinically, he was never immobilized. By clinical criteria as articulated by NEXUS and The Canadian C-Spine Rules, he clearly needed immobilization and imaging. Even more unfortunate is that the patient was in the CT scanner for the head CT. It would not have taken much additional time or effort to scan the cervical spine at the same time.

SOURCE: Klauer (2011)

## Recommended Readings

Bruns, J., and W. A. Hauser. 2003. "The Epidemiology of Traumatic Brain Injury: A Review." *Epilepsia* 44 Suppl (10): 2–10.

Diaz, J. J., C. Gillman, J. A. Morris, A. K. May, Y. M. Carrillo, and J. Guy. 2003. "Are Five-View Plain Films of the Cervical Spine Unreliable? A Prospective Evaluation in Blunt Trauma Patients with Altered Mental Status." *Journal of Trauma* 55: 658–64.

Jackson, A. B., M. Dijkers, M. J. Devivo, and R. B. Poczatek. 2004. "A Demographic Profile of New Traumatic Spinal Cord Injuries: Change and Stability Over 30 Years." *Archives of Physical Medicine and Rehabilitation* 85 (11): 1740–48.

Macciocchi, S., R. T. Seel, N. Thompson, R. Byams, and B. Bowman. 2008. "Spinal Cord Injury and Co-occurring Traumatic Brain Injury: Assessment and Incidence." *Archives of Physical Medicine and Rehabilitation* July 89 (7): 1350–57.

Stiell, I. G., C. M. Clement, B. H. Rowe, M. J. Schull, R. Brison, D. Cass, M. A. Eisenhauer, R. D. McKnight, G. Bandiera, B. Holroyd, J. S. Lee, J. Dreyer, J. R. Worthington, M. Reardon, G. Greenberg, H. Lesiuk, I. MacPhail, and G. A. Wells. 2005. "Comparison of the Canadian CT Head Rule and the New Orleans Criteria in Patients with Minor Head Injury." *Journal of the American Medical Association* 294 (12): 1511–18.

Tagliaferri, F., C. Compagnone, M. Korsic, F. Servadei, and J. Kraus. 2006. "A Systematic Review of Brain Injury Epidemiology in Europe." *Acta Neurochirurgica* 148 (3): 255–68; discussion 268.

CHAPTER 33

# Pulmonary Embolism

**In This Chapter**

- The Magnitude of the Problem
- Strategies for Success: History and Physical Examination
- Strategies for Success: Laboratory
- Strategies for Success: Imaging
- Patient Care Options
- The Role of Executive Leadership
- Case Study
- Strategies for Healthcare Executives

## THE MAGNITUDE OF THE PROBLEM

It has been estimated that 600,000 patients are diagnosed with **pulmonary embolism (PE)** in the United States annually (Fedullo 2003). Of those 600,000, up to 200,000 die because of PE. However, the exact incidence of PE is unknown. Many feel that pulmonary embolism occurs frequently and that many small PEs are naturally broken down by the body's own clot-busting mechanisms. Patients who present to the ED for evaluation are likely to have a more dangerous and clinically significant PE. Another sobering statistic is that 30 percent of PEs are misdiagnosed on the first visit to the ED (Feied 1995). Furthermore, closed claims

> **Pulmonary embolism (PE):** A blood clot to the lungs, which can be life threatening.

history suggests grave outcomes when PEs are missed. The majority of patients with a missed pulmonary embolism die (Agnelli 2010).

The movement toward utilization review and clinical decision tools in the evaluation of venous thromboembolic disease (VTE), primarily PE, aims to reduce the use of CT pulmonary angiogram and to reduce the patient's radiation exposure (Konstantinides 2008). Thinking like a medical economist has its place, but the use of these tools rather than CT pulmonary angiogram comes with a certain percentage of misdiagnoses. Many of the decision rules involve the use of a **D-dimer assay**,

> **D-Dimer assay:** A blood assay that can be used to screen for pulmonary embolism.

which may not have sufficient negative predictive value to rule out VTE disease. Furthermore, even the more accepted rules report a miss rate of up to 5 percent (Ceriani 2010). Caution is urged when applying these money-saving principles to a diagnostic entity that can be, and is often, fatal.

Despite the logic that the risk of misdiagnosis outweighs the cost benefit of reducing utilization, many still argue that the radiation exposure of CT pulmonary angiogram is not benign, and utilization should be reduced for this reason. Healthcare providers need to discuss the benefits and risks of radiation exposure in the context of potential PE and let the patient decide. Any patient who shares concern about PE and wants the CT pulmonary angiogram performed despite the risks of radiation exposure should have the test if PE is in the differential diagnosis.

Misdiagnosis of PE results in grave consequences for the patient and substantial risk for the institution and providers. From a risk management perspective, diagnostic evaluation for PE should be encouraged, as opposed to the current trend to discourage such evaluations.

## STRATEGIES FOR SUCCESS: HISTORY AND PHYSICAL EXAMINATION

The presentation for PE varies. Just as with any disease process, the quality of the history we receive is dependent on the quality and quantity of information provided. Often patients give healthcare providers information that may not clearly lead to the correct diagnosis. The physician should focus less on the minutiae of the history provided and more on the big picture. A patient may report his pain is worse with deep breaths, and he had a cough a week ago. He might also report that he had similar pain with an episode of bronchitis ten years ago. It can be easy for a provider to walk down the wrong path. The fact remains, patients with unexplained pleuritic chest pain should not have their symptoms easily dismissed.

**Exhibit 33.1: Modified Charlotte Criteria**

Unexplained hypoxia < 95%
Unilateral leg swelling
Recent surgery (< 4 weeks)
Hemoptysis
Pregnancy
Age > 70 years
Symptom duration > 4 days

Another issue associated with missed PE is the diagnosis of anxiety in patients with pleuritic chest pain and shortness of breath. Patients with anxiety disorder or panic attacks are known to experience chest pain, often pleuritic, and shortness of breath with their anxiety. Unfortunately, anxiety is a common misdiagnosis for PE, and it is rarely appropriate unless a diagnostic evaluation to rule out more serious pathology is performed first. Several life-threatening diseases provoke the symptom of anxiety; PE is at the top of that list.

## STRATEGIES FOR SUCCESS: LABORATORY

The D-dimer assay is the predominant screening test for PE. However, there is often a misunderstanding of how to apply the test, and it may not function well enough to achieve its intended goals. The test, when applied to the evaluation for VTE, is not designed to identify the presence of the disease, only the absence. Hypothetically, if the test is negative, the patient doesn't have VTE, including PE. Unfortunately, there is enough doubt about the results that D-dimer assays should be used with caution.

When used properly, they are combined with a decision rule, such as the Modified Charlotte rule (Exhibit 33.1), which is designed to identify low-risk patients. Theoretically, low-risk patients with a negative D-dimer can be safely discharged without further evaluation for VTE. If one of the clinical decision rules indicates higher risk, then the patient should have an imaging test.

As stated previously, most decision rules are used in conjunction with a negative D-dimer. However, the D-dimer should be used cautiously, particularly from a risk management point of view. In the last decade, many D-dimer assays have been marketed, and each was reported to have the negative predictive value necessary to exclude VTE. Unfortunately, many have failed in that regard. Finally, the most recent decision tool released by Dr. Jeff Kline, the Pulmonary Embolism Rule-

**Exhibit 33.2: Pulmonary Embolism Rule-Out Criteria (PERC)**

Age < 50 years
Pulse rate < 100 beats per minute
Venous oxygen saturation > 94%
No unilateral leg swelling
No hemoptysis
No recent trauma or surgery
No prior history of VTE
No hormone use

Out Criteria or PERC (Exhibit 33.2), doesn't include the D-dimer. This suggests a paradigm shift in thinking that perhaps the D-dimer should not be included or is not necessary.

Hypothetically, if patients score well on the PERC, further investigation for PE is unnecessary. However, every decision rule will result in some misdiagnoses. Educating patients about the diagnosis and the risk of diagnostics so that they can make an informed decision is perhaps the best route to improve patient care and mitigate risk.

## STRATEGIES FOR SUCCESS: IMAGING

The first line of defense in detecting and treating PE is to order a test, generally a CT pulmonary angiogram. The test previously used for this, a V/Q scan, was not sensitive for smaller PEs. V/Q scans are challenging to read and must be compared to the chest radiograph. The test cannot be done on patients being mechanically ventilated. The radionuclide was often unavailable in the quantities needed to do more than a few studies a day. Finally, V/Q scans provide no opportunity to identify alternate pathology that may explain the patient's symptoms, such as pneumonia or pneumothorax (collapsed lung). Although these limitations to V/Q are more than enough to turn to CT as the primary test, CT may still not detect segmental or subsegmental PE. Patients with high pretest probability of having the disease should still be considered to have PE despite a negative study.

Finally, it is important to mention that VTE is more common in pregnancy. Despite the concerns about fetal radiation exposure, the decision to investigate the possibility of PE should be a much easier one for pregnant patients. V/Q had been the mainstay in pregnancy for years. However, CT may be a better option.

CT results in more maternal radiation exposure but less fetal radiation exposure than V/Q scans. Therefore, CT pulmonary angiograms are appropriate in pregnant patients.

## PATIENT CARE OPTIONS

PE diagnosis is a complex decision-making process and perhaps one of the risk management areas with the gravest consequences when misdiagnosis occurs. Therefore, patients should be informed of the risk of VTE, the risk of the diagnostics being considered, and the risk of following a given decision rule and should be allowed to participate in the decision. Although this should happen with any patient–physician interaction, it often does not. In every high-risk case, these discussions need to take place and should be documented.

It is important to mention that it is appropriate to follow an accepted decision rule. However, the patient must be made aware of the risk of misdiagnosis, and the rule must be strictly followed. Conversely, it is also appropriate to use clinical judgment, erring on the side of treatment when considering PE. Although such an approach will result in more CT scans being ordered, it will also result in fewer missed PEs. The strategy for PE should be standardized for any emergency department.

## THE ROLE OF EXECUTIVE LEADERSHIP

The role of executive leadership is to make certain the appropriate diagnostics are available 24/7. Any limitation in diagnostic access may result in substandard care and a misdiagnosis in this life-threatening disease. The data suggest that the patient, the institution, and the physician are unlikely to get a second chance.

The astute leader will recognize the prevalence and general acceptance of VTE decision rules while recognizing their limitations and encouraging standardization of the institutional approach and of what rule is used. The executive leader may also choose to limit risk by drafting policy that repeat visits for unexplained chest pain, particularly pleuritic in nature, are studied with CT pulmonary angiogram, regardless of any exclusions implied by any decision rule.

A 32-year-old female presented to the ED complaining of left lower chest pain. The pain was mildly pleuritic, but not exertional. She had no medical history or risk factors for VTE. The pain began acutely, without injury, six hours prior to arrival. She was treated with Ibuprofen and Percocet. A chest radiograph and ECG were obtained and normal. She was discharged to follow up with her primary care physician. She was given the diagnosis of "musculoskeletal chest pain." She did follow up with her primary care physician within several days. Her symptoms were persistent. Her prescriptions were refilled. The patient saw another physician two days later, a pathologist, following her cardiopulmonary arrest. He diagnosed her with PE. This patient's vital signs had been normal, and she had no risk factors for VTE. All conventional PE decision tools would have missed this patient's PE. However, performing a CT pulmonary angiogram most likely would have identified the embolus. This unfortunate case illustrates the importance of unexplained pleuritic chest pain and the need to consider PE in such patients.

SOURCE: Slattery (2011).

### Strategies for Healthcare Executives

- Recognize the complexity of the presentations of VTE.
- Recognize the likelihood of misdiagnosis of VTE.
- Understand that misdiagnosed PEs are likely to result in death.
- Provide 24/7 access to all diagnostics needed for the evaluation of VTE.
- Avoid the use of decision rules in patients who have unscheduled returns to the ED with persistent symptoms.
- Support a standardized pathway for evaluating patients for possible PE.

## Recommended Readings

Klauer, K. 2009. "PE Clinical Decision Rules: Worth the Risk?" *Emergency Physicians' Monthly*. Published April 28. www.epmonthly.com/the-literature/evidence-based-medicine/is-a-d-dimer-always-necessary-when-pe-is-being-considered/

Kline, J. A., C. E. Peterson, and M. T. Steuerwald. 2010. "Prospective Evaluation of Real-time Use of the Pulmonary Embolism Rule-out Criteria in an Academic Emergency Department." *Academic Emergency Medicine* 17 (9): 1016–19.

Parent, F., S. Maître, G. Meyer, C. Raherison, H. Mal, R. Lancar, F. Couturaud, D. Mottier, P. Girard, G. Simonneau, and C. Leroyer. 2007. "Diagnostic Value of D-dimer in Patients with Suspected Pulmonary Embolism: Results from a Multicentre Outcome Study." *Thrombosis Research* 120 (2): 195–200.

# CHAPTER 34

# Dangerous Patients

## In This Chapter

- The Magnitude of the Problem
- Risk Factors for Violence: The Patient
- Risk Factors for Violence: The Healthcare/ED Environment
- Risk Factors for Violence: The Facility
- Strategies for Success: Processes and Procedures to Minimize Risk of Violence
- Strategies for Success: Communication Training
- The Role of Executive Leadership
- Case Study
- Strategies for Healthcare Executives

## THE MAGNITUDE OF THE PROBLEM

According to the Occupational Health and Safety Administration (2004) 45 percent of workplace violence occurs in healthcare settings. While workplace violence is reported at a rate of 2 cases per 10,000 workers, in healthcare that rate is 5 times as high and grossly underreported (Duncan, Estabrooks, and Reimer 2000). Healthcare workers are 5 to 12 times as likely to file workers' compensation claims for violence as workers in any other industry. And 9,000 nurses and healthcare workers are injured or threatened every day in the United States (OSHA 2006). The ED and the psychiatric ward are the most frequent locations for workplace violence in healthcare (Welch 2008b).

Yet most emergency departments have been haphazard in their acknowledgment and approach to this problem. Policies and procedures for identifying and managing potentially violent patients have been slow to evolve, and education and training for staff have been equally slow in coming (Welch 2008b). By identifying patients with a high risk of violent behavior, developing action plans for such patients, and educating staff, the number of incidents and injuries can be reduced (Needham et al. 2004). This chapter focuses on identifying high-risk patients and developing strategies for managing violent patients in the ED.

## RISK FACTORS FOR VIOLENCE: THE PATIENT

The literature is replete with articles identifying the characteristics of patients who are likely to behave aggressively or violently (Dunn 2007; Kleepsies 1998). The most important factor in predicting whether or not a patient will be violent is a history of violence. Sadly, most health systems have no mechanism for identifying patients who have had episodes of violence, and in fact often in the name of HIPAA this information is more difficult to obtain than traditional medical records. This information is vital to frontline ED workers, and mechanisms for rapid identification of these high-risk patients should be a priority.

Elements that increase the risk of violent behavior in mental health patients include a history of recent incarceration, probation, police arrest, or elopement from a mental health facility. If these facts are not known, a few questions can get at the propensity for violence in a patient.

---

**Historical Information and Questions Related to Violence**

- What is the most violent thing you have ever done?
- What happened?
- If I were there watching, what would I see?
- Have you ever owned a weapon?
- Do you have any concerns about owning a weapon?

SOURCE: Intermountain Healthcare, Violence Training Module (Welch 2008b).

---

Other characteristics pertinent to the patient that have been associated with violent behavior are listed in the following box.

**Characteristics Associated with a Violent Patient**

- Has a history of violent behavior (strongest indicator)
- Talks loudly and uses profanity or sexual comments
- Blames others
- Demands unnecessary care, makes threats, or holds grudges
- Accuses staff of being against him
- States he is losing control
- Throws or punches inanimate objects
- Paces rapidly, sweats, keeps his head down, or has a furrowed brow
- Challenges authority or makes intimidating comments
- Expresses interest in weapons
- Appears tense and angry
- Appears intoxicated or under the influence of drugs
- Has a romantic obsession with someone
- Has multiple life stressors, such as divorce, death of a loved one, or financial problems

The Broset Violence Checklist is a short-term violence-prediction instrument assessing confusion, irritability, boisterousness, verbal threats, physical threats, and attacks on objects as either present or absent. It has been shown to be highly predictive of violence in the short term when used by nurses (Björkdahl, Olssen, and Palmstierna 2006). This tool may help staff identify the potential for violence in the ED.

A procedure and protocol for identifying and managing dangerous patients is outlined in Exhibit 34.1 with supporting documents that might be adapted to your healthcare setting.

# RISK FACTORS FOR VIOLENCE: THE HEALTHCARE/ED ENVIRONMENT

In addition to the risk of violence from patients, there are characteristics of the healthcare environment that also increase risk. Organizations that have had periods of turmoil or where leadership is in flux seem to have an increased risk of these encounters. Organizations that have not crafted policies or procedures to manage violence or those where verbal hostility is tolerated are also at risk. In addition, understaffing, high activity, long waits, and transporting patients create high-risk

**Exhibit 34.1: Patient Safety Attendant (PSA) Patient Observation Instructions and Checklist**

This form should be returned to ED administration

Patient name: _____

Patient account number: _____

As the Patient Safety Attendant (PSA), you will be required to *continuously observe and visualize* the patient at risk for harming themselves or others. Your specific responsibilities will include:

- Report to the charge nurse and patient care nurse when you arrive on the unit.
- You must be able to continuously observe and visualize the patient at all times. If the patient is under the Aggressive/Assaultive Protocol, notify the RN every 15 minutes of the need for an RN assessment.
- Notify the care nurse or staff as needed.
- Give information when handing off the responsibility to another PSA who is taking over for you.
- Report off to the patient care nurse before leaving if continuous observation is no longer necessary.

If you have any questions about your duties or responsibilities at any time, please ask the patient care nurse or unit charge nurse. You must turn in these instructions with the information you have recorded to the patient care nurse when you have been relieved from observing the patient.

Patient care nurse name: _____

Charge nurse name: _____

Who gave you report? _____

Who did you hand off to? _____ Time: _____

When performing continual observation, you may not have any other responsibilities. Take report from the patient care nurse when beginning patient observation and be sure the following is understood and checked.

**Exhibit 34.1 Patient Safety Attendant (PSA) Patient Observation Instructions and Checklist (continued)**

| | Yes | No |
|---|---|---|
| **Is patient under formal seclusion or aggressive/assaultive restraint procedure?** (If the answer to above is YES, then a nurse is required to assess the patient every 15 minutes and document it on an Aggressive/Assaultive/Seclusion/ Restraint Flow Sheet. You will need to help track the time from the last assessment. A doctor's assessment and order is needed every 4 hours.) | | |
| **Do I understand why this patient requires observation?** (If the answer to above is NO, then clarify this with the patient care nurse.) | | |
| **Is the patient in a gown?** (If the answer to above is NO, then put the patient in a gown. All patients under continuous observation should be in a gown.) | | |
| **Have harmful items been removed from the room?** (If the answer to above is NO, ask the care nurse to help remove any harmful items.) | | |
| **Is there anything that should be avoided to reduce the risk of upsetting the patient? List:** | | |
| **Do I understand what I should do if the patient asks to go to the bathroom, asks for a smoke, wants food or water, or asks for their belongings?** (If the answer to above is NO, then clarify with the patient care nurse.) | | |
| **Do I understand when and how to contact the staff if immediate help is needed?** (If the answer to above is NO, then please clarify with the patient care nurse.) | | |

Time YOU start and end observation     Start Date & Time: _____

End Date & Time: _____

PSA Signature: _____

Print Name: _____

| Stamper Plate |
|---|
| |

conditions for violent outbursts. EDs regularly restrict patients' freedoms, such as eating, drinking, and smoking, which can put patients over the edge and lead to violent outbursts. Overcrowded departments with uncomfortable spaces, conditions where staff work alone, and institutions with no training or procedures for patients who become violent put staff at increased risk.

Most of these factors associated with the ED environment are worth understanding and defining, but until there is more funding to treat mental health patients and to design and build mental health suites in EDs, these constraints will be difficult to change.

## RISK FACTORS FOR VIOLENCE: THE FACILITY

Factors relating to the ED facility itself can also help or hinder in the management of violent episodes.

### Facility Factors That Increase the Risk of Violence

- Poorly lit areas
- Unrestricted movement of visitors
- Inadequate security
- Background noise and chaos

One important and low-cost solution is the distribution of temporary name badges to identify all visitors and patients and their proper locations. Name badges are practical for tracking movement (for instance, Mrs. Wilson's visitor doesn't belong in the trauma suite watching the show!), and badges show that the staff are paying attention to the flow of visitors. Further, staff should be empowered to ask anyone they don't recognize their name and their business in the ED.

Other facility changes—such as brighter lighting, increased security presence, and alarm systems—can improve safety in the ED. In addition keep in mind that furnishings themselves can be used as weapons.

**Security and Safety Changes for the ED**

- Closed-circuit video
- Curved mirrors
- Limited access from the outside
- Bright lights
- Employee safe rooms
- Enclosed nurses' areas
- Silent alarms or panic buttons
- Metal detectors
- Immovable furniture
- Emergency exits
- Security escorts
- Visible security guards
- Flagging the records of violent patients

## STRATEGIES FOR SUCCESS: PROCESSES AND PROCEDURES TO MINIMIZE RISK OF VIOLENCE

Many institutions are educating staff to identify these risk factors at intake and initiate a procedure for managing the potentially violent patient from there (NIOSH 1996). At the very least such patients should be taken to a safe place, be placed in a gown or hospital scrubs, and have all possessions confiscated. Between 4 and 8 percent of patients presenting to a psychiatric ED will bring weapons with them, so this policy is prudent.

At Intermountain Healthcare patients identified in triage as having risk factors for violence (against others or against themselves) are put in a safe room (Welch 2008b). They are identified as emergency patients and are assessed by the physician or the crisis worker as high, medium or low risk. High-risk patient identification activates the "Violent, Self-Destructive, or Suicidal Behavior Procedure." High- to medium-risk patients remain in seclusion, and the physician renews the order every four hours. A patient safety attendant (PSA) is assigned to observe the patient and keep documentation. HCA has similar screening in triage and similar processes in place in its emergency departments. (Note: The Joint Commission has been citing facilities that seclude patients without such a mechanism for observation, so beware of simply locking a patient in a room for hours.) Physicians may order medications that subsequently lessen the risk for violence, allowing the patient's status to be downgraded to low risk. Low-risk patients can be monitored by family, friends, or staff and may not need seclusion or restraints.

---

**Violent, Self-Destructive, or Suicidal Behavior Procedure**

- Intake and initial risk assessment
- Seclusion and safety measures
- Physician and social worker assessment
- Patient safety attendant and protocol implementation

---

The Patient Safety Attendant Observation instructions and checklist have been reproduced in Exhibit 34.1.

## STRATEGIES FOR SUCCESS: COMMUNICATION TRAINING

Training staff in the fundamentals of violence prevention is the responsibility of the organization. The nursing workforce is made up in part of younger clinicians who have no experience in dealing with such difficult patients. Part of the training that staff members should receive includes communication and behavioral training. (Many patients who are under the influence of alcohol and drugs or are acutely psychotic can't be "managed" no matter what communication and behavioral training the staff member has.)

Active listening can often defuse a situation and convince the patient or upset family member that the caregiver is concerned and involved. Using first-person expressions (I or we) is less inflammatory than second-person (you) statements. Scripting can help staff deal with volatile situations.

---

**Examples of Scripting**

- I can see how important this is to you.
- Could you help me understand how...?
- What is it you want to see happen in this situation?
- What else could we do to remedy this situation?

---

In addition it is worth remembering that 80 percent of communication is non-verbal (Borg 2008), and body language can escalate a difficult encounter. Experts recommend that you adopt an open posture as opposed to closing arms across the chest or placing hands on hips (Engleberg 2006). They also caution against pointing at an angry individual. The best stance is with arms at your sides, making eye contact and standing at a slight angle because it is less confrontational.

A technique for disengaging from an angry encounter can also be taught. Experts recommend scripting for this purpose, and the four-step approach is noted in the following list (Tishler 2000).

---

**Disengaging from an Angry Person**

1. Acknowledge: I can see that you are angry with me.
2. Commit involvement: We will talk more about this.
3. State your needs: I need to talk to the charge nurse.
4. State your intention to return: I will be back after I speak with the charge nurse.

SOURCE: Tishler (2000).

---

In summary, our specialty needs education to manage dangerous patients in the ED. We need to acknowledge that we work in a dangerous environment, and we need policies that protect all of us. The ad hoc approach that has been in use for decades needs work. There are data and research to show us the way, but the most successful strategies include adding the following procedures in the ED:

- Performing the high-risk checklist at intake
- Activating the high-risk patient protocol
- Removing belongings and/or clothing from high-risk patients
- Upgrading patients for the crisis worker or physician to see

In addition, staff should have regular training and education on identifying high-risk patients, scripting, body language, and safely extricating themselves from dangerous situations.

# THE ROLE OF EXECUTIVE LEADERSHIP

The collapse of the mental health system in the United States has created an undue share of problems for the EDs in this country. Psychosocial problems now rival chest pain as one of the most common chief complaints presenting to the ED. These patients bring safety issues to the emergency department that need well-crafted strategies. Clinicians are not likely to craft them. The organization that does not have clear strategies for managing this dangerous mental health burden leaves its staff vulnerable to violence.

### Case Study

A 32-year-old man is brought to the ED by police, who found him making threatening comments to passersby leaving the sporting arena downtown. He has a long history of mental health problems, but his records are sequestered and unavailable to the ED.

He is initially placed in a patient care room for evaluation of "confusion." The ED is quite busy, and he is not given any priority in the queue. Increasingly he becomes agitated and eventually throws a chair at a nurse walking by, after upsetting many other patients and their family members.

The physician orders him placed in a locked seclusion room and orders sedation. Before the nurse can administer the medication, the patient sets fire to the floor of the seclusion room with a lighter he had in his pants pocket. His cigarettes were confiscated to keep him from smoking, but his lighter was not taken.

It took this episode to reveal how ad hoc the procedures were at this facility for managing such patients. The incident led to the wholesale crafting of procedures and policies that would minimize the risk of similar incidents.

SOURCE: Welch, QI program case.

## Strategies for Healthcare Executives

- Understand that the work environment in the ED is inherently unsafe.
- Make educating nurses and staff in safety procedures an institutional priority.
- Craft responses for violent or potentially violent episodes on the campus, such as a panic button to call police or a coded message to bring extra staff to the ED.
- Endorse the use of seclusion and sedation in a systematic and standardized way.

## Recommended Readings

Kleepsies, P. M. 1998. *Emergencies in Mental Health Practice: Evaluation and Management.* New York: The Guilford Press.

National Institute for Occupational Safety and Health. 1996. *Violence in the Workplace: Risk Factors and Prevention Strategies.* NIOSH Publication No. 96-100, www.cdc.gov/violcont.html.pdf.

Needham, I., C. Abderhalden, R. Meer, T. Dassen, H. J. Haug, R. J. Halfens, and J. E. Fischer. 2004. "The Effectiveness of Two Interventions in the Management of Patient Violence in Acute Mental Inpatient Settings: Report on a Pilot Study." *Journal of Psychiatric and Mental Health Nursing* 11 (5): 595–601.

Occupational Safety and Health Administration. 2004. *Guidelines for Preventing Workplace Violence for Health Care and Social Workers.* OSHA Publication 3148. www.osha.gov/osha3148.pdf.

# Part IV

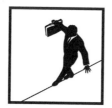

# SURVIVAL STRATEGIES

Part IV describes survival strategies when legal action is imminent, with a detailed look at the judicial process and how it can be fraught with risk for your organization. A strategy for aligning the healthcare provider and the healthcare executive through the legal process is suggested and detailed. Though Part IV might seem to be speaking to physicians, increasingly hospitals are employing physicians or partnering with them in healthcare initiatives. Consequently the healthcare leader must understand how physicians can run afoul of the law and how their missteps may put the organization at risk.

This section also covers the anatomy of a lawsuit (including causation, breach, negligence, and damages), how a provider may lose her license, and how the provider and the organization can get into civil and criminal lawsuits. Protective strategies are presented with an eye toward the ED and its unique set of risks.

# CHAPTER 35

# Anatomy of a Lawsuit

**In This Chapter**

- The Complaint
- Discovery
- Preparing a Defense
- Pretrial Motions
- Settlement Versus Trial
- Appeals
- The Role of Executive Leadership
- Case Study
- Strategies for Healthcare Executives

## THE COMPLAINT

The complaint is the beginning of a lawsuit. The complaint is filed with the court, explaining who the parties are and why the plaintiff is suing the defendant. Simultaneously a summons is usually filed to advise the defendant that she is being sued. For malpractice lawsuits, this may be delivered by a court courier or sheriff's deputy or sent by certified mail. The summons requires a response within a prescribed time line. The response usually consists of an answer, which should address each allegation. The answer will usually state if the defendant admits to or denies the allegations. However, it is acceptable for a defendant to state that she possesses insufficient information to confirm or deny the allegations. Any defenses formulated for the allegations may be noted in the answer.

Another response would be to file a motion to dismiss. This motion would be applicable if there is a clear and compelling reason why the suit should not continue. For instance, if an emergency physician were named as a defendant, but he was not involved in the care of the plaintiff and was erroneously named, it would be reasonable to file a motion to dismiss. If such a motion is filed, the plaintiff must in turn respond.

In some states, additional documentation may be required. For instance, in Pennsylvania, a certificate of merit must be filed within 60 days of filing a lawsuit. The certificate must confirm that a licensed physician has reviewed the case and feels that with reasonable probability, the care rendered fell below the standard of care.

## DISCOVERY

The discovery period provides the opportunity for the plaintiff and defendant to gain a sense of the case the other side will present. Certain disclosures are mandatory, such as those of any witnesses who will be deposed or called to testify. Also, any documents pertinent to the case, such as hospital policies, must be disclosed. Although certain items may slip through this process without being disclosed, it is in both parties' best interest to disclose all pertinent data, as required. If such items are discovered without disclosure, it may appear that they were intentionally withheld, weakening the case of the party who failed to disclose the discovered information.

Several mechanisms exist to obtain additional information during discovery. An *interrogatory* is a written question requiring a response under oath. *Requests for documents* may be made. If one side needs information that the other side possesses but has not provided, a request can and should be made. For example, if a hospital is the defendant, or more likely a codefendant, in a medical malpractice lawsuit and the plaintiff does not have a copy of the medical records, it would be reasonable and appropriate for the plaintiff to request these documents. *Requests for admissions* may also be drafted. These requests are drafted as specific questions that the opposing side must deny or admit. These help clarify questions in preparation for the case if a party is uncertain of a fact or exactly what position the opposition will take on a particular issue.

### Depositions

Depositions are almost universally used in medical malpractice cases. Depositions are interviews under oath; they are court proceedings and recorded documents of the court, despite the fact that they are not conducted in a courtroom. The first step in surviving a deposition is to understand its purpose: to discover evidence. It is a fishing expedition. An attorney can ask nearly anything, provided that the line of questions is reasonably calculated to lead to the discovery of relevant evidence. In other words, the attorney is exploring to see what evidence may justify pursuing the case further. The only information he will obtain will come from those deposed. Therefore, the deponent—an administrator or care provider—must be very careful about what she reveals. In addition to mining for information, a deposition is also used to destroy the credibility of a defendant by showing contradictions in testimony compared to trial testimony. Often, a deposition is performed months prior to trial. This time lapse results in fading recollections, and the defendant will have time to rethink her responses, often subconsciously. Although a defendant may find her more thoroughly considered trial testimony to be protective, if it contradicts that given in the earlier deposition, it is damning.

When the defendant is caught in contradictory answers to the same question, the credibility of all testimony she provided is called into question. This is a huge win for the plaintiff's attorney. The only right answer in trial is the same answer provided in deposition. This is why answers need to be carefully considered, and if clarification of the question is needed prior to answering, it should be asked for. Much time should be spent in prep sessions with an attorney before a deposition. If a statement needs to be revised from the deposition, the defendant's attorney could ask questions in trial that could help to clarify the deposition response. However, this still can be seen as backtracking, diminishing the defendant's credibility with the jury.

When being deposed, it is safest to stick to simple answers. Offering unsolicited information is a common mistake that may open up a new line of questioning the plaintiff's attorney hadn't previously considered. Yes and no answers, when feasible, may help to avoid overdisclosure. However, a plaintiff's attorney may twist this situation to discredit the defendant at a later time. Imagine an attorney trying to relax a defendant by saying, "If this is stressful for you, would you feel comfortable just giving yes or no answers?" If the defendant agrees, she can be limited to yes and no responses, which means she may be asked, "Did Mrs. Smith die because of a pulmonary embolism you misdiagnosed?" If the patient died of a PE, the defendant is now boxed in, and any response provided won't reflect positively on her. Another example, illustrating how a defendant might be trapped is, "Mr. Jones died of an intracranial hemorrhage after receiving t-PA for a stroke, and your policy calls for the administration of thrombolytics to stroke patients. Therefore, didn't following your policy result in his death?"

Another common mistake leading to inadvertent disclosures during deposition testimony is trying to use the deposition as an opportunity to explain one's actions or exonerate oneself. Such efforts only open doors for the plaintiff's attorney that should stay shut. Remember the goal: The plaintiffs are looking for facts that will improve their case and worsen yours. So, even if the defendant successfully explains a fact or issue, she has given the attorney information about what to avoid in the case. She may inadvertently give the plaintiff's attorney information on how better to conduct his case.

The plaintiff's attorney will likely use a reference or "learned treatise" on the topic. He will likely ask the defendant if she is aware of it or if it is a respected textbook. Then, he will ask if she would consider the source "authoritative." This is a legal term. If she has agreed that any source is "authoritative," the attorney will bind her to its contents and standards of care. Recognizing that every case has individual nuances, when being deposed never agree that any source is "authoritative."

Discussing the details of the case with anyone but your attorney may make privileged information discoverable and is not advised. Although most jurisdictions exempt spousal discussions, discussing a case with a coworker, friend, or other individual outside the attorney–client privilege will likely make the information provided discoverable and remove any peer-review protection that may have existed. Furthermore, those who discussed the case can be called to testify.

**Legal representation should be sought for all depositions**. An attorney will protect the defendant's rights during the deposition, submit the appropriate objections to lines of questioning, and advise her whether or not to answer the question posed. Raising the appropriate objections may give the defendant recourse later, as those objections are recorded in the deposition transcript. Even if the defendant ultimately answers the question, the objection should be noted. The defendant's attorney will understand the traps being set and should help the deponent successfully navigate through them. Some may feel that legal representation is not necessary when being deposed about a matter in which the deposed is not the defendant. This may be a fatal mistake, as the deposed may inadvertently become the day's catch while the attorney is fishing for something else. The deposed could suddenly find himself named as a codefendant or as a defendant in a separate lawsuit and cause of action.

Besides representing the deponent at the deposition, an attorney may be able to coach him in preparation for the deposition. Only a fool arrives at the deposition relying on memory, honesty, and luck to get him by. Depositions require preparation and practice. In addition, lawsuits can be stressful life events; litigation support such as counseling should be provided and sought. If such support is provided through the attorney–client privilege, the interactions are protected under that privilege and not discoverable.

---

**Strategies for Surviving a Deposition**

- Do not use a deposition as a chance to exonerate yourself.
- Use simple, brief answers.
- Do not answer questions you do not understand.
- Seek legal representation.
- Prepare for your deposition.
- Do not discuss your case with anyone except your attorney or spouse or significant other.
- Do not agree to yes or no answers only.
- Avoid creating conflicting testimony.

---

## PREPARING A DEFENSE

Preparing a defense has several aspects worth discussing. Initially, the required elements of a negligence lawsuit should be assessed.

---

**Necessary Elements of a Lawsuit for the Tort of Negligence**

- Duty to treat
- Breach of the standard of care in carrying out that duty
- Causation (direct and proximate)
- Damages

---

### Duty to Treat

The element of duty is important but is rarely a factor in medical malpractice claims involving hospitals. For instance, if a patient presented to the ED for treatment, a duty to treat most likely exists. There are some circumstances in which a duty may not be established, and establishing that no duty existed would be a tactic worth pursuing in defense of the allegations.

## Breach of the Standard of Care

Once duty is established, the next question is whether the standard of care was met while fulfilling that duty. The standard of care in medicine in current times is almost always a national standard, defined as what a reasonable provider (physician, nurse, hospital) with similar training in a similar set of circumstances would do. If the provider's actions are deemed to have fallen below the standard of care, negligence will be found.

## Causation

Causation is a bit trickier. Unfortunately, many defenses rest on the merits of causation or lack thereof. The plaintiff's injury or damages must be the direct result of the defendant's negligence. However, the defendant's negligence must also be the *proximate cause* of the injury. Proximate cause makes certain there are no superseding or intervening events that break the chain of causation. In other words, if some other event occurs after the defendant's negligence that may have resulted in the plaintiff's injury or damages, the defendant may not be liable. For example, if a patient is seen at Hospital A's emergency department for chest pain and is discharged inappropriately while experiencing a myocardial infarction and dies, Hospital A and its providers will likely be found negligent—there was a duty to act, the care fell below the standard of care, and their negligence was the direct and proximate cause of the patient's death. But what if the patient went immediately to Hospital B for a second opinion and was correctly diagnosed with an acute myocardial infarction, but died during percutaneous coronary intervention due to hemorrhage resulting from the interventional cardiologist's poor technique? The patient didn't actually die from the missed AMI; the procedural complication was the cause. This will likely relieve Hospital A of its liability.

## Damages

Damages are critical. If the patient does not experience damages (some sort of injury), there is no grounds for a lawsuit. If the patient described above is discharged from Hospital A and goes immediately to Hospital B and has a normal course, it is unlikely any damages occurred from Hospital A's negligence. Thus, there would be no grounds for a lawsuit.

## Reviewing the Case

The claim and allegations must be thoroughly reviewed by an expert panel or committee. Such a review will often provide a good sense of what the cause of action is, such as negligence, and what acts of commission or omissions constitute the plaintiff's negligence claim. The review should focus on the required elements of a negligence lawsuit. An unbiased review of the medical care should be carefully performed by a panel of experts or a committee, or it can be performed by commissioned outside experts. The reviewers should be blinded to the name of the practitioner, location, and outcome of the case. A formal report should be prepared and included in the confidential case file. All discussions need to be held in strict confidence as a work product of the attorney–client privilege, which provides much more powerful protection than any state's peer review statute. The summary should identify strengths and weaknesses of the case. Case attributes may be medical or nonmedical. For instance, if the case involves a child who has died, this is a factor that negatively affects any defendant's case. However, medical facts documenting a stable, well-appearing child at time of discharge are helpful to the defense.

In addition to the medical and nonmedical facts, the damages should be assessed. Reviewing the claimed damages, an estimate can be made of the potential outcome should a case go to trial and end in a plaintiff's verdict. This process may also assist with setting reserves for the case. Reserves are estimates of the judgment that must be set aside to finance the adverse verdict if it occurs.

Assessing the case for defense strategies requires a thorough review of elements of the tort of negligence. Any weaknesses with the elements will guide the defendant in preparing a defense.

Preparation of the defendant as a witness must be considered as well. If the plaintiff will invoke sympathy from the jury or the defendant will not make a good witness for any reason, the defendant may consider a settlement instead of taking a case to trial. Although many malpractice claims do not involve true negligence, the risk of a large jury verdict for the plaintiff may persuade even the most righteous defendant to consider settling a case. If a case proceeds to trial, litigation support should be provided to the defendants. This includes instruction on how to testify as well as instruction on mannerisms, attire, and body language. Responses to anticipated lines of questioning in deposition and in trial should be discussed and rehearsed. Finally, emotional support is frequently necessary but much less often provided.

## PRETRIAL MOTIONS

In addition to the motion to dismiss (discussed on pages 327–28), another pretrial motion the defendant may file is a *motion for summary judgment*. In summary judgment, the judge must rule on the appropriate application of law, not the facts of the case. If there is no reasonable basis in law for the suit following discovery, the case should be dismissed. For example, if the physician was acting as a Good Samaritan and the state offers protections for Good Samaritan actions, a motion for summary judgment may well be granted.

## SETTLEMENT VERSUS TRIAL

The decision to go to trial is one of merit and economics. This is a complicated decision-making process misunderstood by many. It is impossible to make this decision on the medical merits alone. Every provider has a great deal of pride in the care she provides. Furthermore, inappropriate lawsuits filed for economic relief due to bad outcomes without associated negligence should be fought to deter subsequent similar cases. However, when the damages are potentially high, the plaintiff is sympathetic, the defendant may not connect with the jury, and/or the facts of the case pose a risk of a plaintiff's verdict, settling a case is a reasonable consideration. Settling a case that you feel is likely to be lost is usually a good decision for the defense. It will limit the loss, reduce defense expenses, and spare the defendant the emotional strain of enduring a lengthy and often difficult adjudication process. Currently, if a defendant requests to try the case when the insurance company prefers settlement, the physician may be asked to sign an agreement ("bad-faith letter") accepting responsibility for any judgment in excess of what the case could have been settled for. When such forms are presented, the hard financial realities involved in the decision to try or settle a case become very real and personal for the defendant.

The trial itself may only take a week or two. However, the entire process, including pretrial preparation, may take years. The good news is that the majority of cases that go to trial result in a defense verdict (Kirkton 2008).

## APPEALS

Appeals are not uncommon in tort cases. The grounds for an appeal are commonly misunderstood. An appeal cannot be filed on the grounds that you just didn't like how the jury decided the case. A procedural error must have occurred for an appeal to be granted. For instance, the judge giving the jury inappropriate instructions prior to deliberation could be grounds for an appeal. Appeals can take years to complete and are usually expensive. These factors must be weighed when considering whether an appeal is appropriate in a given case or not.

## THE ROLE OF EXECUTIVE LEADERSHIP

Depositions are high-risk legal encounters that often do not get the serious attention they deserve. They place not only the physician or staff member being deposed at risk, but they put the organization at risk. Depositions also increase the stress on all those involved, and these healthcare providers can become impaired by the stress. The healthcare executive can protect the organization and support his staff by offering educational sessions for those being deposed and support services for those in the throes of a lawsuit. From the first inklings of litigation, staff need education on confidentiality during the case and what to expect at each stage of the legal action. This can be a great opportunity for team building, as those involved march through time and tension during a malpractice case.

---

**Case Study**

A hospital-employed mid-level provider is deposed involving the death of a newborn seen in the ED. The mid-level provider goes into the deposition uncoached and unprepared. He is immediately tripped up by the plaintiff's attorney and contradicts himself three times in the first ten minutes of the deposition.

The attorney traps the deponent into saying that he didn't need to call the physician on duty because he was comfortable with his clinical judgment in the case and had no need of the opinion of someone with more training and experience. In addition, and of extreme importance, the attorney brings the hospital into the fray by asking what the supervisory requirements are for a mid-level provider in the emergency department according to the hospital bylaws.

The attorney gets the deponent to say that he is always capable of recognizing an ill infant and that is why he ignored a critical lab value that suggested the child was gravely ill. The attorney then retorts, "Well I guess you can't always recognize a sick infant: You sent this infant home and he died!"

The hospital attorney reports back to the CEO that he feels it would be impossible to recover from the damage done by this deposition, and he urges a meeting with the board to recommend settlement instead of going to trial.

SOURCE: Quality Matters Consulting review case (Welch 2008c).

---

## Recommended Readings

Brenner, I. R. 2010. *How to Survive a Medical Malpractice Lawsuit: The Physician's Roadmap to Success.* Hoboken, NJ: John Wiley & Sons, Inc.

Uribe, C. G. 2000. *The Health Care Provider's Guide to Facing the Malpractice Deposition.* Boca Raton, FL: CRC Press, LLC.

# CHAPTER 36

# How Not to Lose Your License

**In This Chapter**

- State Control of the Practice of Medicine
- Whom Does a State Board Serve?
- Common Themes
- Do You Need a Lawyer?
- Resources for Further Information
- The Role of Executive Leadership
- Case Study
- Strategies for Healthcare Executives

## STATE CONTROL OF THE PRACTICE OF MEDICINE

Every state legislature has created an agency with the authority to control who may practice medicine in that state. Most of these state laws date back to the turn of the twentieth century, when licensure followed the formalization and standardization of medical education. In addition to providing a process for screening applicants for licensure, these agencies carry a duty to monitor doctors in practice and discipline physicians who violate administrative requirements or practice in a manner not conforming to the standards of care in their specialty.

# WHOM DOES A STATE BOARD SERVE?

State legislatures created agencies to protect the public from people posing as doctors and from doctors practicing substandard care. In this context, it should be noted that state control of medical care was in part precipitated by snake oil sellers and other unscrupulous entrepreneurs. The state medical board does protect the economic interests of physicians by limiting competition—if medical boards did not exist, theoretically anyone could start up a physician's practice and take business away from trained physicians. What is interesting, however, is how many physicians believe the state medical board is in place to protect *them*. A look at a sampling of mission statements from four state medical boards reveals how far from the truth that belief really is (Exhibit 36.1).

Each state makes perfectly clear that the board serves the public, yet physicians may become incensed when they perceive the state medical board to be "antiphysician." Understanding the role of the state licensing agency would help many physicians who are subject to disciplinary investigations following a patient's complaint.

## COMMON THEMES

As every state controls the practice of medicine in that state, it is imperative that all physicians look to the licensing agency for guidance in avoiding disciplinary issues.

---

**Exhibit 36.1: Sample State Board Mission Statements**

**Texas: Texas Medical Board**
To protect and enhance the public's health, safety, and welfare by establishing and maintaining standards of excellence used in regulating the practice of medicine and ensuring quality health care for the citizens of Texas through licensure, discipline, and education.

**Massachusetts: Board of Registration in Medicine**
To ensure that only qualified physicians are licensed to practice in the Commonwealth of Massachusetts and that those physicians and health care institutions in which they practice provide to their patients a high standard of care.

**Delaware: Department of State, Division of Professional Regulation**
Our mission is to credential qualified professionals to ensure the protection of the public's health, safety, and welfare.

**Nevada: Nevada State Board of Medical Examiners**
The Nevada State Board of Medical Examiners serves the State of Nevada by ensuring that only well-qualified, competent physicians, physician assistants, and respiratory therapists receive licenses to practice in Nevada.

---

However, certain common themes suggest that the following behavior could result in disciplinary procedures, up to and including suspension or loss of a license to practice medicine.

---

### Behaviors That Will Result in Disciplinary Action Against a Physician

- Not meeting the standard of care in your area of practice
- Sexual impropriety, attacks, or rape (and, in some states, consensual sexual relationships in some areas of practice)
- Impairment (drugs or alcohol) without treatment or with repetitive treatment failures
- Failure to maintain state-required continuing medical education
- Failure to meet state reporting statutes (communicable diseases, wounds, death)
- Inadequate documentation of patient care in patient record
- Inaccurate billing
- Failure to protect patient rights (informed consent, privacy, access to records)
- Practicing beyond scope of practice (in many states, practicing beyond the physician's field of specialty)
- False advertising or declaring an expertise without proper credentials
- Improper patient recruitment (working through "ambulance chasers")
- Unprofessional behavior (threats; intimidation; anger against patients, staff, or other people)
- Failure to maintain licensure
- Repeated claims of negligence
- Violation of state and federal rules pertaining to prescription authority
- Allowing nonlicensed people to practice medicine under the physician's license and with the physician's knowledge
- Falsifying (or withholding) information provided to the state licensing authority
- Failure to properly comply with an investigation by the state licensing authority

---

## DO YOU NEED A LAWYER?

Many physicians are misinformed about the role of the state licensing authority and are not properly concerned when an investigation is initiated, thinking, "These are my people, they will understand." Given that the role of licensing authorities is to protect the *public,* it would be foolhardy to dismiss the importance of any inquiry.

Relatively speaking, physicians are savvy when dealing with medical malpractice suits, but far less so in dealing with their own state licensing authorities. A medical malpractice claim might result in the loss of significant money in the form of damages, but a successful investigation by the state could result in the loss of livelihood.

A lawyer's assistance is obviously mandatory when responding to any inquiry by a state licensing authority. In some cases the cost of the lawyer might be covered by the physician's liability insurance policy; every physician should discuss this matter with her insurance carrier.

## RESOURCES FOR FURTHER INFORMATION

Presumably all physicians are well acquainted with the rules and regulations pertaining to the practice of medicine in their state and know exactly how to reach their state authority if they have any questions about their license. However, the American Medical Association offers a convenient service on its website with access to nonmembers. If a physician wants to know more about the state he is licensed in, or wants to compare other states' rules of practice, he can easily access all licensing authorities through the site.

### AMA Links to State Medical Boards

The process of obtaining a medical license—either initial licensure or a subsequent license in another state—can be challenging. To help physicians navigate the licensure process and to provide up-to-date information on requirements across all US states and jurisdictions, the American Medical Association (AMA) publishes the *State Medical Licensure Requirements and Statistics* annually.

This reference includes data tables on required examinations, training, education (both graduate medical education and continuing medical education), and fees. Data are broken out for US medical school graduates as well as for international medical graduates. Also included are data on the numbers of initial and subsequent licenses awarded by state as well as information on key organizations involved in the licensure process, such as

(continued)

the Federation of State Medical Boards, National Board of Medical Examiners, and Educational Commission for Foreign Medical Graduates. Check out the site at www.ama-assn.org/ama/pub/education-careers/becoming-physician/medical-licensure/state-medical-boards.shtml.

Physicians should monitor their state licensing authority closely; all should be aware of new rules and the trend in investigations in their state. Other support, assistance, and education can be obtained through state professional societies.

## THE ROLE OF EXECUTIVE LEADERSHIP

Many executives in healthcare are directly involved with the ongoing maintenance of the physician licenses in an ED (as well as other licensed professionals). Proper record keeping, including verification of meeting the state CME requirements, is vital. Assisting in the documentation of complaints and the appropriate response to an investigation, in consultation with the subject physician, is an important role for the executive. Even when physicians in an ED are contracted physicians and not employees (which is still the most prevalent staffing model for emergency physicians), the healthcare executive needs to be aware of the licensing requirements in the state as well as the status of any licensing issues with any member of the medical staff.

### Case Study

The manner in which a physician responds to an investigation by the state licensing authority can obviously affect the outcome of the investigation. Without even questioning the merits of the original inquiry, few cases could better illustrate what not to do if you are under state scrutiny than the following 2008 Texas case.

Dr. X was the subject of an investigation based on a complaint that he was prescribing human growth hormone and other substances without medical necessity. The Texas Medical Board (TMB) staff sent several subpoenas to Dr. X requesting the medical records of 13 specified patients as well as various business records. Dr. X's reply to the board stated: "I have reviewed the charts of the following patients.... I find no prescribing irregularities or patient complaints."

(continued)

Dr. X also asked each of the 13 patients to be custodian of her own medical records and had them sign letters stating that they did not want their medical records reviewed by the TMB. Dr. X sent a letter to the board stating that he did not possess any of the items requested by board staff.

The TMB called for two temporary suspension hearings. Dr. X did not attend either hearing, but a representative spoke on his behalf. A panel of the TMB determined that Dr. X's continuation in the practice of medicine presents a continuing threat to the public welfare, and he was suspended. The length of a temporary suspension is indefinite, and it remains in effect until the board takes further action.

SOURCE: Texas Medical Board (2008).

## Strategies for Healthcare Executives

- Know the "hot topics" from the point of view of your state's medical board.
- Require the reporting of any state medical board investigation or sanction to the credentialing and privileging committee and to the medical staff office immediately.
- Consider having personnel documents and other written resources available for physicians, particularly those employed by the organization, undergoing an encounter with the state medical board.

## Recommended Reading

Your state's licensing rules

Alexander, B., B. M. Broccolo, K. F. Conley, A. R. Daniels, M. Dube, R. G. Hoban, C. B. Hutto, C. C. Loepere, D. E. Matyas, T. W. Mayo, J. J. Miles, R. E. Sallade, M. F. Schaff, S. O. Scheutzow, D. J. Schwartz, and E. T. Thomas. 2008. *AHLA Fundamentals of Health Law,* Fourth Edition. Washington, DC: American Health Lawyers Association.

# CHAPTER 37

# How Not to Go to Jail: Criminal Liability in the ED, Part I

**In This Chapter**

- Criminal Versus Civil Liability, Reprise
- Fraudulent Billing
- The Role of Executive Leadership
- Case Study
- Strategies for Healthcare Executives

## CRIMINAL VERSUS CIVIL LIABILITY, REPRISE

As noted in Chapter 15, there is a distinction between *civil* and *criminal* liability in healthcare. However, that distinction is frequently blurred, and often intentionally. Nothing sells quite like fear. Civil laws (e.g., the majority of HIPAA, EMTALA, and Stark) may present significant exposure to fines and other penalties, such as the revocation of a hospital's provider agreement or exclusion from any government program, but they do not include the possibility of incarceration.

This chapter will delve into legal violations that could land a healthcare executive or physician in jail. At the very least, flirtation with any of the following behaviors could result in significant legal fees to stay out of jail. Along those lines, it is important to note that a person cannot be insured for criminal behavior. Criminal financial penalties are supposed to hurt; a person cannot prepay for criminal behavior by purchasing insurance to cover such a penalty.

# FRAUDULENT BILLING

Physicians in an ED are far less likely to run afoul with fraudulent billing, as they are not as involved in the billing process as their colleagues in private practice. Having said that, anyone involved in the billing process for ED services could participate in activities that rise to the level of criminal activity.

## A Long Line of Legislative Initiatives and the Impact of HIPAA

Shortly after the government became a payer for healthcare, Congress started passing laws warning against defrauding the government for healthcare services. Year after year Congress issued warnings that did not appear to stem the tide of billing irregularities.

---

### Long Line of Legislative Initiatives*

- 1972: Amendment of Social Security Act
- 1977: Medicare and Medicaid Antifraud and Abuse
- 1981: Medicare and Medicaid Antifraud and Abuse
- 1986: False Claims Act
- 1987: Medicare and Medicaid Patient and Program Protection Act
- 1996: Health Insurance Portability and Accountability Act (HIPAA)
- 1997: Balanced Budget Act

*This list is not all-inclusive.

---

It was HIPAA in 1996 that set fraud and abuse investigations on a new course. Although HIPAA is most commonly associated with patient privacy protections, the law made significant contributions to the government's endeavors to detect, investigate, and punish fraudulent billing activity.

The focus on fraudulent billing of governmental payers should not be construed as a lack of liability when falsely billing private payers. In fact, private companies and third-party payers maintain their own internal antifraud units and may cooperate with government investigations in combating healthcare fraud (Matyas and Valiant 2006). Activities that violate other federal laws (e.g., the antikickback statute and Stark) may dovetail with questionable billing practices and be combined with a False Claims Act violation (OIG 2010).

## Fraud and Abuse, Defined

According to the False Claims Act (31 U.S.C. § 3729–3733), any provider, including a physician, that "knowingly presents, or causes to be presented, a false or fraudulent claim for payment or approval, or knowingly makes, uses, or causes to be made or used, a false record or statement material to a false or fraudulent claim" can be prosecuted for filing a false claim against the government.

The risks of fraudulent billing are great. Civil monetary penalties (CMP) include a possible penalty of $11,000 per false claim, plus up to three times the amount of the claim. Each item or service billed constitutes a claim under the False Claims Act, so fines can add up quickly (OIG 2010).

Under the False Claims Act a person who has submitted a false bill may be fined, even if the filing was not an intentional fraud, because "no specific intent to defraud is required" (OIG 2010). For those billing practices that rise to criminal intent, incarceration and/or criminal penalties may result.

The Office of Inspector General (OIG 2010) has released an excellent resource, *A Roadmap for New Physicians: Avoiding Medicare and Medicaid Fraud and Abuse*. Aimed at physicians entering the workforce but appropriate for all providers, the guide provides succinct, clear descriptions of all the laws that might be violated as a result of billing practices and provides guidance on how to best avoid activity that could be construed as fraud and abuse. It is available for free download at the OIG website (http://oig.hhs.gov/compliance/physician-education/index.asp).

## How Honest People Can Find Themselves Under Investigation

The stated intent of authorities is to uncover truly fraudulent billing activity, but in the process of that pursuit a lot of perfectly honest providers find themselves under investigation. All payers, public and private, compare the billings from one provider against other providers who are similarly situated. An ED should be aware, therefore, that an unusually high volume of claims, an unusually high number of claims for a particular intervention, and billing for services not generally offered by EDs could raise suspicion.

An investigation might also be precipitated by a complaint from a member of the public (such as a Medicare beneficiary who reports he does not agree with the bill as evidenced by the explanation of benefits), a disgruntled former employee reporting to the authorities that the ED is involved in fraudulent billing practices, or a **qui tam** action initiated by an employee in administration or

> **Qui tam:** A suit brought by an individual on behalf of the US government seeking to expose the misuse or waste of federal funds.

the business office. Documentation that explains and confirms any bill submitted for payment is critical.

## Penalties

All people make mistakes, and even the most scrupulous healthcare providers will have errors on their books if someone looks hard enough. An investigation precipitated by a confused patient or a disgruntled former employee could, therefore, result in significant civil penalties.

Criminal violations require intent and are the result of behavior that cannot be construed as a mistake. Providers should be warned that doing bad things while remaining deliberately ignorant will still be sufficient to show criminal intent. However, the greatest danger on either the civil or criminal side of the law is for most providers the threat of exclusion from government health programs. Even a conscientious biller can be excluded for obstructing or interfering with an investigation. Under the Social Security Act, "an individual owner, officer, or managing employee of a sanctioned entity" may be individually excluded for "their role or interest in a company that is excluded or is convicted of certain offenses. These exclusions are permissive, that is, the Secretary has the discretion whether to exclude or not to exclude. OIG's exercise of this discretion is not subject to administrative or judicial review" (OIG 1997).

The threat of exclusion increases as the billing activities that precipitate an investigation become more egregious. The penalty of exclusion is not limited to fraudulently billing Medicare; HIPAA and the Balanced Budget Act of 1997 expanded the OIG's sanction authorities so that exclusion may now be imposed for improper billing from all federal healthcare programs (OIG 1999).

The penalty of exclusion is so significant that some providers may feel compelled to slip an excluded provider some patient referrals. To ward against such Good Samaritans within the healthcare community, the government created a $10,000 penalty under the Balanced Budget Act of 1997 that may be levied against any provider participating with an excluded colleague or institution. To assist people in the healthcare community in knowing whom they should not do business with, the US Department of Health and Human Services provides an online database of sanctioned providers that is updated daily.

# THE ROLE OF EXECUTIVE LEADERSHIP

A crucial role for leaders in healthcare is to consistently address rumors and unfounded fears of criminal liability in their workforce and among their peers. Far too many people have a vested interested in creating commotion among providers; leaders can help others maintain an educated distinction between civil and criminal liabilities.

At the same time, any suggestion of criminal activity must be dealt with immediately and aggressively. A zero-tolerance policy should extend not only to employees but to colleagues as well.

---

### Case Study

The owner and the vice president of a Detroit-area physical therapy clinic were convicted by a federal jury for their roles in a $23 million Medicare fraud scheme. After a six-day trial, the jury convicted Bernice Brown of ten counts of healthcare fraud and one count of conspiracy to commit healthcare fraud. Daniel Smorynski was convicted of six counts of healthcare fraud and one count of conspiracy to commit healthcare fraud. Each substantive healthcare fraud charge and the conspiracy charge carry a maximum penalty of ten years in prison and a $250,000 fine.

Evidence at trial established that Bernice Brown was the owner and president of Wayne County Therapeutic Inc. (WCT) in Livonia, Michigan. Daniel Smorynski was the vice president. WCT purported to be an outpatient clinic that specialized in physical and occupational therapy. Evidence at trial established that Brown purchased fake physical and occupational therapy files from certain third-party contractors, and she and Smorynski billed the services reflected in the files to Medicare as if WCT therapists had provided the services. Brown instructed her staff to create false documents and to add those documents to medical files to make it appear that the WCT therapists, who were licensed in the state and enrolled with Medicare, had performed the services, when she knew they had not. According to evidence presented at trial, Smorynski was in charge of billing at WCT and aided in the submission of claims for services he knew WCT did not provide. Between approximately October 2002 and September 2006, Brown and Smorynski submitted approximately $23.2 million in claims to Medicare for physical and occupational therapy services that were never provided. Medicare paid approximately $6.5 million of those claims.

Evidence at trial showed that Brown and Smorynski, in addition to submitting claims for nonexistent physical and occupational therapy, caused WCT to submit fraudulent claims for psychotherapy services. In January 2006, when Congress enacted a cap on physical and occupational therapy services to control costs,

(continued)

Brown and Smorynski devised a scheme to avoid the cap by billing for psycho-therapy services. Evidence at trial showed that Brown and Smorynski launched a lobbying effort to repeal the cap, which included WCT staff drafting letters and petitions to Congress purportedly on behalf of Medicare patients. Brown and Smorynski then instructed WCT staff to bill Medicare for their lobbying efforts as psychotherapy evaluations and visits. In 2006, WCT billed $493,200 to Medicare for psychotherapy services that were not necessary and not provided, and Medicare paid approximately $121,921 of those claims.

CMS, working in conjunction with the OIG, are taking steps to increase accountability and decrease the presence of fraudulent providers.

SOURCE: Office of Public Affairs, US Department of Justice (2010b).

### Strategies for Healthcare Executives

- Ensure that staff are well trained to handle the complexities of billing and coding.
- Commit to regular training courses for the people managing billing and coding.
- Demand excellence, and conduct in-house audits regularly.

## Recommended Readings

Alexander, B., B. M. Broccolo, K. F. Conley, A. R. Daniels, M. Dube, R. G. Hoban, C. B. Hutto, C. C. Loepere, D. E. Matyas, T. W. Mayo, J. J. Miles, R. E. Sallade, M. F. Schaff, S. O. Scheutzow, D. J. Schwartz, and E. T. Thomas. 2008. *AHLA Fundamentals of Health Law,* Fourth Edition. Washington, DC: American Health Lawyers Association.

Matyas, D., and C. Valiant. 2006. *Legal Issues in Healthcare Fraud and Abuse: Navigating the Uncertainties,* Third Edition. Washington, DC: American Health Lawyers Association.

Office of Inspector General. 2010. *A Roadmap for New Physicians: Avoiding Medicare and Medicaid Fraud and Abuse.* http://oig.hhs.gov/compliance/physician-education/index.asp.

Wing, K., and B. Gilbert, B. 2006. *The Law and the Public's Health* Seventh Edition. Particularly Chapter 8: "The Antitrust Laws: Government Enforcement of Competition." Chicago: Health Administration Press.

# CHAPTER 38

# How Not to Go to Jail: Criminal Liability in the ED, Part II

## In This Chapter

- Kickbacks
- Antitrust
- Criminal Penalties Under HIPAA
- Rape and Assault
- Homicide and Criminal Negligence
- The Role of Executive Leadership
- Case Study
- Strategies for Healthcare Executives

## KICKBACKS

Any time any financial incentive is given for prescribing any medical treatment—including money exchanged in return for filling a hospital bed, obtaining a diagnostic service, prescribing a certain medication, or using certain durable medical equipment—the specter of a **kickback** is raised.

Most of the reported investigations for kickback schemes involve doctors out in the community, as opposed to within the hospital. Physicians with hospital privileges who are in a position to determine what prosthetics are used in surgery (orthopedic surgery), what high-end equipment is purchased (radiology, neurosurgery), and what medications are stocked (oncology, cardiol-

> **Kickback:** Any inducement, solicitation, receipt, offer, or payment of any kind in return for referrals or for recommending, ordering, leasing, or purchasing a service or item that may be at least partially paid for through a federal program.

ogy) may all be prey to kickback scenarios within a hospital, but the ED physicians are less likely to be subject to illegal schemes and bribery.

If a kickback is proven, both parties involved are subject to significant repercussions, including up to five years in prison and/or a $25,000 fine, which is not covered by any insurance policy because offering or accepting a kickback is a felony.

Certain activities that on the surface appear to be kickbacks may be permitted, particularly if patient access to healthcare is improved or quality of care is enhanced. "Safe harbors" have been identified by the government to allow for innovation and economies of scale. The designation of a safe harbor is, however, fact specific. Any ED that would like to participate in activity that could be questioned needs to obtain an advisory opinion, available through the Office of Inspector General (OIG), to first determine if the arrangement the ED proposes will pass scrutiny. Advisory opinions are available for a relatively small investment of time and money, but they should be pursued only with appropriate legal counsel.

The scenario that is most likely to raise suspicion in the ED is paying doctors to provide on-call coverage. As discussed in Chapter 19, this practice has become common, but that does not mean it is universally accepted. The two advisory opinions released by the OIG on this issue have demonstrated that paying physicians to accept responsibility for patients in the ED must not result in double payment, must not involve federal money, and must be motivated by increasing access for the public (OIG 2008, 2006).

The determining factor in any kickback inquiry, including payment for on-call services, is whether the amount exchanged constitutes fair market value. Currently the amount of money paid for on-call services is ratcheting up in most communities, as the physicians demanding payment set the market. This does not mean that the level of payment would pass government inquiry (McConnell et al. 2007). The amount of money involved in the two reimbursement plans submitted for advisory opinions was miniscule compared to current payments rumored to be common in the healthcare community. In both opinions, fair market value had been established by third parties retained by the hospitals in question; it remains to be seen how high federal law enforcement will allow payment for on-call coverage to climb.

## ANTITRUST

Antitrust legislation was originally passed in 1890 and 1914 to control anticompetitive behavior in the manufacturing and industrial communities. The "learned professions," including medicine, were exempt until the 1970s. Since then antitrust liability, including criminal penalties, has been an increasing concern in healthcare.

Antitrust actions could be brought by federal authorities or by state law enforcement under anticompetitive state statutes. Criminal penalties are usually the threat if a government is involved, but a private party (e.g., a physician denied credentials) may bring an antitrust action seeking triple civil damages for harm caused by anticompetitive activity. One set of facts could, therefore, result in simultaneous suits by both the federal and state governments, although they are likely to coordinate efforts, and a completely separate private action in civil court.

Other activities that could be considered antitrust would more likely involve the hospital administration than individual physicians in an ED. These uncompetitive activities include horizontal price fixing, market splitting, boycotts, or tying the purchase of one product or service with another. Any predatory conduct of this nature could result in significant fines and penalties, including incarceration. However, the good news for EDs is that the nature of the emergency patient makes illegal prearrangements of this nature less possible than with the elective patient population.

## HCQIA and Antitrust Protection

The risk for antitrust actions within the ED is lower than it is in more competitive departments of the hospital. Allegations might arise, however, in the hiring of ED medical personnel and could include any effort to deny mid-level practitioners employment opportunities within their scope of practice under state law. Physicians in an ED must also be sure that any peer review process follows the Health Care Quality Improvement Act of 1986 (HCQIA) to the letter, as that law provides the only true protection against antitrust allegations related to credentialing and peer review. All medical personnel should seek direction from the hospital attorney and hospital bylaws when they participate in any credentialing or peer-review functions.

Most antitrust actions in the healthcare industry start with the threat of jail, but they are resolved by settlement through a consent decree. These will invariably involve extensive financial penalties and some level of court supervision of the provider for a number of years.

# CRIMINAL PENALTIES UNDER HIPAA

As discussed in Chapter 15, the vast majority of HIPAA penalties do not involve jail, as they are lapses on the civil side of the law. If, however, someone is participating in "wrongful conduct that involves the intent to sell, transfer, or use identifiable health information for commercial advantage, personal gain, or malicious harm," she could be subject to criminal penalties, including incarceration (US Congress 42 U.S.C. 1320d–6).

## RAPE AND ASSAULT

Any action that would be criminal on the street would, of course, be criminal in an ED as well. Assault or sexual attack, such as rape, would be subject to the state law and enforcement pertaining to that crime. The real concern in an ED is not preventing these crimes by hospital personnel but preventing false allegations by patients and the public. Both male and female personnel in an ED must be vigilant in maintaining procedures meant to help them, such as the presence of a chaperone during any intimate examination.

Finally, and of particular concern, is the growing possibility of violence by the public against personnel in the ED. Hospitals were put on alert early in 2010 by The Joint Commission that violence in hospitals was increasing; those concerns escalated significantly with the shooting of a physician at Johns Hopkins Hospital on September 16, 2010. All departments should be evaluating security precautions; this is particularly true of EDs, which are closest to the street and remain the most likely location in a hospital for violence against providers. (More is said about this in Chapter 34).

## HOMICIDE AND CRIMINAL NEGLIGENCE

Medical malpractice lawsuits are meant to address negligence in the delivery of healthcare. These cases arise under state law, in state courts, and in accordance with state precedence. Successful claims of medical malpractice result in the award of damages to the plaintiff and often also include injunctions and court orders for institutional and individual providers to change their behavior and practices. Similar civil court proceedings are available under federal civil law to patients who claim to have been injured in federal facilities.

An argument can be made that the medical malpractice liability system works. Heaven knows there are angry people on both sides arguing against the system. One side would like greater liability and more patient protections, while the other side argues for tort reform, citing abuses of the system, frivolous suits, and increased costs due to defensive medicine. All of these arguments for revision occur on the civil side of the law.

Medical malpractice suits frequently involve claims for life-altering disability, dismemberment, or death. Many of these lawsuits invoke feelings of sadness and even anger. The civil courts—with the award of damages, punitive damages, and injunctions—are designed to deal effectively with even the most egregious outcomes. Unfortunately, there are times when the public, made aware of an injured patient by local media, will express outrage and demands for "justice" that if brought to that conclusion might involve incarceration of physicians or other healthcare executives.

Egregious care calls for egregious damages, as allowed for under the civil rules. Licensure should also be questioned in many cases; the system is designed to deny truly bad providers access to patients. The concern is that public furor will increasingly blur the line between civil and criminal claims, which will undoubtedly result in more errors going underground. Adding the threat of incarceration to the delivery of care will not advance society's quality objectives.

To prevent further criminalization of medical malpractice, state law enforcement must resist the calls of public mobs. Our communities need to be taught that no one benefits from bringing healthcare into the criminal sphere.

## THE ROLE OF EXECUTIVE LEADERSHIP

We may be on the cusp of a new era of healthcare criminal liability. The public is angry about the costs and delivery issues in healthcare and may begin pushing prosecutors to act. The prudent executive leader is aware of this changing landscape and seeks to minimize risk on all fronts.

### Case Study

In 2006 a jury declared the death of a heart attack victim, who spent almost two hours in an ED waiting room, to be a homicide. Beatrice Vance, 49, died of a heart attack, but the jury at a coroner's inquest ruled that her death also was "a result of gross deviations from the standard of care that a reasonable person would have exercised in this situation."

Vance had waited almost two hours for a doctor to see her after complaining of classic heart attack symptoms—nausea, shortness of breath, and chest pains—deputy coroner Robert Barrett testified. She was seen by a triage nurse about 15 minutes after she arrived, and the nurse classified her condition as "semi-emergent," Barrett said. He said Vance's daughter twice asked nurses after that

(continued)

when her mother would see a doctor. When her name was finally called, a nurse found Vance slumped unconscious in a waiting room chair without a pulse. Barrett said. She was pronounced dead shortly afterward.

Eventually the state's attorney dropped criminal charges after insufficient evidence was found to support the criminal charges, but the case stands as a cautionary tale for how egregious negligence coupled with public outrage can result in criminal liability.

SOURCE: Peterson (2007).

### Strategies for Healthcare Executives

- Ensure that informed legal counsel looks at all financial arrangements with a keen eye for possible kickback and antitrust violations.
- Institute sound and decisive programs for credentialing and performance evaluation.
- Make patient safety rounds a regular part of the executive leader's work.
- Institute policies and procedures regarding violent persons on hospital property and educate all staff in them.

## Recommended Readings

Alexander, B., B. M. Broccolo, K. F. Conley, A. R. Daniels, M. Dube, R. G. Hoban, C. B. Hutto, C. C. Loepere, D. E. Matyas, T. W. Mayo, J. J. Miles, R. E. Sallade, M. F. Schaff, S. O. Scheutzow, D. J. Schwartz, and E. T. Thomas. 2008. AHLA *Fundamentals of Health Law* Fourth Edition. Washington, DC: American Health Lawyers Association.

Matyas, D., and C. Valiant. 2006. *Legal Issues in Healthcare Fraud and Abuse: Navigating the Uncertainties,* Third Edition. Washington, DC: American Health Lawyers Association.

Wing, K., and B. Gilbert, B. 2006. *The Law and the Public's Health,* Seventh Edition. Particularly Chapter 8: "The Antitrust Laws: Government Enforcement of Competition." Chicago: Health Administration Press.

# Glossary

Adnexal mass: A mass in the space in and around the fallopian tube or ovary, that is suggestive of an ectopic pregnancy. It may also be a malignancy, a complex ovarian cyst, or an infectious process.

Advanced triage protocols: Chief complaint-based, nurse-driven order sets that allow the nurse to begin diagnostic and therapeutic interventions from triage, before the physician sees the patient.

Adverse drug event (ADE): An injury associated with administration of a medication, which may include a drug reaction, drug–disease interaction, drug–drug interaction, allergic reaction, or medication side effects.

Aortic aneurysm: A ballooning or widening of the main artery (the aorta) as it courses down through the body. The aneurysm weakens the wall of the aorta and can result in the aorta dissecting or rupturing with catastrophic consequences. These are typically found in the abdomen.

Aortic dissection: A separation of the layers of the arterial wall. This may occur in conjunction with aneurysm formation. This typically occurs in the chest, in the thoracic aorta.

Apnea: A period of time during which breathing stops or is markedly reduced.

Case fatality: The ratio of deaths within a designated population of people with a particular condition over a certain period of time. An example of a fatality rate would be 9 deaths per 10,000 people at risk per year. This means that within a given year, out of 10,000 people formally diagnosed with a disease, 9 died.

Core measures: A set of quality indicators defined by The Joint Commission. There are 33 core measures in 4 categories (acute myocardial infarction, community-acquired pneumonia, congestive heart failure, and surgical care improvement project). Under each category, key actions are listed that represent the most widely accepted, research-based care processes for appropriate care in that category.

D-dimer assay: A blood assay that can be used to screen for pulmonary embolism.

Decompensation: A catastrophic disruption of an organ system with progression to organ system failure.

Deep venous thrombosis (DVT): Blood clots, typically in the legs, sometimes developed by postoperative patients. By applying compression stockings and getting patients moving early in the post-op period, this risk is reduced.

Done nomogram: A chart used to predict serious aspirin overdose using blood levels of aspirin and the time from ingestion.

Door-to-balloon time: The time from arrival at the emergency department to angioplasty in the cardiac catheterization lab for patients with an acute ST elevation myocardial infarction.

Dyspnea: Difficulty breathing, shortness of breath.

Elopement: Unauthorized departure of a patient.

ED ultrasonography: Also called "bedside ultrasound," this procedure refers to testing done in the ED with a machine trundled to the bedside.

Epididymitis: Inflammation or infection of the epididymis, the long coiled tube attached to the upper part of each testicle.

Iatrogenic: An illness or symptoms induced in a patient as the result of a physician's words or actions (e.g., as a consequence of taking a prescribed drug).

Implied consent: Signs, actions, or facts, or an inaction or silence, that raise a presumption that consent has been given.

Intrapartum: Related to the birth process.

Ischemia: Inadequate blood flow to tissues or organs.

Kickback: Any inducement, solicitation, receipt, offer, or payment of any kind in return for referrals or for recommending, ordering, leasing, or purchasing a service or item that may be at least partially paid for through a federal program.

Medication error: Any preventable event that may cause or lead to inappropriate medication use or patient harm while the medication is in the control of the healthcare professional, patient, or consumer.

Neonate: An infant in the first 28 days of life.

Nosocomial infection: Hospital-acquired infection.

Paresis: Weakness or loss of strength.

Paresthesia: Decrease or loss of sensation.

Pulmonary embolism: A blood clot to the lungs, which can be life threatening.

Pulsatile abdominal mass: A characteristic of an abdominal aneurysm. The mass can be felt because the aorta has ballooned out and pulses with arterial blood.

Pyuria: Pus cells in the urine.

Qui tam: A suit brought by an individual on behalf of the US government seeking to expose the misuse or waste of federal funds.

Radiology ultrasonography: A procedure performed by a technician in the ultrasound department and read by a trained radiologist.

Rales: A recognizable sound on pulmonary exam indicating fluid in the lungs.

Sentinel event: Any unanticipated event in a healthcare setting not related to the natural course of the patient's illness resulting in death or serious physical or psychological injury to a patient.

Sepsis: The presence of bacteria or other infectious organisms or their toxins in the blood stream or in other tissues of the body. Sepsis can be life threatening, requiring urgent and comprehensive care.

Silent myocardial infarction: Heart attacks that present with vague or atypical complaints such as sweating, nausea, or jaw pain instead of the typical chest pains.

Situation awareness (SA): Being aware of what is happening around you and understanding what the information means to you now and in the future.

STEMI (ST segment elevation myocardial infarction): These heart attacks are more easily diagnosed and treated because findings are readily visible on the ECG. The evidence is clearest on how to manage these patients.

Subdural hematoma: A collection of blood on the surface of the brain that may cause pressure on the cerebral cortex.

$10^{-1}$: A reliability level of 80 to 90 percent; referred to as "ten to the minus one."

Thrombolytic therapy: Any of the "clot-busting" drugs that have been administered in cardiovascular and cerebrovascular disease.

Transient ischemic attack (TIA): A neurological event that shares the signs and symptoms of a stroke but is reversible. Also called a mini-stroke, TIAs typically last 2 to 30 minutes and can produce problems with vision, dizziness, weakness, or speaking. If not treated, a patient has a high risk of having a major stroke in the near future.

# References

Abaris Group. 2011. "On Call and Fair Market Strategies for Physicians." Presented at The Advanced ED Management Course, Las Vegas, March 9.

Alberti, M. 2011. "Warnings of Doctor Shortage Go Unheeded." [Online article; retrieved 4/21/11.] www.remappingdebate.org/article/warnings-doctor-shortage-go-unheeded?page=0,0.

Acheson, A. G., A. N. Graham, C. Weir, and B. Lee. 1998. "Prospective Study on Factors Delaying Surgery in Ruptured Abdominal Aortic Aneurysms." *Journal of the Royal College of Surgeons of Edinburgh* 43 (3): 182–84.

Agnelli, G. 2010. "Acute Pulmonary Embolism." *New England Journal of Medicine* 363 (3): 266–74.

Al-Orifi, F., D. McGillivray, S. Tange, and M. S. Kramer. 2000. "Urine Culture from Bag Specimens in Young Children: Are the Risks Too High?" *Journal of Pediatrics* 200 (137): 221–26.

Allshouse, K. D. 1993. "Treating Patients as Individuals." In *Through the Patient's Eyes: Understanding and Promoting Patient-Centered Care*, edited by M. Gerteis, S. Edgman-Levitan, J. Daley, and T. L. Delbanco, 19–44. San Francisco: Jossey-Bass.

Amal, M., and G. Deepi. 2007. "Evaluation and Management of Patients with Chest Syndromes." *Emergency Medicine: Avoiding the Pitfalls and Improving the Outcomes.* Malden, MA: Blackwell.

American College of Emergency Physicians (ACEP). n.d. "Evaluation and Management Documentation Requirements—CMS vs. CPT." [Online information; retrieved 4/12/11.] http://my.acep.org/Content.aspx?id=30416.

————. 2008. "Clinical Policy: Neuroimaging and Decisionmaking in Adult Mild Traumatic Brain Injury in the Acute Setting." [Online information; retrieved 7/12/11.] www.acep.org/WorkArea/DownloadAsset.aspx?id=8814.

————. 2006. "Critical Issues in the Evaluation and Management of Adult Patients with Non-ST-Segment Elevation Acute Coronary Syndromes." [Online information; retrieved 5/14/11.] www.acep.org/MobileArticle. aspx?id=48387&coll_id=618&parentid=740.

————. 2002. "Use of Intravenous tPA for the Management of Acute Stroke in the Emergency Department." [Online information; retrieved 5/14/11.] www.acep.org/content.aspx?id=29936.

American Health Lawyers Association, Task Force of the Physician Organizations Practice Group. 2009. *AHLA Representing Physicians Handbook*, 2nd ed. Washington, DC: American Health Lawyers Association.

American Heart Association. 2010. "Heart Disease and Stroke Statistics 2010 at a Glance." [Online information; retrieved 5/14/11.] www. americanheart.org/downloadable/heart/1265665152970DS-3241%20 HeartStrokeUpdate_2010.pdf.

American Hospital Association (AHA). 2008. Letter from AHA to CMS opposing the curbing of nurse-initiated orders in the ED. [Online document; retrieved 6/4/11.] www.aha.org/aha/letter/2008/080411-let-pollack-weems. pdf.

American Medical Association (AMA). 2008. "Medical Liability Reform— NOW!" [Online information; retrieved 3/13/11.] www.ama-assn.org/ama1/ pub/upload/mm/-1/mlrnow.pdf.

Anderson, G. F., P. S. Hussey, B. K. Frogner, and H. R. Waters. 2005. "Health Spending in the United States and the Rest of the Industrialized World." *Health Affairs* 24 (4): 903–14.

Anderson-Berry, A. 2010. "Neonatal Sepsis." Medscape.com. Published February 23, 2010. http://emedicine.medscape.com/article/978352-overview.

*APS Update.* 2007. "Optimizing Revenue for Evaluation and Management Services: Does Your Documentation Measure Up?" [Online article; retrieved 6/4/11.] www.apsmedbill.com/images/Dec_07.pdf.

Arendt, W., A. T. Sadosty, A. L. Weaver, C. R. Brent, and E. T. Boie. 2003. "The Left-Without-Being-Seen Patients: What Would Keep Them from Leaving?" *Annals of Emergency Medicine* 42: 317–23.

Arizona Hospital and Healthcare Association (AZHHA). 2008. "Medical Screening Examination for Behavioral Health Patients." [Online information; retrieved 4/23/11.] www.azhha.org/educational_services/documents/MedScreenExamforBHPts.pdf.

Artman, H. 2000. "Team Situation Assessment and Information Distribution." *Ergonomics* 43 (8): 1111–28.

Baker, G. R., P. G. Norton, V. Flintoft, R. Blais, A. Brown, J. Cox, E. Etchells, W. A. Ghali, P. Hébert, S. R. Majumdar, M. O'Beirne, L. Palacios-Derflingher, R. J. Reid, S. Sheps, and R. Tamblyn. 2004. "The Canadian Adverse Events Study: The Incidence of Adverse Events Among Hospitalized Patients in Canada." *Canadian Medical Association Journal* 170: 1678–86.

Barada, J. H., J. L. Weingarten, and W. J. Cromie. 1989. "Testicular Salvage and Age-Related Delay in the Presentation of Testicular Torsion." *Journal of Urology* 142: 746–48.

Bard, M., and M. Nugent. 2011. *Accountable Care Organizations: Your Guide to Strategy, Design, and Implementation* Chicago: Health Administration Press.

Bates, D. W. 1996. "Medication Errors. How Common Are They and What Can Be Done to Prevent Them?" *Drug Safety* 15 (5): 303–10.

Beckman, H. B., K. M. Markakis, A. L. Suchman, and R. M. Frankel. 1994. "The Doctor-Patient Relationship and Malpractice: Lessons from Plaintiff Depositions." *Archives of Internal Medicine* 154 (12): 1365–70.

Björkdahl, A., D. Olsson, and T. Palmstierna. 2006. "Nurses' Short-Term Prediction of Violence in Acute Psychiatric Intensive Care." *Acta Psychiatrica Scandinavica* 113 (3): 224–29.

Bonacum, D., and M. Leonard. 2004. "SBAR Technique for Communication: A Situational Briefing Model." [Online information; retrieved 4/22/11.] http://www.ihi.org/IHI/topics/patientsafety/safetygeneral/tools/SBARTechniqueforCommunicationASituationalBriefingModel.htm.

Bonsu, B. K. 2003. "Identifying Febrile Young Infants with Bacteremia: Is the Peripheral White Blood Cell Count an Accurate Screen?" *Annals of Emergency Medicine* 42 (2): 216–25.

Boothman, R. 2006. "Apologies: A Strong Defense at the University of Michigan Health System." *Physician Executive* (March–April): 7–10.

Borg, J. 2008. *Body Language: 7 Easy Lessons to Master the Silent Language.* Upper Saddle River, NJ: Prentice Hall Life.

Borowsky, M., and J. Gaynor. 2002. "What's More Dangerous? Airplane Versus Automobile Accidents." [Online article; retrieved 3/19/11.] http://findarticles.com/p/articles/mi_m0FKE/is_4_47/ai_86504189/.

Botwinick, L., M. Bisognano, and C. Haraden. 2006. *Leadership Guide to Patient Safety.* IHI Innovation Series white paper. Cambridge, MA: Institute for Healthcare Improvement.

Boudreaux, E. D., and E. L. O'Hea. 2004. "Patient Satisfaction in the Emergency Department: A Review of the Literature and Implications for Practice." *Journal of Emergency Medicine* 26: 13–26.

Boudreaux, E., S. D'Autremont, K. Wood, and G. N. Jones. 2004a. "Predictors of Emergency Department Patient Satisfaction: Stability over 17 Months." *Academic Emergency Medicine* 11: 51–58.

Boudreaux, E., J. Friedman, M. E. Chansky, and B. M. Baumann. 2004b. "Emergency Department Patient Satisfaction: Examining the Role of Acuity. *Academic Emergency Medicine* 11: 162–68.

Boudreaux, E., R. Ary, C. V. Mandry, and B. McCabe. 2000. "Determinants of Patient Satisfaction in a Large Municipal ED: The Role of Demographic Variables, Visit Characteristics and Patient Perceptions." *American Journal of Emergency Medicine* 18: 394–400.

BrainandSpinalCord.org. 2011. "Spinal Cord Injury Statistics." [Online information; retrieved 5/15/11.] www.brainandspinalcord.org/spinal-cord-injury/statistics.htm.

Brandt, M. L. 2003. "Researchers ID Best Hours to Sleep when Time Is Limited: People Who rest in the Early Morning Do Better than Those Who Sleep Late at Night." [Online report; retrieved 3/14/11.] http://news.stanford.edu/news/2003/may28/sleep.html.

Brooks-Buza, H., R. Fernandez, and J. P. Stenger. 2001. "The Use of In Situ Simulation to Evaluate Teamwork and System Organization During a Pediatric Dental Clinic Emergency." *Simulation in Healthcare* 6 (2): 101–8.

Brown, L., T. Shaw, and W. A. Wittlake. 2005. "Does Leucocytosis Identify Bacterial Infections in Febrile Neonates Presenting to the Emergency Department?" *Emergency Medicine Journal* 22 (4): 256–59.

Bukata, R. 2011. "The Power of the Pen." Presented at Taking Your ED From Good to Great conference, Las Vegas, March 7.

Burgess, K. n.d. "Physician Self-Referral (Stark Law)." [Online article; retrieved 4/23/11. www.ahcancal.org/facility_operations/ComplianceProgram/Pages/PhysicianSelf-ReferralStarkLaw.aspx.

Bursch, B., J. Beezy, and R. Shaw. 1993. "Emergency Department Satisfaction: What Matters Most?" *Annals of Emergency Medicine* 22: 586–91.

Cadotte, D. W., S. Vachhrajani, and F. Pirouzmand. 2011. "The Epidemiologic Trends of Head Injury in the Largest Canadian Adult Trauma Center from 1986 to 2007." *Journal of Neurosurgery* 114 (6): 1502–09.

Canadian CT Head and C-Spine (CCC) Study Group. 2002. "Canadian C-Spine Rule Study for Alert and Stable Trauma Patients." *Canadian Journal of Emergency Medicine* 4 (2): 84–90.

Capella, J. 2010. "Teamwork Training Improves the Clinical Care of Trauma Patients." Journal of Surgical Education 67 (6): 439–43.

Caspe, W. B. 1983. "The Evaluation and Treatment of the Febrile Infant." *Pediatric Infectious Disease Journal* 2 (2): 131–35.

Celizic, M. 2008. "John Ritter's Widow: 'The Jury has Spoken.'" [Online article; retrieved 5/13/11.] http://today.msnbc.msn.com/id/23723123/ns/today-today_people/t/john-ritters-widow-jury-has-spoken/

Center for Emergency Medical Education (CEME). 2011. "Extremity Injuries." Presented at The High Risk Emergency Medicine Course, Las Vegas, May 11.

———. 2010. "Medication Errors." Presented at The High Risk Emergency Medicine Course, Las Vegas, March 7.

Centers for Medicare & Medicaid Services. 2010a. "Appendix V—Interpretive Guidelines—Responsibilities of Medicare Participating Hospitals in Emergency Cases." [Online information; retrieved 4/23/11.] https://www.cms.gov/manuals/downloads/som107ap_v_emerg.pdf.

———. 2010b. "Revisions to Appendix V-Interpretive Guidelines—Responsibilities of Medicare Participating Hospitals in Emergency Cases." [Online information; retrieved 4/23/11.] https://www.cms.gov/transmittals/downloads/R60SOMA.pdf.

———. 2003. "Medicare Program; Clarifying Policies Related to the Responsibilities of Medicare-Participating Hospitals in Treating Individuals With Emergency Medical Conditions." [Online information; retrieved 7/18/11.] http://federalregister.gov/a/03-22594.

————. 1997. "1997 Documentation Guidelines for Evaluation and Management Services." [Online information; retrieved 6/4/11.] https://www.cms.gov/MLNProducts/Downloads/MASTER1.pdf.

————. 1995. "1995 Documentation Guidelines for Evaluation & Management Services." [Online information; retrieved 6/4/11.] www.cms.gov/mlnproducts/downloads/referenceI.pdf.

Ceriani, E. 2010. "Clinical Prediction Rules for Pulmonary Embolism: A Systematic Review and Meta-analysis." *Journal of Thrombosis and Haemostasis* 8 (5): 957–70.

Chande, V. T., M. S. Bhende, and H. W. Davis. 1991. "Pediatric Emergency Department Complaints: A Three-Year Analysis of Sources and Trends." *Annals of Emergency Medicine* 20: 1014–16.

Chisholm, C. D. 2001. "Work Interrupted: A Comparison of Workplace Interruptions in Emergency Departments and Primary Care Offices." *Annals of Emergency Medicine* 38 (2): 146–51.

————. 2000. "Emergency Department Workplace Interruptions: Are Emergency Physicians 'Interrupt-Driven' and 'Multi-tasking'"? *Academic Emergency Medicine* 7 (11): 1239–43.

————. 1998. "How Do Physicians and Nurses Spend Their Time in the Emergency Department?" *Annals of Emergency Medicine* 31 (1): 87–91.

Chisholm, C. D., C. S. Weaver, L. Whenmouth, and B. Giles B. 2011. "A Task Analysis of Emergency Physician Activities in Academic and Community Settings." [Online article; retrieved 6/4/11.] www.annemergmed.com/article/S0196-0644(10)01823-8/abstract.

Cheung, D. 2011. Strategies to Improve ED Intake Poster Competition, February 25-26, sponsored by AHRQ, Salt Lake City, UT.

Cincinnati Children's Hospital Medical Center, FUS Team. 2010. "Evidence-Based Clinical Care Guideline for Fever of Uncertain Source in Infants 60 Days of Age or Less." [Online information; retrieved 6/6/11.] www.cincinnatichildrens.org/svc/alpha/h/health-policy/ev-based/default.htm.

CitronLegal.com. 2009. "University of Chicago ER Sends Kid Mauled by Pit Bull Home." [Online article; retrieved 6/6/11.] http://citronlegal.wordpress.com/2009/02/27/university-of-chicago-er-sends-kid-mauled-by-pit-bull-home/.

Claudius, I. 2010. "Pediatric Emergencies Associated with Fever." *Emergency Medicine Clinics of North America* 28 (1): 67–84, vii–viii.

Cohen, M. R., ed. 2007. *Medication Errors*, 613–15. Washington, DC: American Pharmacists Association.

Constantine, M., and A. Jagoda. 2009. "Revised Clinical Policy: Neuroimaging and Decisionmaking in Adult Mild TBI in Acute Settings." [Online information; retrieved 5/15/11.] www.acep.org/content.aspx?id=45443.

Cooper, G. E., M. D. White, and J. K. Lauber, eds. 1980. "Resource Management on the Flightdeck." [Online information; retrieved 3/19/11.] www.crewresourcemanagement.net/.

Cooper, J. B., R. S. Newbower, and R. J. Kitz. 1984. "An Analysis of Major Errors and Equipment Failures in Anesthesia Management: Considerations for Prevention and Detection." *Anesthesiology* 60 (1): 34–42.

Cooper, S., R. Cant, J. Porter, F. Bogossian, L. McKenna, S. Brady and S. Fox-Young. 2011. "Simulation Based Learning in Midwifery Education: A Systematic Review." [Online article; retrieved 6/4/11.] www.sciencedirect.com/science/article/pii/S1871519211000266.

Cox, W. 2007. "The Five A's: What Patients Want After an Adverse Event. *Journal of Healthcare Risk Management* 27 (3): 25–29.

Crain, E. F., and J. C. Gershel. 1988. "Which Febrile Infants Younger than Two Weeks of Age Are Likely to Have Sepsis? A Pilot Study." *Pediatric Infectious Disease Journal* 7 (8): 561–64.

Crain, E. F., and S. P. Shelov. 1982. "Febrile Infants: Predictors of Bacteremia." Journal of Pediatrics 101 (5): 686–89.

Croskerry, P. 2003. "The Importance of Cognitive Errors in Diagnosis and Strategies to Minimize Them." *Academic Emergency Medicine* 78 (8): 775–80.

Croskerry, P., and D. Sinclair. 2001. "Emergency Medicine: A Practice Prone to Error?" *Canadian Journal of Emergency Medicine* 3 (4): 271–76.

Croskerry, P., K. S. Cosby, S. M. Schenkel, and R. L. Wears. 2009. *Patient Safety in Emergency Medicine*, 334. Philadelphia, PA: Wolters Kluwer.

Davis, L., and P. F. Jacques. 2008. "Heuristics in the Emergency Room." *Journal of Physician Assistant Education* 19 (2): 52–54.

Dent, A. W., T. J. Weiland, L. Vallender, and N. E. Oettel. 2007. "Can Medical Admission and Length of Stay Be Accurately Predicted by Emergency Staff, Patients or Relatives?" *Australian Health Review* 31 (4): 633–41.

Diaz, J. J., Jr., C. Gillman, J. A. Morris, Jr., A. K. May, Y. M. Carrillo, and J. Guy. 2003. "Are Five-View Plain Films of the Cervical Spine Unreliable? A Prospective Evaluation in Blunt Trauma Patients with Altered Mental Status." *Journal of Trauma* 55 (4): 658–63.

Diercks, D. B., E. Boghos, H. Guzman, E. A. Amsterdam, and J. D. Kirk. 2005. "Changes in the Numeric Descriptive Scale for Pain After Sublingual Nitroglycerin Do Not Predict Cardiac Etiology of Chest Pain." *Annals of Emergency Medicine* 45 (6): 581.

Duncan, S., C. A. Estabrooks, and M. Reimer. 2000. "Violence Against Nurses." *Alta RN* 56 (2): 13–14.

Dunn, S. G. 2007. "Safe Strategies for Potentially Violent Patients. Part I." Journal of Medical Practice Management 23 (2): 86–89.

Durston, W., M. L. Carl, and W. Guerra. 1999. "Patient Satisfaction and Diagnostic Accuracy with Ultrasound by Emergency Physicians." *American Journal of Emergency Medicine* 17: 642–46.

Emtala.com. n.d.(a). "Definitions." Section (b) of EMTALA statute, 42 USC 1395dd. [Online information; retrieved 4/23/11.] www.emtala.com/law/b. htm.

———. n.d.(b). "Special Note—What Is the 250-Yard Rule and How Does It Affect These Issues?" [Online information; retrieved 4/23/11.] www.emtala. com/250yard.htm.

Engel, B. 2001. *The Power of Apology*. New York: John Wiley & Sons.

Engleberg, I. N. 2006. "Working in Groups: Communication Principles and Strategies." My Communication Kit series, p. 137. Boston: Allyn & Bacon.

Fairbanks, R. J., and A. W. Gellatly. 2009. "Human Factors Engineering and Safe Systems," chap. 14. In *Patient Safety in Emergency Medicine*, edited by P. Croskerry, K. S. Cosby, S. M. Schenkel, and R. L. Wears. Philadelphia, PA: Wolters Kluwer.

Fazel, R. 2009. "Exposure to Low Dose Ionizing from Medical Imaging Procedures." *New England Journal of Medicine* 361 (9): 849–857.

Fedullo, P. F. 2003. "Clinical Practice. The Evaluation of Suspected Pulmonary Embolism." *New England Journal of Medicine* 349 (13): 1247–56.

Feied, C. F. 1995. "Chronic Pulmonary Embolism. Often Misdiagnosed, Difficult to Treat." *Postgraduate Medicine* 97 (1): 75–78, 81–84.

Fosmire, M. S. 2009. "Frequently Asked Questions About the Emergency Medical Treatment and Active Labor Act (EMTALA)." [Online information; retrieved 4/23/11.] www.emtala.com/faq.htm.

Fosnocht, D. E., M. B. Hollifield, and E. R. Swanson. 2004. "Patients' Preference for Route of Pain Medication Delivery." *Journal of Emergency Medicine* 26: 7–11.

Fosnocht, D. E., and E. R. Swanson. 2007. "Use of a Triage Pain Protocol in the ED." *American Journal of Emergency Medicine* 25 (7): 791–93.

Frei, S. P., W. F. Bond, R. K. Bazuro, D. M. Richardson, G. M. Sierzega, and J. F. Reed. 2008. "Appendicitis Outcomes with Increasing Computed Tomographic Scanning." *American Journal of Emergency Medicine* 26 (1): 39–44.

Frew, S., and K. Giese. 2008. *EMTALA Field Guide: Quick Risk and Compliance Answers*, 2nd ed. Madison, WI: Johnson Insurance Services.

Gallagher, T., and M. H. Lucas. 2005. "Should We Disclose Harmful Medical Errors to Patients? If So, How?" *Journal of Clinical Outcomes Management* 12 (5): 251–53.

Ganguli, S., V. Raptopoulos, F. Komlos, B. Siewert, and J. B. Kruskal. 2006. "Right Lower Quadrant Pain: The Value of the Non-visualized Appendix in Patients with Multidetector CT." *Radiology* 241 (1): 175–80.

Garra, G. 2005. "Reappraisal of Criteria Used to Predict Serious Bacterial Illness in Febrile Infants Less than 8 Weeks of Age." *Academic Emergency Medicine* 12 (10): 921–25.

Garvey, D. 2010. Personal communication regarding the "T-system," August 7.

George, J. C., and G. D. Dangas. 2010. "Focused Updates to Guidelines in ST-Elevation Myocardial Infarction and Percutaneous Coronary Intervention." *Journal of the American College of Cardiology Interventions* 2010 (3): 256–58.

Giannarosi, R. 1989. "Exercise Induced ST Depression in the Diagnosis of Coronary Artery Disease." *Circulation* 80 (1): 87–98.

Government Accountability Office (GAO). 2003. *Medical Malpractice Insurance: Multiple Factors Have Contributed to Increased Premium Rates*. [Online report; retrieved 3/12/11.] www.gao.gov/new.items/d03702.pdf.

Graber, M. A., J. Pierre, and M. Charlton. 2003. "Patient Opinions and Attitudes Toward Medical Student Procedures in the Emergency Department." *Academic Emergency Medicine* 10: 1329–33.

Greenes, D. S., and S. A. Schutzman. 1999. "Clinical Indicators of Intracranial Injury in Head-Injured Infants." *Pediatrics* 104 (4, Pt. 1): 861–67.

Griffith, J. R., and K. R. White. 2006. *The Well-Managed Healthcare Organization*, 6th ed. Chicago: Health Administration Press.

Grout, J. 2007. *Mistake-Proofing the Design of Health Care Processes.* Chapter 1, "What is Mistake Proofing?" AHRQ Publication No. 07-0020. Rockville, MD: Agency for Healthcare Research and Quality.

Gumenyuk, V., T. Roth, O. Korzyukov, C. Jefferson, A. Kick, L. Spear, N. Tepley, and C. L. Drake. 2010. "Shift Work Sleep Disorder Is Associated with an Attenuated Brain Response of Sensory Memory and an Increased Brain Response to Novelty: An ERP Study." *Sleep* 33 (5): 703–13.

Hall, M. F., and I. Press. 1996. "Keys to Patient Satisfaction in the Emergency Department: Results of a Multiple Facility Study." *Hospitals & Health Services Administration* 41: 515–32.

Handel, D. A., R. Fu, M. Daya, J. York, E. Larson, and K. John McConnell. 2010. "The Use of Scripting at Triage and Its Impact on Elopements." *Academic Emergency Medicine* 17 (5): 495–500.

Hays, D. P. 2007. "Clinical Pharmacy Services in the Emergency Department." [Online slide presentation; retrieved 4/26/11.] www.ahrq.gov/about/annualmtg07/0927slides/hays/Hays-7.html.

Hazen, S., and J. Cookson. 1990. "A Database Tool for Centralized Analysis of Untoward Health Care Events." *Military Medicine* 155 (10): 492–97.

He, W., M. Sengupta, V. A. Velkoff, and K. A. DeBarros. 2005. *65+ in the United States.* [Online report; retrieved 4/22/11.] http://www.census.gov/prod/2006pubs/p23-209.pdf.

*Health Business Daily.* 2010. "Hospital Settles Stark Case on Leases; Real Estate Director Was Whistleblower." [Online article; retrieved 3/23/10.] www.aishealth.com/Bnow/hbd032310.html.

Hedges, J. R., A. Trout, and A. R. Magnusson. 2002. "Satisfied Patients Exiting the Emergency Department (SPEED) Study. *Academic Emergency Medicine* 9: 15–21.

Helmreich, R. L. 1997. "Managing Human Error in Aviation." *Scientific American* (May): 62–67.

Helmreich, R. L., and H. C. Foushee. 1993. "Why Crew Resource Management? Empirical and Theoretical Bases of Human Factors Training in Aviation." In *Cockpit Resource Management*, edited by E. L. Weiner, B. G. Kanki, and R. L. Helmreich, 3–45. San Diego: Academic Press.

Helmreich, R. L., A. C. Merritt, and J. A. Wilhelm. 1999. "The Evolution of Crew Resource Management Training in Commercial Aviation." *International Journal of Aviation Psychology* 9 (1): 19–32.

Henrikson, C. A., E. E. Howell, D. E. Bush, J. S. Miles, G. R. Meininger, T. Friedlander, A. C. Bushnell, and N. Chandra-Strobos. 2003. "Chest Pain Relief by Nitroglycerin Does Not Predict Active Coronary Artery Disease." *Annals of Internal Medicine* 139 (12): 979.

Henry, G., and R. Bukata. 2011. Personal communication, March 13.

Henson, J. 2011. "Missed Test Results Cause Patient Harm." [Online article; retrieved 2/28/11.] www.hcqualitynews.com/home/2011/2/28/missed-test-results-cause-patient-harm.html.

Higashida, R. T. 2003. "Trial Design and Reporting Standards for Intra-arterial Cerebral Thrombolysis for Acute Ischemic Stroke." *Stroke* 34 (8): e109–e137.

Hoffman, J. R., W. R. Mower, A. B. Wolfson, K. H. Todd, and M. I. Zucker. 2000. "Validity of a Set of Clinical Criteria to Rule Out Injury to the Cervical Spine in Patients with Blunt Trauma. National Emergency X-Radiography Utilization Study Group." *New England Journal of Medicine* 343 (2): 94–99.

Hollander, J. E., and H. I. Litt. 2006. "Computerized Tomographic Coronary Angiography for the Evaluation of ED Patients with Potential Acute Coronary Syndromes." [Online article; retrieved 6/6/11.] www.emcreg.org/pdf/monographs/cta.pdf.

Holmes, J. F., and R. Akkinepalli. "Computed Tomography Versus Plain Radiography to Screen for Cervical Spine Injury: A Meta-analysis." *Journal of Trauma* 58 (5): 902–5.

Hsiao, C.-J., D. K. Cherry, P. C. Beatty, and E. A. Rechtsteiner. 2010. "National Ambulatory Medical Care Survey: 2007 Summary." [Online information; retrieved 4/22/11.] http://www.cdc.gov/nchs/data/nhsr/nhsr027.pdf.

Hughes, R. G. 2005. "First Do No Harm." *American Journal of Nursing* 105 (5): 79–84.

Hull, L. 2011. "Observational Teamwork Assessment for Surgery: Content Validation and Tool Refinement." *Journal of the American College of Surgeons* 212 (2): 234–43.

Institute for Healthcare Improvement (IHI). 2003. *Move Your Dot™: Measuring, Evaluating, and Reducing Hospital Mortality Rates (Part 1).* IHI Innovation Series white paper. Boston: IHI.

Isselbacher, E. M. 2005. "Thoracis and Abdominal Aneurysms." *Circulation* 111 (6): 816–28.

*Jacovach v. Yocum,* 237 N. W. 444, Iowa (1931).

James, B. 2006. *Advanced Training Program (ATP) Course Manual.* Salt Lake City, UT: Intermountain Institute for Health Care Delivery Research.

Jazayeri, A. 2008. "Surgical Management of Ectopic Pregnancy." http://emedicine.medscape.com/article/267384-overview, posted January 7.

Jensen, K., T. A. Mayer, S. J. Welch, and C. Haraden. 2007. *Leadership for Smooth Patient Flow: Improved Outcomes, Improved Service, Improved Bottom Line.* Chapter 2, "The Benefits of Flow." Chicago: Health Administration Press.

Jiang, H. J., C. Lockee, K. Bass, and I. Fraser. 2009. "Board Oversight of Quality: Any Differences in Process of Care and Mortality?" *Journal of Healthcare Management* 54 (1): 15–29.

———. 2008. "Board Engagement in Quality: Findings of a Survey of Hospital and System Leaders." *Journal of Healthcare Management* 53 (2): 121–34.

Johnson, B. A., and T. S. Schroeder. 2011. "Stark Rules Change—Again." [Online article; retrieved 4/23/11.] www.envoynews.com/rtacpa/e_article001197838.cfm?x=b11,0,w.

Johnston, S. C., D. R. Gress, W. S. Browner, and S. Sidney. 2000. "Short-Term Prognosis After Emergency Department Diagnosis of TIA." *Journal of the American Medical Association* 284 (22): 2901–06.

Joint Commission, The. 2011. "Sentinel Event Data: Root Cause by Event Type." [Online slide presentation; retrieved 3/19/11.] www.jointcommission.org/assets/1/18/Root_Causes_by_Event_Type_2004-4Q2010.pdf.

————. 2010. "Preventing Violence in the Health Care Setting." [Online information; retrieved 6/9/11.] http://www.jointcommission.org/sentinel_event_alert_issue_45_preventing_violence_in_the_health_care_setting_/.

————. 2002. "Delays in Treatment." [Online information; retrieved 5/5/11.] www.jointcommission.org/assets/1/18/SEA_26.pdf.

————. 1998. "Accreditation Committee Approves Examples of Voluntarily Reportable Sentinel Events." [Online information; retrieved 4/2/11.] www.jointcommission.org/assets/1/18/SEA_4.pdf.

Jones, J. S., M. S. Young, R. A. LaFleur, and M. D. Brown. 1997. "Effectiveness of an Organized Follow-Up System for Elder Patients Released from the Emergency Department." *Academic Emergency Medicine* 4 (12): 1147–52.

Joshi, M. S., and S. C. Hines. 2006. "Getting the Board on Board: Engaging Hospital Boards in Quality and Patient Safety." *Joint Commission Journal on Quality and Patient Safety* 32 (4): 179–87.

JuryVerdictReview.com. n.d. "Resources for the Tort Litigator: Massachusetts (48725)." www.jvra.com/Verdict_Trak/article.aspx?id=48725.

Kanegave, J. T. 2005. "Improved Documentation of Wound Care with a Structured Encounter Form in the Pediatric Emergency Department." *Ambulatory Pediatrics* 5 (4): 253–57.

Kaveler, F., and A. Spiegel. 2003. *Risk Management in Health Care Institutions: A Strategic Approach*, 2nd ed., p. 4. Sudbury, MA: Jones and Bartlett.

Kim, C. 2001. "Pharmacologic Stress Testing for Coronary Artery Disease Diagnosis: A Meta-analysis." *American Heart Journal* 142 (6): 934–44.

King, J. C., E. D. Berman, and P. F. Wright. 1987. "Evaluation of Fever in Infants Less than 8 Weeks Old." Southern Medical Journal 80 (8): 948–52.

Kirkton, J. L. 2008. "Medical Negligence Litigation in Illinois: Facts and Figures." [Online article; retrieved 5/25/11.] www.lawbulletin.com/assets/documents/medical_negligence_article.pdf.

Klauer, K. 2011. "Neuro Nightmares." Presented at The High Risk Emergency Medicine Course, Las Vegas, May.

Kleepsies, P. M. 1998. *Emergencies in Mental Health Practice*. New York: Guilford Press.

Klein Hesselink, J. K., J. de Leede, and A. Goudswaard. 2010. "Effects of the New Fast Forward Rotating Five-Shift Roster at a Dutch Steel Company." *Ergonomics* 53 (6): 727–38.

Konstantinides, S. 2008. "Clinical Practice. Acute Pulmonary Embolism." *New England Journal of Medicine* 359 (26): 2804–13.

Kuan, S., and J. J. O'Donnell. 2007. "Medical Students in the Emergency Department: How Do Patients View Participation in Clinical Teaching?" *Irish Medical Journal* 100: 560–61.

Kuppermann, N., J. F. Holmes, P. S. Dayan, J. D. Hoyle, S. M. Atabaki, R. Holubkov, F. M. Nadel, D. Monroe, R. M. Stanley, D. A. Borgialli, M. K. Badawy, J. E. Schunk, K. S. Quayle, P. Mahajan, R. Lichenstein, K. A. Lillis, M. G. Tunik, E. S. Jacobs, J. M. Callahan, M. H. Gorelick, T. F. Glass, L. K. Lee, M. C. Bachman, A. Cooper, E. C. Powell, M. J. Gerardi, K. A. Melville, J. P. Muizelaar, D. H. Wisner, S. J. Zuspan, J. M. Dean, S. L. Wootton-Gorges, for the Pediatric Emergency Care Applied Research Network (PECARN). 2009. "Identification of Children at Very Low Risk of Clinically-Important Brain Injuries After Head Trauma: A Prospective Cohort Study." *Lancet* 3374 (9696): 1160–70.

Landro, L. 2008. "Hospitals Tackle High Risk Drugs to Reduce Errors." *Wall Street Journal* March 5.

Lazare, A. 2004. *On Apology.* New York: Oxford University Press.

Leape, L. L. 2005. "Understanding the Power of Apology: How Saying 'I'm Sorry' Helps Heal Patients and Caregivers." *Focus on Patient Safety* 8 (4): 1–3.

———. 1994. "Error in Medicine." *Journal of the American Medical Association* 272: 1851–57.

Leape, L. L., T. A. Brennan, N. Laird, A. G. Lawthers, A. R. Localio, B. A. Barnes, L. Hebert, J. P. Newhouse, P. C. Weiler, and H. Hiatt. 1991. "The Nature of Adverse Events in Hospitalized Patients. Results of the Harvard Medical Practice Study II." *New England Journal of Medicine* 324 (6): 377–84.

Leonard, M., A. Frankel, T. Simmonds, with K. Vega. 2004. *Achieving Safe and Reliable Healthcare: Strategies and Solutions.* Chicago: Health Administration Press.

Liang, B. A. 2008. "Empirical Characteristics of Litigation Involving Tissue Plasminogen Activator and Ischemic Stroke." *Annals of Emergency Medicine* Volume 52 (2): 160–64.

———. 2002. "A System of Error Disclosure." *Quality & Safety in Health Care* 11: 64–68.

Loren, D. J., J. Garbutt, W. C. Dunagan, K. M. Bommarito, A. G. Ebers, W. Levinson, A. D. Waterman, V. J. Fraser, E. A. Summy, and T. H. Gallagher. 2010. "Risk Managers, Physicians, and Disclosure of Harmful Medical Errors." *Joint Commission Journal on Quality and Patient Safety* 36 (3): 101–8.

Louis Harris and Associates. 1997. "Public Opinion of Patient Safety Issues Research Finding." Presented to National Patient Safety Foundation at the American Medical Association, Rochester, NY, September.

LSU Law Center. 1993. "Nursing Practice." [Online information; retrieved 4/26/11.] http://biotech.law.lsu.edu/books/lbb/x410.htm.

Macciocchi, S., R. T. Seel, N. Thompson, R. Byams, and B. Bowman 2008. "Spinal Cord Injury and Co-occurring Traumatic Brain Injury: Assessment and Incidence." *Archives of Physical Medicine and Rehabilitation* 89 (7): 1350–57.

Mack, J. L., and K. M. File. 1995. "Factors Associated with Emergency Room Choice Among Medicare Patients." *Journal of Ambulatory Care Marketing* 6: 45–49.

Mack, J. L., K. M. File, and J. E. Horwitz. 1995. "The Effect of Urgency on Patient Satisfaction and Future Emergency Department Choice." *Health Care Management Review* 20: 7–15.

Mador, R. L. 2009. "The Impact of a Critical Care Information System (CCIS) on Time Spent Charting and in Direct Patient Care by Staff in the ICU: A Review of the Literature." *International Journal of Medical Informatics* 78 (7): 435–45.

Maister, D. 1985. "The Psychology of Waiting Lines." [Online article; retrieved 9/25/09.] http://davidmaister.com/articles/5/52/.

Marsich, V. 2009. "Paying for On-Call Coverage—Here We Go Again!" [Online article; retrieved 6/4/11.] www.michiganhealthlawlink.com/tags/oig/.

Marston, W. A., R. Ahlquist, G. Johnson, Jr., and A. A. Meyer. 1992. "Misdiagnosis of Ruptured Abdominal Aortic Aneurysms." *Journal of Vascular Surgery* 16 (1): 17–22.

Marx, D. 2001. "Patient Safety and the "Just Culture": A Primer for Health Care Executives." [Online article; retrieved 4/22/11.] www.mers-tm.org/support/ Marx_Primer.pdf .

Matteson, J. R. 2001. "Medicolegal Aspects of Testicular Torsion." *Urology* 57 (4): 783–86; discussion 786–87.

Mattu, A., and D. Goyal. 2007. *Emergency Medicine: Avoiding the Pitfalls and Improving the Outcomes.* Chapter 1, "Evaluation and Management of Patients with Chest Syndromes." Malden, MA: Blackwell Publishing.

Matyas, D., and C. Valiant. 2006. *Legal Issues in Healthcare Fraud and Abuse: Navigating the Uncertainties*, 3rd ed. Washington, DC: American Health Lawyers Association.

Mayer, T. 2004. *Leadership for Great Customer Service: Satisfied Patients, Satisfied Employees.* Chicago: Health Administration Press.

McAnaney, K. (ed.). 2009. *Complete Connected Stark Laws & Regulations CD-ROM*, 2nd ed. Washington, DC: American Health Lawyers Association.

McCaig, L. F., and E. W. Nawar. 2006. "National Hospital Ambulatory Medical Care Survey: 2004 Emergency Department Summary." [Online information; retrieved 6/4/11.] www.cdc.gov/nchs/data/ad/ad372.pdf.

McConnell, K. J., L. A. Johnson, N. Arab, C. F. Richards, C. D. Newgard, and T. Edlund. 2007. "The On-Call Crisis: A Statewide Assessment of the Costs of Providing On-Call Specialist Coverage." *Annals of Emergency Medicine* 49 (6): 727–33.

McDonnell, W. M. 2006. "Deficits in EMTALA: Knowledge Among Pediatric Physicians." *Pediatric Emergency Care* (22) 8: 555–61.

McDowell, T. 1989. "Physician Self Referral Arrangements: Legitimate Business or Unethical Entrepreneurialism." *American Journal of Law & Medicine* 15 (1): 61–109.

McGrayne, J. 2005. "Outstanding ED Performance." Presented at ED Benchmarks 2005, Orlando, FL, March 5.

Meade, C. M., J. Kennedy, and J. Kaplan. 2010. "The Effects of Emergency Department Staff Rounding on Patient Safety and Satisfaction." *Journal of Emergency Medicine* 38 (5): 666–74.

Medical Malpractice Today. 2003. "Health Care Providers Win Most Cases." [Online article; retrieved 5/25/11.] www.medicalmalpracticetoday.com/medicalmalpracticestats-hcpwinmore.html.

Miaoulis, G., Jr., J. Gutman, and M. M. Snow. 2009. "Closing the Gap: The Patient-Physician Gap." *Health Marketing Quarterly* 26: 56–68.

Miner, J. R., J. Moore, R. O. Gray, L. Skinner, and M. H. Biros. 2008. "Oral Versus Intravenous Opioid Dosing for the Initial Treatment of Acute Musculoskeletal Pain in the Emergency Department." *Academic Emergency Medicine* 14: 1234–40.

Morey, J. C., R. Simon, G. D. Jay, R. L. Wears, M. Salisbury, K. A. Dukes, and S. D. Berns. 2002. "Error Reduction and Performance Improvement in the Emergency Department Through Formal Teamwork Training: Evaluation Results of the MedTeams Project." *Health Services Research* 37 (6): 1553–81.

Mustard, L. W. 2003. "Improving Patient Satisfaction Through the Consistent Use of Scripting by the Nursing Staff." *JONA's Healthcare Law, Ethics, and Regulation* 5 (3): 68–72.

Najaf-Zadeh, A., F. Dubos, M. Aurel, and A. Martinot. 2008. "Epidemiology of Malpractice Lawsuits in Paediatrics." *Acta Paediatrica* 97 (11): 1486–91.

Nance, J. 2008. *Why Hospitals Should Fly*. Bozeman, MT: Second River Healthcare Press.

Naoum, J. J., W. J. Mileski, J. A. Daller, G. A. Gomez, D. C. Gore, T. D. Kimbrough, T. C. Ko, A. P. Sanford, and S. E. Wolf. 2002. "The Use of Abdominal Computed Tomography Scan Decreases the Frequency of Misdiagnosis in Cases of Suspected Appendicitis." *American Journal of Surgery* 184 (6): 587–89; discussion 589–90.

National Institute for Occupational Safety and Health (NIOSH). 1996. *Violence in the Workplace: Risk Factors and Prevention Strategies*. [Online report; retrieved 6/8/11.] www.cdc.gov/niosh/violcont.html.

National Quality Forum. 2009. *Safe Practices for Better Healthcare—2009 Update*. [Online report; retrieved 4/22/11.] www.qualityforum.org/Publications/2009/03/Safe_Practices_for_Better_Healthcare%e2%80%932009_Update.aspx.

———. 2003. *Safe Practices for Healthcare—A Consensus Report*. Washington DC: National Quality Forum.

National Sleep Foundation. Shift Work and Sleep, [Online article; retrieved 3/14/11.] http://www.sleepfoundation.org/article/sleep-topics/shift-work-and-sleep.

Nebraska Hospital Association. n.d. "HIPAA Communication Guide for News Media." [Online information; retrieved 4/21/11.] www.nhanet.org/pdf/hipaa/hipaamediaguide.pdf.

Needham, I., C. Abderhalden, R. Meer, T. Dassen, H. J. Haug, R. J. Halfens, and J. E. Fischer. 2004. "The Effectiveness of Two Interventions in the Management of Patient Violence in Acute Mental Inpatient Settings: Report on a Pilot Study." *Journal of Psychiatric and Mental Health Nursing* 11 (5): 595–601.

Nicastro, D. 2010. "HIPAA Faces HITECH-Empowered State AGs." [Online article; retrieved 4/2/11.] www.healthleadersmedia.com/content/LED-254310/HIPAA-Faces-HITECHEmpowered-State-AGs.

Nipomnick E. 2009. "Ectopic Pregnancy." Presented at the High Risk Emergency Medicine Course, March 5. Las Vegas, NV.

Nolan, T. 2000. "System Changes to Improve Patient Safety." *British Medical Journal* 320 (7237): 771–73.

Nolan, T., R. Resar, C. Haraden, and F. Griffin. 2004. *Improving the Reliability of Healthcare.* [Online report; retrieved 4/22/11.] www.ihi.org/IHI/Results/WhitePapers/ImprovingtheReliabilityofHealthCare.htm.

Norman, D. A. 1989. *The Design of Everyday Things.* New York: Doubleday.

Occupational Safety and Health Administration (OSHA). 2006. *OSHA Regional News Release.* Region 4. Washington, DC: OSHA.

———. 2004. *Guidelines for Preventing Workplace Violence for Health Care and Social Workers.* [Online information; retrieved 6/8/11.] www.osha.gov/Publications/OSHA3148/osha3148.html.

Odle-Dusseau, H. N., J. L. Bradley, and J. J. Pilcher. 2010. "Subjective Perceptions of the Effects of Sustained Performance Under Sleep-Deprivation Conditions." *Chronobiology International* 27 (2): 318–33.

Office of Inspector General (OIG), US Department of Health and Human Services. 2010. "A Roadmap for New Physicians: Avoiding Medicare and Medicaid Fraud and Abuse." [Online information; retrieved 6/8/11.] http://oig.hhs.gov/compliance/physician-education/index.asp.

————. 2009. Letter re: OIG Advisory Opinion No. 09-05. [Online information; retrieved 6/4/11.] http://oig.hhs.gov/fraud/docs/advisoryopinions/2009/AdvOpn09-05.pdf.

————. 2008. Letter re: OIG Advisory Opinion No. 08-07. [Online information; retrieved 6/9/11.] http://oig.hhs.gov/fraud/docs/advisoryopinions/2008/AdvOpn08-07.pdf.

————. 2007. Letter re: OIG Advisory Opinion No. 07-10. [Online information; retrieved 6/4/11.] http://oig.hhs.gov/fraud/docs/advisoryopinions/2007/AdvOpn07-10A.pdf.

————.2006. Letter re: OIG Advisory Opinion No. 06-10. [Online information; retrieved 6/9/11.] http://oig.hhs.gov/fraud/docs/advisoryopinions/2006/AdvOpn06-10A.pdf.

————. 1999. "Special Advisory Opinion: The Effect of Exclusion From Participation in Federal Health Care Programs." Washington, DC: OIG.

————. 1997. "Guidance for Implementing Permissive Exclusion Authority." [Online information; retrieved 6/8/11.] http://oig.hhs.gov/fraud/exclusions/files/permissive_excl_under_1128b15_10192010.pdf

————. 1989. *Financial Arrangements Between Physicians and Health Care Businesses.* Washington, DC: HHS.

Office of Public Affairs, US Department of Justice. 2010a. "Chicago Hospital to Pay More Than $1.5 Million to Resolve Medicare False Claims Act Allegations." [Online information; retrieved 3/9/11.] www.justice.gov/opa/pr/2010/March/10-civ-240.html.

————. 2010b. "Detroit-Area Medical Clinic Owner and Vice President Convicted in $23 Million Medicare Fraud Scheme." [Online article; retrieved 6/6/11.] www.justice.gov/opa/pr/2010/June/10-crm-730.html.

Ohayon, M., M. Smolensky, and T Roth. 2010. "Consequences of Shiftworking on Sleep Duration, Sleepiness, and Sleep Attacks." *Chronobiology International* 27 (3): 575–89.

Orlikoff, J., and G. B. Landau. 1981. "Why Risk Management and Quality Assurance Should Be Integrated." *Hospitals* 55 (11): 54–55.

Oser, R. L., E. Salas, D. C. Merket, and C. A. Bowers. 2001. "Applying Resource Management Training in Naval Aviation: A Methodology and Lessons Learned." In *Improving Teamwork in Organizations: Applications of Resource Management Training*, edited by E. Salas, C. A. Bowers, and E. Edens, 283–301. Mahwah, NJ: Erlbaum.

Ottolini, M. C. 2003. "Utility of Complete Blood Count and Blood Culture Screening to Diagnose Neonatal Sepsis in the Asymptomatic At Risk Newborn." *Pediatric Infectious Disease Journal* 22 (5): 430–34.

Owens, P., and A. Elixhauser. 2006. "Hospital Admissions That Began in the Emergency Department, 2003." [Online article; retrieved 5/3/11.] www.hcup-us.ahrq.gov/reports/statbriefs/sb1.pdf.

Pelt, J. L., and L. P. Faldmo. 2008. "Physician Error and Disclosure." *Clinical Obstetrics and Gynecology* 51 (4): 700–708.

Peterson, A. 2007. "Insufficient Evidence: State's Attorney's Office Drops Vance Death Probe." *News Sun*, February 27.

Petinaux, B., R. Bhat, K. Boniface, and J. Aristizabal. 2011. "Accuracy of Radiographic Readings in the Emergency Department." *American Journal of Emergency Medicine* 29 (1): 18–25.

Peto, R. R., L. M. Tenerowicz, E. M. Benjamin, D. S. Morsi, and P. K. Burger. 2009. "One System's Journey in Creating a Disclosure and Apology Program." *Joint Commission Journal on Quality and Patient Safety* 35 (10): 487–96.

Pettiker, C. M. S. F. Thung, C. A. Raab, K. P. Donohue, J. A. Copel, C. J. Lockwood, and E. F. Funai. 2011. "A Comprehensive Obstetrics Patient Safety Program Improves Safety Climate and Culture." *American Journal of Obstetrics and Gynecology* 204 (3): 216.e1–6.

Petty, M. M., G. W. McGee, and J. W. Cavender. 1984. "A Meta-analysis of the Relationships Between Job Satisfaction and Individual Performance." *Academy of Management Review* 9: 712–21.

Physician Insurers Association of America (PIAA). 2006. *2005 Claims Trend Analysis: A Comprehensive Analysis of Malpractice Cases*, exhibit 6-v. Rockville, MD: Physician Insurers Association of America.

Pines, J. M. 2006. "Profiles in Patient Safety: Confirmation Bias in Emergency Medicine." *Academic Emergency Medicine* 13 (1): 90–94.

Press, I. 2005. *Patient Satisfaction: Understanding and Managing the Experience of Care*, 2nd ed. Chicago: Health Administration Press.

———. 2002. *Patient Satisfaction: Defining, Measuring and Improving the Experience of Care*. Chicago: Health Administration Press.

Reason, J. 2000. "Human Error: Models and Management." *Western Journal of Medicine* 172 (6): 393–96.

Rehmani, R., and A. Norain. 2007. "Trends in Emergency Department Utilization in a Hospital in the Eastern Region of Saudi Arabia." *Saudi Medical Journal* 28 (2): 236–40.

Resar, R. K. 2006. "Making Noncatastrophic Health Care Processes Reliable: Learning to Walk Before Running in Creating High-Reliability Organizations." *Health Services Research* 41 (4, Pt. II): 1677–89.

Retezar, R. 2011. "The Effect of Triage Diagnostic Standing Orders on Emergency Department Treatment Time." *Annals of Emergency Medicine* 57 (2): 89–99.

Rhee, K. J., and J. Bird. 1996. "Perceptions and Satisfaction with Emergency Department Care." *Journal of Emergency Medicine* 14: 679–83.

Risser, D. T., M. M. Rice, M. L. Salisbury, R. Simon, G. D. Jay, and S. D. Berns. 1999. "The Potential for Improved Teamwork to Reduce Medical Errors in the Emergency Department." *Annals of Emergency Medicine* 34 (3): 373–83.

Robert Wood Johnson Foundation. 2006. "Scripting." *Urgent Matters Program Toolkit*. [Online information; retrieved 4/22/11.] www.rwjf.org/about/product.jsp?id=56517.

Roberts, J. 2011. Personal communication, April 25.

Robinson, P. J., G. Culpan, and M. Wiggins. 1999. "Interpretation of Selected Accident and Emergency Radiographic Examinations by Radiographers: A Review of 11000 Cases." *British Journal of Radiology* 72 (858): 546–51.

Rocker, G., D. Cook, P. Sjokvist, B. Weaver, S. Finfer, E. McDonald, J. Marshall, A. Kirby, M. Levy, P. Dodek, D. Heyland, G. Guyatt, Level of Care Study Investigators, and Canadian Critical Care Trials Group. 2004. "Clinician Predictions of Intensive Care Unit Mortality." *Critical Care Medicine* 32 (5): 1149–54.

Ruiz, R. 2008. "What Doctor Shortages Mean for Health Care." *Forbes* December 2.

Runciman, W. B. 2003. "Adverse Drug Events and Medication Errors in Australia." *International Journal for Quality in Health Care* 15 (Suppl. 1): i49–i59.

Russ, S. 2010. "Placing Physician Orders at Triage: The Effect on Length of Stay." *Annals of Emergency Medicine* 56 (1): 27–33.

Sabatine, M. S., D. A. Morrow, J. A. de Lemos, C. M. Gibson, S. A. Murphy, N. Rifai, C. McCabe, E. M. Antman, C. P. Cannon, and E. Braunwald. 2002. "Multimarker Approach to Risk Stratification in Non-ST Elevation Acute Coronary Syndromes: Simultaneous Assessment of Troponin I, C-reactive Protein, and B-type Natriuretic Peptide." *Circulation* 105: 1760.

*St. Joseph's Medical Center, Respondent, v. The Inspector General.* US Department of Health and Human Services, Departmental Appeals Board, Civil Remedies Division. 2009. [Online document; retrieved 6/21/11.] www.hhs. gov/dab/decisions/civildecisions/2009/CR1895.pdf.

Santen, S. A., R. R. Hemphill, C. M. Spanier, and M. D. Fletcher. 2005. "'Sorry, It's My First Time!' Will Patients Consent to Medical Students Learning Procedures?" *Medical Education* 39: 365–69.

Scheer, F., and J. Bass. 2009. "Night Shift Work Hard on the Heart." [Online information; retrieved 3/23/11.] http://news.health.com/2009/03/03/night-shift-work-hard-on-heart.

*Schloendorff v. Society of New York Hospital*, 211 N.Y. 125, 105 N.E. 92 (1914).

Schwartz, L. R., and D. T. Overton. 1987. "Emergency Department Complaints: A One-Year Analysis." *Annals of Emergency Medicine* 16: 857–61.

Sexton, J. B., R. Helmreich, P. J. Pronovost, and E. Thomas. n.d. "Safety Climate Survey." [Online survey; retrieved 3/19/11.] www.rmf.harvard.edu/files/documents/Mod7doclink3.pdf.

Sexton, J. B., R. L. Helmreich, T. B. Neilands, K. Rowan, K. Vella, J. Boyden, P. R. Roberts, and E. J. Thomas. 2006. "The Safety Attitudes Questionnaire: Psychometric Properties, Benchmarking Data, and Emerging Research." *BMC Health Services Research* 6: 44.

Sexton, J. B., J. A. Wilhelm, R. L. Helmreich, A. C. Merritt, and J. R. Klinect. 2001. "Flight Management Attitudes & Safety Survey (FMASS): A Short Version of the FMAQ." University of Texas at Austin Human Factors Research Project Technical Report 01-01. Austin: University of Texas.

Sexton, J. B, E. J. Thomas, and R. L. Helmreich. 2000. "Error, Stress, and Teamwork in Medicine and Aviation: Cross Sectional Surveys." *British Medical Journal* 320: 745–49.

Simmons, J. 2010. "Some Hospitals Falling Short of Protecting for Gay Patients." [Online article; retrieved 4/2/11.] www.healthleadersmedia.com/content/QUA-252125/Some-Hospitals-Falling-Short-of-Protecting-for-Gay-Patients.

Sinuff, T., N. K. Adhikari, D. J. Cook, H. J. Schünemann, L. E. Griffith, G. Rocker, and S. D. Walter. 2006. "Mortality Predictions in the Intensive Care Unit: Comparing Physicians with Scoring Systems." *Critical Care Medicine* 34 (3): 878–85.

Slattery, D. 2011. "Pulmonary Embolism." Presented at High Risk Emergency Medicine Course, Las Vegas, April 11.

Smith-Jentsch, K. A., D. P. Baker, E. Salas, and J. A. Cannon-Bowers. 2001. "Uncovering Differences in Team Competency Requirements: The Case of Air Traffic Control Teams." In *Improving Teamwork in Organizations: Applications of Resource Management Training*, edited by E. Salas, C. A. Bowers, and E. Edens, 31–54. Mahwah, NJ: Erlbaum.

Social Security Administration. 2011. "Examination and Treatment for Emergency Medical Conditions and Women in Labor." Section 1867 of EMTALA. [Online information; retrieved 4/23/11.] www.ssa.gov/OP_Home/ssact/title18/1867.htm.

Somani, B. K., G. Watson, and N. Townell. 2010. "Testicular Torsion." *BMJ* 341: c3213.

Søreide, O. 1984. "Appendicitis—A Study of Incidence, Death Rates, and Consumption of Hosptial Resources." *Postgraduate Medical Journal* 60 (703): 341–45.

Soremekun, O. A., J. K. Takayesu, and S. J. Bohan. 2011. "Framework for Analyzing Wait Times and Other Factors that Impact Patient Satisfaction in the Emergency Department." *Journal of Emergency Medicine* March 24.

Sorrel, A. L. 2009. "OIG Approves Hospital Plan to Pay for Emergency Call." [Online article; retrieved 4/21/11.] www.ama-assn.org/amednews/2009/06/08/gvsc0608.htm.

Spinal Cord Injury Information Network. 2009. "National Spinal Cord Injury Database." [Online information; retrieved 5/15/11.] www.spinalcord.uab. edu/show.asp?durki=24480.

Spinal Cord Injury Information Pages. 2010. "Spinal Cord Injury Facts & Statistics." [Online information; retrieved 5/14/11.] www.sci-info-pages. com/facts.html.

Sprivulis, P. 2004. "A Pilot Study of Emergency Department Workload Complexity." *Emergency Medicine* 16: 59–64.

Staiger, D. O., D. I. Auerbach, and P. I. Buerhaus. 2010. "Trends in the Work Hours of Physicians in the United States." *Journal of the American Medical Association* 303 (8): 747–53.

StarkLaw.org. 2010. "Stark Law FAQ's." [Online article; retrieved 4/22/11.] http://starklaw.org/stark-law-faq.htm.

Steele, R., T. McNaughton, M. McConahy, and J. Lam. 2006. "Chest Pain in Emergency Department Patients: If the Pain Is Relieved by Nitroglycerin, Is It More Likely to Be Cardiac Chest Pain?" *Canadian Journal of Emergency Medicine* 8 (3): 164.

Steiger, B. 2006. "Survey Results: Doctors Say morale Is Hurting." *Physician Executive* 32 (6): 6–12.

*Stephen Kozup, et al., Appellant, v. Georgetown University*, d/b/a Georgetown University Medical Center, et al. 851 F.2d 437 (1988).

Stiell, I. G. 2001. "The Canadian CT Head Rule for Patients with Minor Head Injury." *Lancet* 357 (9266): 1391–96.

Stone-Griffith, S. 2011. Personal communication. March 8.

Strangely, M. 2009. "Night Shift Health Risks." [Online article; retrieved 4/22/11.] www.associatedcontent.com/article/1661200/night_shift_health_ risks.html?cat=5.

Studdert, D. M., M. M. Mello, A. A. Gawande, T. K. Gandhi, A. Kachalia, C. Yoon, A. L. Puopolo, and T. A. Brennan. 2006. "Claims, Errors, and Compensation Payments in Medical Malpractice Litigation." *New England Journal of Medicine* 354 (19): 2024–33.

Sun, B. C., J. G. Adams, and H. R. Burstin. 2001. "Validating a Model of Patient Satisfaction with Emergency Care." *Annals of Emergency Medicine* 38 (5): 527–32.

Sun, B., J. Adams, E. J. Orav, D. W. Rucker, T. A. Brennan, and H. R. Burstin. 2000. "Determinants of Patient Satisfaction and Willingness to Return with Emergency Care." *Annals of Emergency Medicine* 35: 426–34.

Sullivan, W., and J. DeLucia. 2010. "2+2=7? Seven Things You May Not Know About Press Ganey Statistics. [Online article; retrieved 3/27/10.] www.epmonthly.com/features/current-features/227-seven-things-you-may-not-know-about-press-gainey-statistics.

Tanabe, P., R. Myers, A. Zosel, J. Brice, A. H. Ansari, J. Evans, Z. Martinovich, K. H. Todd, and J. A. Paice. 2007. "Emergency Department Management of Acute Pain Episodes in Sickle Cell Disease." *Academic Emergency Medicine* 14: 419–25.

Tayal, V. S., H. Cohen, and H. J. Norton. 2004. "Outcome of Patients with an Indeterminate Emergency Department First-Trimester Pelvic Ultrasound to Rule Out Ectopic Pregnancy." *Academic Emergency Mecidine* 11 (9): 912–17.

Taylor, T. 2010. "Solutions to the On-Call Crisis." Advanced ED Operations Course, Las Vegas, March.

Texas Medical Board. "Medical Board Continues Licensure Suspension of Charles R. Massey Jr., M.D., of Fredericksburg." [Online press release; posted August 25, 2008.] www.tmb.state.tx.us/news/press/2008/082508b.php.

Thomalla, G. 2007. "Two Tales: Hemorrhagic Transformation But Not Parenchymal Hemorrhage After Thrombolysis Is Related to Severity and Duration of Ischemia: MRI Study of Acute Stroke Patients Treated with Intravenous Tissue Plasminogen Activator Within 6 Hours." *Stroke* 38 (2): 313–18.

Thomas, C., and C. Power. 2010. "Shift Work and Risk Factors for Cardiovascular Disease: A Study at Age 45 Years in the 1958 British Birth Cohort." *European Journal of Epidemiology* 25 (5): 305–14.

Tishler, C. L. 2000. "Managing the Violent Patient: A Guide for Psychologists and Other Mental Health Professionals." *Professional Psychology: Research and Practice* 31 (1): 34–41.

Todd, K. H. 1996. "Pain Assessment and Ethnicity." *Annals of Emergency Medicine* 27: 1421–1423.

Todd, K. H., N. Samaroo, and J. R. Hoffman. 1993. "Ethnicity as a Risk Factor for Inadequate Emergency Department Analgesia." *Journal of the American Medical Association* 69: 1537–39.

Trimble, T. 1998. "Night Shift Survival Tips." [Online article; retrieved 4/22/11.] http://enw.org/NightShift.htm.

Turner, G.-M. 2002. "HIPAA and the Criminalization of American Medicine." [Online article; retrieved 4/2/11.] www.cato.org/pubs/journal/cj22n1/cj22n1-9.pdf.

US Congress. "Wrongful Disclosure of Individually Identifiable Health Information." 42 U.S.C. 1320d–6 §177(b)(3). [Online information; retrieved 4/2/11.] www.ssa.gov/OP_Home/ssact/title11/1177.htm.

———. 1996. Health Insurance Portability and Accountability Act, 42 U.S.C. 1320d–6 §177.

———. 1986. Emergency Medical Treatment and Active Labor Act, 42 U.S.C.A. §1395dd(a).

———. 1863. False Claims Act, 31 U.S.C. § 3729(a)(1)(A),(B).

US Department of Health and Human Services. n.d. (a). "A Health Care Provider's Guide to the HIPAA Privacy Rule: Communicating with a Patient's Family, Friends, or Others Involved in the Patient's Care." [Online information; retrieved 4/21/11.] www.hhs.gov/ocr/privacy/hipaa/understanding/coveredentities/provider_ffg.pdf.

———. n.d. (b). "Fast Facts for Covered Entities." [Online information; retrieved 4/2/11.] www.hhs.gov/ocr/privacy/hipaa/understanding/coveredentities/cefastfacts.html.

———. n.d. (c). "Is the HIPAA Privacy Rule Suspended During a National or Public Health Emergency?" [Online information; retrieved 4/2/11.] www.hhs.gov/ocr/privacy/hipaa/faq/disclosures_in_emergency_situations/1068.html.

———. 2006a. "Can Health Care Providers Engage in Confidential Conversations with Other Providers or with Patients, even if There Is a Possibility That They Could Be Overheard?" [Online information; retrieved 4/22/11.] www.hhs.gov/ocr/privacy/hipaa/faq/smaller_providers_and_businesses/196.html.

————. 2006b. "Does the HIPAA Privacy Rule Require Hospitals and Doctors' Offices to be Retrofitted, to Provide Private Rooms, and Soundproof Walls to Avoid Any Possibility That a Conversation Is Overheard?" [Online information; retrieved 4/22/11.] www.hhs.gov/ocr/privacy/hipaa/faq/safeguards/197.html.

————. 2003. "Summary of the HIPAA Privacy Rule." [Online information; retrieved 4/21/11.] www.hhs.gov/ocr/privacy/hipaa/understanding/summary/privacysummary.pdf.

Vila-de-Muga, M. 2011. "Factors Associated with Medication Errors in the Pediatric Emergency Department." *Pediatric Emergency Care* 27 (4): 290–94.

Vincent, C., M. Young, and A. Phillips. 1994. "Why People Sue Doctors: A Study of Patients and Relatives Taking Legal Action." *Lancet* 343: 1609–13.

Vinogradova, I. A., V. N. Anisimov, A. V. Bukalev, A. V. Semenchenko, and M. A. Zabezhinski. 2009. "Circadian disruption Induced by Light-at-Night Accelerates Aging and Promotes Tumorigenesis in Rats." *Aging* 1 (10): 855–65.

Von Thaden, T., M. Hoppes, L. Yongjuan, N. Johnson, and A. Schriver. 2006. "The Perceptions of Just Culture Across Disciplines in Healthcare." [Online article; retrieved 4/22/11.] www.humanfactors.illinois.edu/Reports&PapersPDFs/humfac06/The%20Perception%20of%20Just%20Culture%20Across.pdf.

Vukimer, R. B. 2006. "Customer Satisfaction with Patient Care: 'Where's the Beef?'" *Journal of Hospital Marketing & Public Relations* 17: 79–107.

Wang, R., T. A. Reynolds, H. H. West, D. Ravikumar, C. Martinez, I. McAlpine, V. L. Jacoby, and J. C. Stein. 2011. "Use of a β-hCG Discriminatory Zone with Bedside Pelvic Ultrasonography." [Online article; retrieved 6/4/11.] www.ncbi.nlm.nih.gov/pubmed/21310509.

Wardlaw, J. M. 1997. "Systematic Review of Evidence on Thrombolytic Therapy for Acute Ischaemic Stroke." *Lancet* 350 (9078): 607–14.

Wasserman, G. M., and C. B. White. 1990. "Evaluation of the Necessity for Hospitalization of the Febrile Infant Less than Three Months of Age." *Pediatric Infectious Disease Journal* 9 (3): 163–69.

Weakliem, D. L., and S. J. Frenkel. 2006. "Morale and Workplace Performance," *Work and Occupations* 33 (3): 335–61.

Weant, K. A. 2010. "Effect of Emergency Medicine Pharmacists on Medication Error Reporting in an Emergency Department." *American Journal of Health-System Pharmacy* 67 (21): 1851–55.

Weizberg, M. B. Cambria, Y. Farooqui, B. Hahn, F. Dazio, E. M. Maniago, N. Berwald, D. Kass, and B. Ardolic. 2009. "Pilot Study on Documentation Skills: Is There Adequate Training in Emergency Medicine Residency?" [Online information; retrieved 6/4/11.] www.sciencedirect.com/science/article/pii/S0736467909008166.

Welch, R. D., R. J. Zalenski, P. D. Frederick, J. A. Malmgren, S. Compton, M. Grzybowski, S. Thomas, T. Kowalenko, N. R. Every, and National Registry of Myocardial Infarction 2 and 3 Investigators. 2001. "Prognostic Value of a Normal or Nonspecific Initial Electrocardiogram in Acute Myocardial Infarction." *Journal of the American Medical Association* 286 (16): 1977.

Welch, S. J. 2010a. "Beyond Scribes: A Better Idea on the Horizon." [Online article; retrieved 4/21/11.] http://journals.lww.com/em-news/Fulltext/2010/01000/Beyond_Scribes__A_Better_Idea_on_the_Horizon.8.aspx.

———. 2010b. "Driving Hospital Quality and Safety Improvement." Presented at American College of Emergency Physicians Scientific Assembly, Las Vegas, September 30.

———. 2010c. "Quality Matters: Night Warriors." *Emergency Medicine News* 32 (10): 18.

———. 2010d. "Quality Matters: Smile for the Camera." *Emergency Medicine News* 32 (11): 4.

———. 2010e. "Medication Errors." Presented at the High Risk Emergency Medicine Course, Las Vegas, March 8.

———. 2009a. "Intake." In *Quality Matters: Solutions for the Safe and Efficient Emergency Department.* Oakbrook Terrace, IL: Joint Commission Resources.

———. 2009b. "Priority One Protocol Relieves ED of Critical Care Burden." *Emergency Medicine News* 31 (4): 15–18.

———. 2009c. *Quality Matters: Solutions for a Safe and Efficient Emergency Department.* Oakbrook Terrace, IL: Joint Commission Resources.

———. 2008a. "Community Acquired Pneumonia: Perfect Performance." *Emergency Medicine News* 30 (9): 9.

————. 2008b. "Dangerous Liaisons: Managing Dangerous Psych Patients." *Emergency Medicine News* 30 (11): 20, 24.

————. 2008c. "Error Reduction: Tools and Techniques for the Pit Boss." Presented at American College of Emergency Physicians Scientific Assembly 2008, Chicago, October 28.

————. 2007. "The Case for Standardization in Emergency Medicine." *Emergency Medicine News* 29 (6): 7.

————. 2006. Unpublished quality improvement data, LDS Hospital.

Welch, S., and S. Fontenot. 2011. "Risky Business: How Top-Performing Organizations Manage Risk in the ED." Presented at American College of Healthcare Executives Congress on Healthcare Leadership, Chicago, March 22.

————. 2010. "Quality Matters: Hang onto That Whiteboard." *Emergency Medicine News* 32 (12): 22–23.

Welch, S., and K. Jensen. 2007. "The Concept of Reliability in Emergency Medicine." *American Journal of Medical Quality* 22 (1): 50–58.

Welch, S. J., B. A. Asplin, S. Stone-Griffith, S. J. Davidson, J. Augustine, and J. Schuur. 2010. "Emergency Department Operational Metrics, Measures and Definitions: Results of the Second Performance Measures and Benchmarking Summit." [Online article; retrieved 4/22/11.] http://www.annemergmed.com/article/S0196-0644(10)01498-8/abstract.

Welch, S.J., J. Augustine, L. Dong, L. Savitz, and B. James. Under review. "Size Matters: Census and Acuity Predict Emergency Department Performance on Some Metrics." *Joint Commission Journal of Quality and Patient Safety*.

Welch, S., J. Augustine, C. A. Camargo, Jr., and C. Reese. 2006. "Emergency Department Performance Measures and Benchmarking Summit." *Academic Emergency Medicine* 13 (10): 1074–80.

Wiler, J. 2010. "Optimizing Emergency Department Front-End Operations." *Annals of Emergency Medicine* 55 (2): 142–60.

Williams, G. R. 2001. "Incidence and Characteristics of Total Stroke in the US." *BioMedCentral Neurology* (1): 2.

————. 1999. "Incidence and Occurrence of Total Stroke." *Stroke* 30: 2523–28.

Williams, S. M., D. J. Connelly, S. Wadsworth, and D. J. Wilson. 2000. "Radiological Review of Accident and Emergency Radiographs: A 1-Year Audit." *Clinical Radiology* 55 (11): 861–65.

Witman, A. M., D. M. Park, and S. B. Hardin. 1996. "How Do Patients Want Physicians to Handle Mistakes? A Survey of Internal Medicine Patients in an Academic Setting." *Archives of Internal Medicine* 156: 2565–69.

Wojcieszak, D., J. Banja, and C. Houk. 2006. "The Sorry Works! Coalition: Making the Case for Full Disclosure." *Joint Commission Journal on Quality and Patient Safety* 32 (6): 344–50.

Woo, C. K. 2009. "High Risk Chief Complaints 1: Chest Pain—the Big Three." *Emergency Medicine Clinics of North America* 27 (4).

Woods, M. 2007. *Healing Words: The Power of Apology in Medicine,* 82–83. Oakbrook Terrace, IL: Joint Commission Resources.

Worthington, K. 2004. "Customer Satisfaction in the Emergency Department." *Emergency Medicine Clinics of North America* 22: 87–102.

Zane, R. D. 2009. "The Legal Process." *Emergency Medicine Clinics of North America* 27 (4): 583–92.

# Index

American Hospital Association, 120–21, 207

American Medical Association: concern with medical liability environment, 14; *State Medical Licensure Requirements and Statistics* of, 340–42

American Recovery and Reinvestment Act, 144, 146–47

American Red Cross, 142, 227

Analgesia, oral *versus* intravenous, 91–92

Anesthesia: safety of, 55, 59; standardization in, 59

Anesthesia Patient Safety Foundation, 59

Anger management, 318–19, 321

Antacids, as chest pain treatment, 271

Antelope Valley Medical Center, 201

Antibiotics, adverse reactions to, 234

Anticoagulant therapy: adverse reactions to, 234, 236, 298; outpatient, 59

Anticompetition statutes, of states, 351

Anticonvulsants, adverse reactions to, 234

Antidepressants, adverse reactions to, 236

Antihypertensives, adverse reactions to, 234

Antikickback legislation, 184, 188. *See also* Kickbacks: differentiated from Stark Law, 155

Antitrust legislation, 350–51; Health Care Quality Improvement Act and, 351

Anxiety, 307; in night-shift workers, 46

Aortic aneurysm and dissection, 255–60; definition of, 255, 256, 355; misdiagnosis of, 256–57, 259

Apnea, 355

Apology, 97-105. *See also* Empathy: benefits of, 98; constraints to, 98–100; as disclosure component, 100; five Rs of, 101; as risk-management component, 102, 103–04; scripting for, 102–103, 105

"Apology Laws," 99

Apparent life-threatening events (ALTEs), 275

Appendicitis, 241–46; misdiagnosis of, 241, 242–43

Archives of Physical Medicine and Rehabilitation, 296

Arrival time, 28

Arrival-to-provider time, 29

Arrival-to–treatment space time, 29

Aspirin, 236, 285, 298

Assaults, reporting of, 124

Association of American Medical Colleges, 7

Associative activation, 42

ATMs, error prevention in, 36

At-risk behavior, 79

Atrophy, cerebral, 297–98

Attitudinal surveys, 79–81

Attorneys. *See* Legal representation

Availability heuristic, 43

Aviation industry: accidents in, 67–68; crew resource management in, 68; safety in, 33, 34, 62; standardization in, 57–58, 61; teamwork training in, 69

## B

Baby-boomer generation, 7

Bacteremia, 276

Bacterial infections, neonatal, 275–80

"Bad-faith letters," 334

Balanced Budget Act, 344, 346

Balanced scorecards, 108

Banner Health System, Arizona, 202

Baptist Health Care of Pensacola, Florida, 15

Barrett, Robert, 353–54

Baxter Pharmaceuticals, 235, 238

Bed assignment interval, 30

Beecher, Henry, 55

Behavioral training, for violence prevention, 318–19, 321

Benchmarking, data required for, 19

Benzodiazepines, adverse reactions to, 234

Beth Israel Hospital, New York City, 290

Bias, confirmation, 43

Billing: charting for, 194–97, 198–99; fraudulent. *See* Fraud and abuse

Biomarkers, for myocardial infarction, 269–70

Bioterrorism, implication for HIPAA Privacy Rule waivers, 141–43

Bloodbloc label system, 54

Blood transfusions, HIV-contaminated, 227–28

Boards. *See* Governing boards

Body language, 319, 321

Brain death, 225–26

Brain injuries, 295-304. *See also* Head injuries: misdiagnosis of, 295; as mortality cause, 295

Brost Violence Checklist, 315

Brown, Bernice, 347–48

Brown, Mark, 201

Brown University, 74

Bukata, Richard, 200, 201

## C

Call-backs, 44, 71, 233–34

Call-back systems, 89

Call list, 169

Camera telephones, 146, 147–48

Canada, malpractice lawsuits in, 14

Canadian C-Spine Rules, 299, 300, 302

Canadian CT Head Rule, 298–99

Cardiac arrest, emergency care for, 233–34

Cardiac medications, adverse reactions to, 234

Cardiovascular disease. *See also* Myocardial infarction, acute: in night-shift workers, 46

Cardozo, Benjamin N., 223

Caregivers, multiple, 44

Case fatality, 296, 355

Causation, of negligence, 332

CBC (complete blood count), for neonatal sepsis diagnosis, 278

Cedars Sinai Medical Center, Los Angeles, 238

Celebrity patients, 137–38

Census data, 19–20, 23, 24–25

Center for Emergency Medical Education, "High Risk Emergency Medicine" course offered by, 234–35

Centers for Disease Control and Prevention (CDC), 278

Centers for Medicare & Medicaid Services (CMS): core measures of, 19; EMTALA enforcement role of, 165; fraud and abuse prevention role of, 348; Hospital Compare data of, 111–12; opposition to nurse-initiated care, 207; pay-for-performance program of, 24; statement on EMTALA, 163; value-based purchase scheme of, 20

Certificates of merit, 328

Cervical spinal injuries, 298; imaging of, 298, 299–301, 302, 303

Chain of command, 233–34

Change package, 25

Chaperones, 352

Charting: for billing and coding, 194–97, 198–99; case study of, 200–01; for communication, 198–99; cost of, 195; for foreign body detection, 263; functions of, 193–94; "hybrid," 198, 200; inadequate, 195; to limit risk, 200–01; of orders, 208; template, 198–99, 200, 262; with time stamping, 200; in wound management, 261, 262

Charts, transcription of, 198

Chest pain: acute coronary syndrome-related, 267–68, 270, 271–72; aortic aneurysm-related, 257, 259; as chief complaint, 321–22; diagnostic errors regarding, 307; frequency of, 4; musculoskeletal, 307, 310; pleuritic, unexplained, 306–07, 310; psychological, 272

Chest x-rays, for aortic aneurysm or dissection diagnosis, 259, 260

Cheung, Dickson, 220

Chief executive officers (CEOs), as governing board members, 108

Children. See Pediatric patients

Chisholm, C.D., 195

Cincinnati Children's Medical Center, 278

Clergy, 138

Clinical decision support, 37

CMS. See Centers for Medicare & Medicaid Services

Coding, charting for, 194–97

Cognition: errors and, 52–54; three-tiers of, 41–42

Communication. See also Scripting: during apologies, 102; call-backs, 44, 71, 233–34; for error prevention, 71, 73, 233–34; of personal health information, 133–35; physician–patient, 14; repeat-backs, 44, 62–63, 71, 233–34

Communication errors: as airline accident cause, 67–68; case study of, 74–75; in healthcare, 68–69

Communication training, 16; for violence prevention, 318–19, 321

Compartment syndrome, 264

Compensation. See also Reimbursement: fair market value of, 154, 186; for governing board members, 108; for night-shift workers, 47, 48; for on-call coverage, 184–90, 350

Competition, limitation by state medical boards, 338

Complaint management, 15, 94

Complaint ratios, 20, 30

Complaints: about EMTALA noncompliance, 155; about fraudulent billing, 345–46; as basis for lawsuits, 327–28; scripting for, 16; use in risk identification, 118, 119

Compliance: feedback on, 35; implication for patient satisfaction, 86

Complications, anesthesia-related, 55

Computed tomography (CT) coronary angiography, 270

Computed tomography (CT) pulmonary angiography, 306, 308–09, 310

Computed tomography (CT) scans, 8–9; for aortic aneurysm evaluation, 258, 259, 260; for appendicitis evaluation, 243, 245; for cervical spinal injury evaluation, 299–301; cranial, in adult patients, 302; cranial, in pediatric patients, 298–99, 300, 302; for foreign body detection, 263; for head injury evaluation, 296–97, 298–301; radiation exposure during, 298; for spinal cord injury evaluation, 298, 301; for stroke evaluation, 285

Computer technology, for error prevention, 53–54

Connecticut, HIPAA Privacy Rule enforcement in, 146–47

Consent. See also Informed consent: for access to personal health information, 135, 136, 138; implied, 225, 227–28, 356; for incompetent patients, 224–25; for photographs, 146, 148; right to, 223–24

Consolidated Omnibus Budget Reconciliation Act (COBRA), 160

Consultation interval, 29

Consultations: difficulty in obtaining, 7; neurological, 282; payment for, 188;

**E**

# H

Hand-surgery coverage, 264

Hand-tendon injuries, 264

Harvard Brain Death Criteria, 225

Harvard Medical Practices study, 51

HCA (Hospital Corporation of America), 9–10, 220

Head injuries: computed tomography scans of, 296–97, 298–301; minor, 296–98

*Healing Words: The Power of Apology in Medicine* (Woods), 97

Healthcare Cost and Utilization Project, 111–12

Healthcare executives, risk management roles of, 125–27; apology and disclosure, 103–05; documentation, 201; EMTALA compliance, 169–70, 172, 179–80, 181; HIPAA Privacy Rule compliance, 147; licensure, 341, 342; malpractice lawsuit prevention, 335; med teams training, 74, 75; patient satisfaction, 92–94; quality improvement, 25, 27, 125; reliability, 38; standardization, 64, 212

Health Care Quality Improvement Act (HCQIA), 351

Healthcare system, unreliability of, 32–33

Health Information Technology for Economic and Clinical Health (HITECH) Act, 144

Health insurance companies, antifraud units of, 344

Health Insurance Portability and Accountability Act (HIPAA), 131; criminal penalties under, 351–52; impact on fraud and abuse, 344, 346; implication for patient violence, 314

Health Insurance Portability and Accountability Act Privacy Rule, 131–39, 150; case study of, 139, 147–48; challenges to, 145–46; enforcement of, 143–47; healthcare executives' role in compliance with, 147; implication for family and loved ones, 135–38; information sources about, 132–33; misinformation about, 131–33, 143–45; during national or public health emergencies, 141–43; penalties for violations of, 143–45, 146–47; purpose of, 131–32

Health Insurance Portability and Accountability Act Security Rule, 150

Health Net, 146–47

Hematoma, subdural, 357

Hemolytic transfusion reactions, 124

Henry Ford Hospital, 46

Heparin, 235, 238

Hip fractures, 263–64

HIPAA. *See* Health Insurance Portability and Accountability Act

Hiroshima survivors, 298

Homicide: medical malpractice-related, 352–54; reporting of, 124

Hospital campus, definition of, 163–64

Hospital Compare data, 111–12

Hospital Corporation of America (HCA), 9–10, 220

Hospitals. *See also names of specific hospitals:* volume bands of, 9, 23–24

Human chorionic gonadotropin hormone (hCG), 248, 252

Human factors engineering (HFE), 44–48; error prevention systems design in, 45

Hypertension: acute coronary syndrome-associated, 271; in night-shift workers, 46

# I

Iatrogenic, definition of, 51, 356

Illnesses, presentation of, 4–5

Imaging. *See also* Computed tomography (CT) scans; Magnetic resonance imaging (MRI); X-rays: of acute coronary syndrome, 270; of aortic aneurysm, 258, 259, 260; of appendicitis, 242–43, 245; of cervical spinal injuries, 298, 299, 302, 303; of foreign bodies, 263; of limb injuries, 263–64; of pulmonary embolism, 308–309

Imaging interval, 29–30

Immunosuppressants, adverse reactions to, 234

Incarceration, for HIPAA Privacy Rule violations, 143, 144–45

Incident reporting, 62, 78, 118, 119, 122–23, 237

Incompetence, 224–25

Infants: cranial computed tomography scans in, 298–99, 300; head injuries in, 297; lumbar puncture in, 278, 279; sepsis in, 275–80; testicular torsion in, 291

Infections, of wounds, 261, 262

Information dispensation, 88, 89, 92

Information overload, 8–9

Information technology: use in dosage calculations, 45; use in reliability improvement, 37

Informed consent, 90; for head injury imaging, 298, 302; implication for malpractice lawsuits, 13; right to, 223–24; for tissue plasminogen activator administration, 284, 285

Inpatient Prospective Payment Proposed Rule, 149–50

Institute for Healthcare Improvement, 7, 31; Emergency Department Innovation Community of, 25, 60; 100,000 Lives Campaign of, 51; "The Two Challenge Rule" communication technique of, 71, 73

Institute of Medicine, 97

Instruction manuals, 53

Insulin, 235

Insurance coverage, for criminal behavior, 343

Intensive care units (ICUs): admission to, 26; error rate in, 33

Intermountain Healthcare, 317–18, 319–20

Intermountain Institute for Health Care Delivery Research, 205, 206

Intermountain Medical Center, 26

Internal Revenue Service (IRS), 165, 171

Interpreters, 138

Interrogatories, 328

Interruptions, 5, 59–60, 199–200, 232

Interviews, with patient safety personnel, 78

Intrapartum, definition of, 124, 356

Ireland, 90

## J

James, Brent, 205, 206

Johns Hopkins Hospital, 352

Joint Commission: high-risk process analysis requirement of, 125; hospital violence alert from, 352; occurrence reporting guidelines of, 123–24; Ongoing Practice Performance Evaluation by, 22; opposition to nurse-initiated care, 207; patient privacy requirement of, 132; restraint use monitoring by, 118–19; sentinel events policy of, 123–24; sentinel events reports of, 33, 68, 69; violent patient management regulations of, 317

*Journal of Healthcare Management,* 111

*Journal of the American Medical Association,* 7–8

*Journal of Trauma,* 300

"Just culture," 55, 77–84; accountability and, 78–79; attitudinal surveys and, 79–81; promotion of, 127

335; impact on physician practice, 14; implication for patient satisfaction, 86; initiation of, 327–28; interrogatories in, 328; involving pediatric patients, 275; motions for summary judgments in, 334; patient privacy violations-related, 143; preparation of defense for, 331–34; pretrial motions for, 334; prevalence of, 14; radiology-related, 264–65; requests for admission in, 328; requests for documents in, 328; retained foreign bodies-related, 262; settlements *versus*, 334; strategies for dealing with, 336; strategies for prevention of, 15–16; stroke-related, 282, 286; testicular torsion misdiagnosis-related, 290, 292; tissue plasminogen activator administration-related, 284–85

Malpractice risk, *versus* other insurance risk, 11–12

Marfan's syndrome, 256

Marx, David, 78–79

Massachusetts, Board of Registration in Medicine of, 338

Mayo Clinic, 33

Media, HIPAA guidelines regarding, 137–38

Medical culture, 62

Medical errors. *See also* Misdiagnoses; Missed diagnoses; Reliability: accepting responsibility for, 101, 103; apologies for, 97–105; "bad apple" approach to, 77–78; case study of, 48, 238; of commission, 44–45, 45, 62; communication-based prevention of, 233–234; definition of, 231; description-type, 42; diagnostic, 43; disclosure of, 100, 103–04; ectopic pregnancy-related, 250; in execution, 53; healthcare executives' role in prevention of, 237, 238; inadvertent, 79; incompetence-related, 52; of intent, 53; levels of, 32; as mortality cause, 51,

231, 232; during the night shift, 231; of omission, 45, 62; predisposing factors for, 233; prevalence of, 32–33, 231; rates of, 44–45; scripting for, 102–03, 105; as slips, 42–43; standardization-related reduction of, 59; strategies for prevention of, 237, 238; "Swiss cheese" model of, 33–34; system-derived, 52; systems-related approach to, 77–78; teamwork training-related reduction in, 70

Medical history, elements of, 194–97

Medical records. *See also* Charting; Documentation: functions of, 193–94

Medical screening examinations (MSEs), 159–60, 161–62, 173–74, 175, 178, 180, 181; differentiated from triage, 174

Medical students, 90

Medical teams. *See* Med teams

Medicare, fraudulent claims submitted to, 156, 347–48

Medicare and Medicaid Antifraud and Abuse Acts, 344

Medicare and Medicaid Patient and Program Protection Act, 344

Medicare Conditions of Participation (COP), 164

"Medicare Death Penalty," 166

Medicare Modernization Act, 149–50

Medicare participation: Conditions of Participation (COP), 164; exclusion from, 165, 166, 346

Medicare patients, choice of emergency department by, 86–87

Medication errors: communication-based prevention of, 71, 73; definition of, 356; high-risk medications for, 44, 53, 234–37; probability of, 62; rate of, 45; reporting of, 124; system changes-based prevention of, 62–63

Med teams: advantages of, 74; communication within, 71–73

Med teams training, 69–70, 74; in communication skills, 71–73; healthcare executives' role in, 74, 75

Meningitis, neonatal, 275, 276

Mental health assessments, 174, 175

Mental health emergencies, 162

Mercy Health, Philadelphia, 199

Mercy Medical Center, Cedar Rapids, Iowa, emergency department protocols of, 208, 209–12

Methotrexate, as ectopic pregnancy treatment, 250–52, 253

"Mini-strokes." *See* Transient ischemic attacks (TIAs)

Minority-group patients, pain undertreatment in, 91–92

Misdiagnoses, 43; of acute coronary syndrome, 271; of aortic aneurysm and dissection, 256–57, 259; of appendicitis, 241, 242–43; of brain injuries, 295; of epididymitis, 290, 291–92; of neonatal sepsis, 277; of pulmonary embolism, 305–06, 307, 309–10; of stroke, 282; of testicular torsion, 289–92, 293; of transient ischemic attacks, 282, 286

Missed diagnoses, 33; of ectopic pregnancy, 247–48, 249; of limb injuries, 263–64

Mission statements, of state medical boards, 338

Mistake proofing, 53; by design, 54

Mistakes, 42; apologies for, 97–105; as errors of intent, 53; knowledge-based, 43; risk factors for, 44; rule-based, 43

*Modern Healthcare,* Excellence in Healthcare Award of, 15

Modified Charlotte rule, 307, 308

Mortality: acute coronary syndrome-related, 267; aviation-related, 57–58; brain injury-related, 295; ectopic pregnancy-related, 247; healthcare-related, 51–52; maternal, reporting of, 124; medical error-related, 51, 231, 232; missed diagnoses-related, 33; perinatal, reporting of, 124; pulmonary embolism-related, 305–06; sepsis-related, 275; stroke-related, 281

Mortality rate, as performance measure, 112–13

Motor vehicle accidents, as spinal cord injury cause, 296

Multitasking, 5, 232

Myocardial infarction, acute, 267–68; biomarkers for, 269–70; electrocardiogram-based diagnosis of, 268; NSTEMI, 269; silent, 267–68, 357; STEMI, 268–69, 357; in women, 271–72

Myocardial perfusion imaging, 270

Myoglobin, as cardiac disease biomarker, 269

## N

Name badges, 316

Narcan, 235

Narcotics, adverse reactions to, 234

NASA, 68

National Board of Medical Examiners, Educational Commission for Foreign Medical Graduates of, 340–41

National emergencies, HIPAA Privacy Rule waivers during, 141–43

National Emergency X-ray Utilization Study (NEXUS), 299, 301, 302

National Patient Safety Foundation, 51

National Quality Forum, 248

National Spinal Cord Injury Database, 295–96

Navicular fractures, 263

Neck injuries. *See* Cervical spinal injuries

Negligence: causation of, 332; civil *versus* criminal nature of, 352–54; under

EMTALA, 180; state medical boards' response to, 339; torts of, 331

Neonates: definition of, 276, 357; sepsis in, 275–80

Nevada, State Board of Medical Examiners of, 338

NEXUS (National Emergency X-ray Utilization Study), 299, 301, 302

Night shift, adverse health effects of, 46

Night-shift workers, strategies for, 46–48

Noise, in the emergency department, 42, 43

Nolan, Thomas, 31

Nonsteroidal anti-inflammatory drugs (NSAIDs), adverse reactions to, 234, 236

Northeastern Vermont Regional Hospital, 38

Nosocomial infections, 124, 357

Nuclear power plants, 33, 34

Nurses: order set initiation by, 206–07; questioning of physicians' orders by, 71, 73

## O

Obesity, in night-shift workers, 46

Obstetric/gynecological services, 252-53. *See also* Labor and delivery; Pregnancy

Occupational Safety and Health Administration (OSHA), 313

Occurrence reporting, 118, 119, 123–24

Occurrence screening, 124–25

Office for Civil Rights, 143–44, 165

Office of Inspector General, 149, 154, 165, 346, 347; on-call coverage reimbursement opinions of, 184–89; *Roadmap for New Physicians: Avoiding Medicare and Medicaid Fraud and Abuse,* 345; safe harbor opinions of, 350

Omnibus Reconciliation Act (1989). *See* Stark law

On-call coverage: compensation for, 184–90, 350; hospital by-laws regarding, 184, 190; physicians' refusal to participate in, 183–84

On-call crisis, 7, 8

On-call physicians: call list of, 169; EMTALA noncompliance by, 167–69

100,000 Lives Campaign, 51

Operating characteristics, 19, 23, 24

Operating rooms, errors in, 55

Operational data, 22

Operational errors, 33

Opiates, 235

Orders sets, standardized. *See* Standardized order sets

Orlikoff, James, 120–21

Otis elevator brakes, 54

Outcomes: 100% goal for, 60–61; prediction of, 43

Outliers, 60

## P

Pain management, 64, 117; correlation with patient satisfaction, 88, 91–92

Panic attacks, 307

Paralysis, 298

Parents, divorced, 224–25

Paresis, 298, 357

Paresthesia, 298, 357

Patient(s): celebrities as, 137–38; characteristics of, 4; "horizontal," 5; "vertical," 5

Patient advocates, 92

Patient expectations, 5; failure to meet, 101; implication for malpractice lawsuits, 13

Patient safety: continuum of, 17, 18; governing board's promotion of, 110–11, 114; white board use and, 135, 139

Patient safety attendants (PSAs), observation instructions for, 317–18, 319–20

Patient safety committees, 110–111

Patient safety culture, 78

Patient satisfaction: correlates of, 88–92; *versus* customer service, 85–86; definition of, 86; demographic factors affecting, 87–88; healthcare executives' role in, 92–94; implication for malpractice lawsuits, 14, 15; importance of, 86–87; measurement of, 85, 86; as risk management strategy, 85–95; staff turnover effects of, 86; surveys of, 86, 92–93, 118, 119; technical issues in, 88, 90–91

Patient transfers. *See* Transfers, of patients

Patient volume: pediatric, 19; relationship to patient satisfaction, 87–88

Pediatric patients. *See also* Infants; Neonates: adverse drug reactions in, 236–37, 238; appendicitis diagnosis in, 243; cervical spinal imaging in scans in, 301; consent for, 224–25, 227–28; cranial imaging in, 298–99, 300, 302; malpractice lawsuits related to, 275; testicular torsion in, 289, 291

Pediatric volume, 19

Peer review, in occurrence screening, 124

Pennsylvania, certificates of merit in, 328

"Per-click" reimbursement, 153

"Perfect storm," in emergency medicine, 6–9

Performance measures, 20–22, 23

Performance Measures and Benchmarking Summit, Second, 20

Photographs, 137–38, 146, 147–48

Physician(s): female, 8; on-call, 167–69; primary care, 8; shortage of, 7–8, 14; young, 7–8

Physician Insurance Association of America, 11, 12

Physician-patient relationship, 5; communication in, 14; implication for malpractice lawsuit risk, 100; trust in, 98

Pilots, physicians as, 62

Pilot studies: for quality improvement, 25; for reliability improvement, 36–37

Plavix, 298

Pneumonia: community-acquired, core measures for, 38; neonatal, 276

Polypharmacy, 236

Potassium chloride, 235

*Power of Apology, The* (Engel), 101

Prednisone, 236

Pregnancy: computed tomography angiography during, 309; ectopic, 37, 247–54; heterotopic, 248, 249; venous thromboembolism during, 309

Pregnancy tests, 248, 252, 253

Pregnant women, EMTALA-mandated treatment for, 160, 162–63

Presidential declarations, of national disasters or emergencies, 142

Press Ganey surveys, 86, 92–93

Primary care physicians, shortage of, 8

Private payers, fraudulent billing practices of, 344

Procedures: lack of standardization of, 59–60; performed on wrong patient, body side, or organ, 124

Process failure, designing for, 62–64

Professional courtesy, 153

Project BioShield Act, 142

Proportion metrics, 30

Protocols, 205–21; case study of, 220; deviation from, 207; examples of, 208–19; nurse-initiated, 207; review and approval of, 207

Protocols and Process Improvement Workgroup, 60

Provider contact time, 28

Shortness of breath. *See* Dyspnea

Shoulder dislocations, 264

Situation awareness, 70, 357

*Sleep,* 46

Sleep deprivation, in night-shift workers, 46–47

Slips, 42–43, 53

Smorynski, Daniel, 347–48

SOAP notes, 199

Social media policies, 148

Social Security Act, 346; 1972 Amendments to, 344; Section 1135 (b) (7) of, 142

Souter, Steve, 26

Specialties, malpractice litigation rate in, 12

Spinal cord injuries, 295–304;

Sprivulis, Peter, 7

Staff. *See also* Nurses; Physician(s): experience levels of, 90

Staff satisfaction, 86

Standardization, 57–65; in aviation, 57–58; benefits of, 58–60; case study of, 64, 220; concepts behind, 61; customization of, 60, 61; in ectopic pregnancy diagnosis and treatment, 252; for error prevention, 35; healthcare executives' role in, 64, 212; importance of, 205; lack of, 44; for process failure prevention, 62–64; pushback against, 60–61

Standardized order sets, 63-64, 205-21. *See also* Advanced triage order sets/ protocols: for foreign body removal, 262; legal considerations concerning, 206–07; nurse-initiated, 206–07; strategies for implementation of, 220

Standards of care, breaches of, 332

Stanford University, 46

Standing orders, for urine pregnancy tests, 248, 252, 253

Stark, Peter, 149

Stark Final Regulations, 149–50

Stark law, 149–57; case study of, 156; confusion regarding, 150–51; definitions of, 149, 151–52; exceptions to, 153–54; False Claims Act and, 156; *versus* kickbacks, 155; penalties under, 154–55; strategies for compliance with, 157

State medical boards, 337–42; case study of, 341–42; disciplinary actions by, 338–40; investigations by, 339–42; mission statements of, 338

*State Medical Licensure Requirements and Statistics* (American Medical Association), 340–42

States. *See also names of specific states:* anti-competition statutes of, 351; apology laws of, 99

State University of New York at Albany, 46

STAT response, 164

STEMI myocardial infarction, 268–69, 357

Stiell, Ian, 296

Stone-Griffith, Suzanne, 10

Strategic planning, 114

Stress: as error cause, 45; experienced by patients, 4

Stroke, 281–87; case study of, 286; as mortality cause, 281; tissue plasminogen activator therapy for, 283–85

Stroke policies, 284–85

Subcycle time intervals, 22, 23

Substance abuse: as emergency medical condition, 162; EMTALA-mandated assessment of, 174

Suicidal behavior, 317, 318

Suicides, reporting of, 124

Summons, 327

"Swiss cheese model," of errors, 33–34

## T

Tasks, steps in, 52–53

Teaching hospitals, patient satisfaction surveys of, 87–88

Team approach, to medical care, 59

Teamwork, 67–76; advantages of, 74; for communication improvement, 68; communication in, 71–73; crew resource management approach to, 67–68; elements of, 71; *versus* group work, 70–71

Technology. *See also* Computer technology; Information technology: impact on emergency medical care, 8–9

Telephone consultations, 285, 286

$10^{-1}$, 32, 358

Testicular torsion, 289–94; management of, 292; misdiagnosis of, 289–92, 293

Tetraplegia, 296

Texas Medical Board, 338, 341–42

Third-party payers, antifraud units of, 344

Thought, three tiers of, 41–42

Thrombolytic therapy, 282, 283–85, 358

Throughput for processes, 20

Throughput times, quality improvement programs for, 93–94

Time intervals, 20, 21, 22, 29

Time measures, 20–22

Time pressure, as error risk factor, 44

Time stamps, 20, 21, 22, 28, 200

Time-to-pain-treatment, 20

Tissue plasminogen activator therapy, for stroke, 283–85

Torts, of negligence, 331

Training: in communication techniques, 16, 318–19, 321; of med teams, 69–70, 71–73, 74; in patient satisfaction strategies, 16

Transfer certificates, 179

Transfer rate, 19

Transfers, of patients: EMTALA requirements regarding, 160, 165, 166–67,
168, 169, 175–76; guidelines for, 176–77, 179; hospitals' refusal of, 177

Transient ischemic attacks, 281, 283; definition of, 283, 358; misdiagnosis of, 282, 286

Trauma care, 59

Trauma centers, patient satisfaction surveys of, 87–88

Traumatic brain injuries. *See* Brain injuries

Treatment space, 28

Treatment space time, 28

Triage, differentiated from medical screening examinations (MSEs), 174

Triage interval, 29

Triage order sets/protocols, advanced, 62–64, 206–08, 355; examples of, 208–19

Triage system, wait time in, 89–90

Troponins, cardiac, 269–270

Trust, 98

Turnover, effect of patient satisfaction on, 86

"Two Challenge Rule" communication technique, 71, 73

## U

Ultrasonography: for aortic aneurysm diagnosis, 258, 260; for appendicitis diagnosis, 242–43; bedside, 249, 258, 260; bedside *versus* radiologic, 90, 91; for ectopic pregnancy diagnosis, 248, 249, 250–51, 252; for foreign body detection, 263; radiology, 263, 357; scrotal, in testicular torsion, 291, 292

Unconscious patients, photographs of, 138

Under-arrangements, 153

Uninsured patients, patient satisfaction of, 87

United Airlines, 67, 68

U.S. Department of Health and Human Services, 132, 133, 346. *See also* Centers for Medicare & Medicaid Services (CMS): Office for Civil Rights, 143–44, 165; Office of Inspector General, 149, 154, 165, 345, 346, 347, 350; Secretary of, HIPAA waivers from, 142

U.S. Department of Labor, 171

University of Chicago Hospital, 170

University of Michigan Health System, 100, 102

University of Utah, 64

Urinalysis: for abdominal pain evaluation, 58; for neonatal sepsis diagnosis, 278

Urinary tract infections, in infants and neonates, 276, 278

Urine collection, 62–64

Urine cultures, 33

## V

Vahedian, Mahmood, 202

Vance, Beatrice, 353–54

Venous thromboembolic events, 306, 307–08

Ventilation/perfusion (V/Q) scans, 308–09

Veterans Administration Center/Hospital, Lexington, Kentucky, 100, 104

VHA, 63

Violence, in the emergency department, 313–23, 352; risk factors for, 314–17; as spinal cord injury cause, 296

Violent patients: communication with, 318–19, 321; identification of, 314–15, 317; management of, 317–22

Volume bands, 9, 23–24

Volunteers, as patient advocates, 92

Vomiting, 59–60

V/Q scans, 308–09

## W

Wait time, correlation with patient satisfaction, 87–88, 89–90

Walkaways, 20

Wayne County Therapeutic Inc., 347–48

Weapons, patients' possession of, 317

Wheelchairs, brakes on, 54

White boards, 63, 135, 139, 146

Williamsport Regional Medical Center, Williamsport, Pennsylvania, emergency department protocols of, 209, 215–19

Withdrawal, from alcohol or drugs, 174, 178

Women: appendicitis diagnosis in, 241, 243; myocardial infarction in, 271–72; pain undertreatment in, 91–92

Woods, Michael, 97

Workers' compensation claims, 313

Work flow: centralized, 45; effect of charting on, 199–200, 201

Work hours, of physicians, 7–8

Wound management, 261–63

## X

X-rays: of cervical spinal injuries, 300; chest, for aortic aneurysm or dissection diagnosis, 259, 260; of foreign bodies, 262; of limb injuries, 263–66; of spinal cord injuries, 298; "wet reads" of, 264, 265

# About the Authors

**Shari Welch, MD, FACEP,** received her doctor of medicine from the University of Rochester and completed an emergency medicine residency at Emory University in Atlanta, where she was chief resident. She is board certified by the American Board of Emergency Medicine and a fellow of the American College of Emergency Physicians and the American Academy of Emergency Medicine. She has 24 years of experience in clinical emergency medicine, both in community hospitals and academic medical centers. In 2009 she also passed the American College of Healthcare Executives exam and is board certified in healthcare management. She anticipates induction as a Fellow in 2012.

Dr. Welch was formerly the quality improvement director for the emergency department at LDS Hospital, the flagship hospital for Intermountain Healthcare. She has served as a quality improvement consultant for Salt Lake Emergency Physicians, Utah Emergency Physicians, VHA, and the Abaris Group. In 2010 she founded Quality Matters Consulting, a firm dedicated to improving ED operations, quality, safety, and efficiency. She is a board member of the Emergency Department Benchmarking Alliance and was appointed to the faculty of the Institute for Healthcare Improvement in 2006. In addition she has served as a technical expert in ED quality improvement for the Centers for Medicare & Medicaid Services and for the Canadian Health System.

Dr. Welch writes a regular column in *Emergency Medicine News* titled "Quality Matters." She has written three books on ED operations and management and has been widely published in the emergency medicine and the healthcare quality literature. She also produces *ED Leadership Monthly,* a monthly CD and newsletter subscription designed for ED leaders, directors, and managers.

Dr. Welch serves as a research fellow at the Intermountain Institute for Health Care Delivery Research. She has a faculty appointment at the University of Utah School of Medicine and is a practicing emergency physician with Utah Emergency Physicians. In 2010 she received a grant from the Agency for Healthcare Research and Quality to study ED intake models.

**Kevin Klauer, DO, EJD, FACEP,** is chief medical officer for Emergency Medicine Physicians, Ltd., based in Canton, Ohio. He serves as the director of the Center for Emergency Medical Education and on the boards of directors for Physicians Specialty Limited Risk Retention Group, Emergency Medicine Physicians, Ltd., and the National Emergency Medicine Political Action Committee. He has received the ACEP National Faculty Teaching Award and the EMRA Robert J. Dougherty Teaching Fellowship Award. He is an assistant clinical professor at the Michigan State University College of Osteopathic Medicine, and he is the former chair of the national ACEP Finance Committee. Dr. Klauer serves as editor-in-chief of *Emergency Physicians Monthly*. He graduated with honors from Concord Law School in 2011.

**Sarah Freymann Fontenot, JD,** is a lawyer and a nurse. Ms. Fontenot taught hospital law and public health law in the Department of Epidemiology and Public Health at Yale Medical School for two years. She has been an adjunct faculty member at Trinity University in San Antonio, Texas, since 1997, where she has been selected "Most Outstanding Professor" by the students. She teaches extensively for Texas Medical Association, Southern Medical Association, Arkansas Medical Society, and the American College of Physician Executives. She has served as faculty for many other national provider groups, including the Physician Insurers Association of America and the Medical Group Management Association. Since 2007 Ms. Fontenot has served as a faculty member for the American College of Healthcare Executives (ACHE); she currently teaches both the health law and ethics portions of ACHE's Board of Governor's examination review course, as well as ACHE's six-week online health law program. *Risky Business*, a course co-taught by Dr. Shari Welch and Ms. Fontenot, will launch as an ACHE Cluster program in 2011.